Funded by
MISSION COLLEGE
VTEA
Carl D. Perkins Vocational and Technical Education Act Grant

The Health of Lesbian, Gay, Bisexual, and Transgender People

Building a Foundation for Better Understanding

Committee on Lesbian, Gay, Bisexual, and Transgender Health Issues and Research Gaps and Opportunities

Board on the Health of Select Populations

INSTITUTE OF MEDICINE
OF THE NATIONAL ACADEMIES

THE NATIONAL ACADEMIES PRESS
Washington, D.C.
www.nap.edu

THE NATIONAL ACADEMIES PRESS • 500 Fifth Street, N.W. • Washington, DC 20001

NOTICE: The project that is the subject of this report was approved by the Governing Board of the National Research Council, whose members are drawn from the councils of the National Academy of Sciences, the National Academy of Engineering, and the Institute of Medicine. The members of the committee responsible for the report were chosen for their special competences and with regard for appropriate balance.

This study was supported by Contract No. N01-OD-4-2139 between the National Academy of Sciences and the National Institutes of Health. Any opinions, findings, conclusions, or recommendations expressed in this publication are those of the author(s) and do not necessarily reflect the view of the organizations or agencies that provided support for this project.

Library of Congress Cataloging-in-Publication Data

The health of lesbian, gay, bisexual, and transgender people : building a foundation for better understanding / Committee on Lesbian, Gay, Bisexual, and Transgender Health Issues and Research Gaps and Opportunities, Board on the Health of Select Populations, Institute of Medicine of the National Academies.
p. ; cm.
Includes bibliographical references and index.
ISBN 978-0-309-21061-4 (hardcover) — ISBN 978-0-309-21062-1 (pdf)
1. Gays—Medical care—United States. 2. Bisexuals—Medical care—United States.
3. Transgender people—Medical care—United States. I. Institute of Medicine (U.S.). Committee on Lesbian, Gay, Bisexual, and Transgender Health Issues and Research Gaps and Opportunities.
[DNLM: 1. Health Status—United States. 2. Minority Health—United States.
3. Bisexuality—United States. 4. Health Services Research—United States. 5. Homosexuality—United States. 6. Transsexualism—United States. WA 300 AA1]
RA564.9.H65H44 2011
362.1086'64—dc23

2011017453

Additional copies of this report are available from the National Academies Press, 500 Fifth Street, N.W., Lockbox 285, Washington, DC 20055; (800) 624-6242 or (202) 334-3313 (in the Washington metropolitan area); Internet, http://www.nap.edu.

For more information about the Institute of Medicine, visit the IOM home page at: **www.iom.edu.**

Printed in the United States of America

The serpent has been a symbol of long life, healing, and knowledge among almost all cultures and religions since the beginning of recorded history. The serpent adopted as a logotype by the Institute of Medicine is a relief carving from ancient Greece, now held by the Staatliche Museen in Berlin.

Cover design by LeAnn Locher.

Suggested citation: IOM (Institute of Medicine). 2011. *The Health of Lesbian, Gay, Bisexual, and Transgender People: Building a Foundation for Better Understanding*. Washington, DC: The National Academies Press.

"Knowing is not enough; we must apply.
Willing is not enough; we must do."
—Goethe

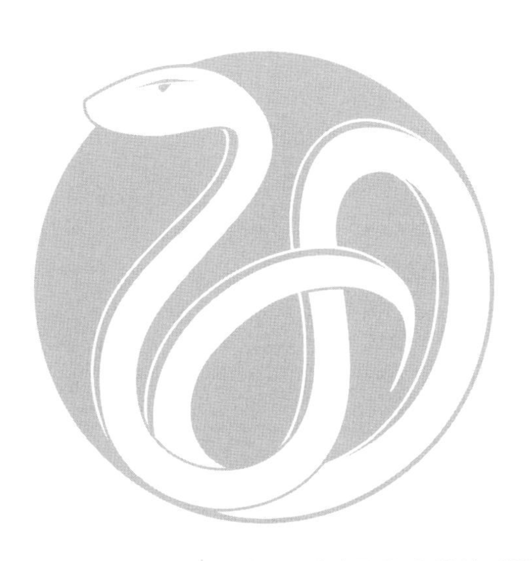

INSTITUTE OF MEDICINE
OF THE NATIONAL ACADEMIES

Advising the Nation. Improving Health.

THE NATIONAL ACADEMIES

Advisers to the Nation on Science, Engineering, and Medicine

The **National Academy of Sciences** is a private, nonprofit, self-perpetuating society of distinguished scholars engaged in scientific and engineering research, dedicated to the furtherance of science and technology and to their use for the general welfare. Upon the authority of the charter granted to it by the Congress in 1863, the Academy has a mandate that requires it to advise the federal government on scientific and technical matters. Dr. Ralph J. Cicerone is president of the National Academy of Sciences.

The **National Academy of Engineering** was established in 1964, under the charter of the National Academy of Sciences, as a parallel organization of outstanding engineers. It is autonomous in its administration and in the selection of its members, sharing with the National Academy of Sciences the responsibility for advising the federal government. The National Academy of Engineering also sponsors engineering programs aimed at meeting national needs, encourages education and research, and recognizes the superior achievements of engineers. Dr. Charles M. Vest is president of the National Academy of Engineering.

The **Institute of Medicine** was established in 1970 by the National Academy of Sciences to secure the services of eminent members of appropriate professions in the examination of policy matters pertaining to the health of the public. The Institute acts under the responsibility given to the National Academy of Sciences by its congressional charter to be an adviser to the federal government and, upon its own initiative, to identify issues of medical care, research, and education. Dr. Harvey V. Fineberg is president of the Institute of Medicine.

The **National Research Council** was organized by the National Academy of Sciences in 1916 to associate the broad community of science and technology with the Academy's purposes of furthering knowledge and advising the federal government. Functioning in accordance with general policies determined by the Academy, the Council has become the principal operating agency of both the National Academy of Sciences and the National Academy of Engineering in providing services to the government, the public, and the scientific and engineering communities. The Council is administered jointly by both Academies and the Institute of Medicine. Dr. Ralph J. Cicerone and Dr. Charles M. Vest are chair and vice chair, respectively, of the National Research Council.

www.national-academies.org

COMMITTEE ON LESBIAN, GAY, BISEXUAL, AND TRANSGENDER HEALTH ISSUES AND RESEARCH GAPS AND OPPORTUNITIES

ROBERT GRAHAM (*Chair*), Professor of Family Medicine and Robert and Myfanwy Smith Chair, Department of Family Medicine, University of Cincinnati College of Medicine, Ohio
BOBBIE A. BERKOWITZ, Dean and Mary O'Neil Mundinger Professor, Columbia University School of Nursing; Senior Vice President, Columbia University Medical Center, New York, New York
ROBERT BLUM, William H. Gates, Sr. Professor and Chair, Department of Populations, Family and Reproductive Health, Johns Hopkins Bloomberg School of Public Health, Baltimore, Maryland
WALTER O. BOCKTING, Associate Professor, Program in Human Sexuality, Department of Family Medicine and Community Health, University of Minnesota Medical School, Minneapolis
JUDITH BRADFORD, Co-Chair, The Fenway Institute; Director, Center for Population Research in Lesbian, Gay, Bisexual and Transgender Health, Boston, Massachusetts
BRIAN de VRIES, Professor of Gerontology, San Francisco State University, California
ROBERT GAROFALO, Associate Professor of Pediatrics, Northwestern University's Feinberg School of Medicine, and Director, Adolescent HIV Services, Children's Memorial Hospital, Chicago, Illinois
GREGORY HEREK, Professor of Psychology, Department of Psychology, University of California, Davis
ELIZABETH A. HOWELL, Associate Professor, Departments of Health Evidence and Policy and Obstetrics, Gynecology, and Reproductive Science and Psychiatry, Mount Sinai School of Medicine, New York, New York
DANIEL KASPRZYK, Vice President and Director, Center for Excellence in Survey Research, National Opinion Research Center at the University of Chicago, Bethesda, Maryland
HARVEY J. MAKADON, Clinical Professor of Medicine, Harvard Medical School and Director of Professional Education and Training, The Fenway Institute, Boston, Massachusetts
CHARLOTTE J. PATTERSON, Professor of Psychology, Department of Psychology, University of Virginia, Charlottesville
JOHN L. PETERSON, Professor, Department of Psychology, Georgia State University, Atlanta
CAITLIN C. RYAN, Director, Family Acceptance Project at the Marian Wright Edelman Institute, San Francisco State University, San Francisco, California

MARK A. SCHUSTER, William Berenberg Professor of Pediatrics, Harvard Medical School, and Chief, Division of General Pediatrics, Children's Hospital, Boston, Massachusetts
LOWELL J. TAYLOR, Professor of Economics, Heinz College, Carnegie Mellon University, Pittsburgh, Pennsylvania
RUTH E. ZAMBRANA, Professor of Women's Studies and Director of the Consortium on Race, Gender and Ethnicity, University of Maryland, College Park

Study Staff

MONICA N. FEIT, Study Director
JOSHUA JOSEPH, Associate Program Officer
JON Q. SANDERS, Program Associate
KAREN M. ANDERSON, Senior Program Officer
ANDREA COHEN, Financial Associate
FREDERICK (RICK) ERDTMANN, Director, Board on the Health of Select Populations
SARAH ISQUICK, Christine Mirzayan Science and Technology Policy Graduate Fellow, Fall 2010

Consultants

RONA BRIERE, Briere Associates, Inc., Felton, Pennsylvania
JOHN D'EMILIO, University of Illinois at Chicago
RONALD C. FOX, Saybrook University, San Francisco, California
CARLOS GODOY, Rensselaer Polytechnic Institute, Troy, New York
ROBERT BRADLEY SEARS, The Williams Institute on Sexual Orientation and Gender Identity Law and Public Policy, UCLA School of Law, California

Reviewers

This report has been reviewed in draft form by individuals chosen for their diverse perspectives and technical expertise, in accordance with procedures approved by the National Research Council's Report Review Committee. The purpose of this independent review is to provide candid and critical comments that will assist the institution in making its published report as sound as possible and to ensure that the report meets institutional standards for objectivity, evidence, and responsiveness to the study charge. The review comments and draft manuscript remain confidential to protect the integrity of the deliberative process. We wish to thank the following individuals for their review of this report:

Thomas J. Coates, David Geffen School of Medicine, University of California, Los Angeles
Anthony R. D'Augelli, Pennsylvania State University
Lisa M. Diamond, University of Utah
Angela Diaz, Mount Sinai School of Medicine
Jamie Feldman, Program in Human Sexuality, University of Minnesota
Karen Fredriksen-Goldsen, University of Washington School of Social Work
Gary Gates, The Williams Institute, University of California, Los Angeles School of Law
Susan R. Johnson, University of Iowa
David E. Kanouse, The RAND Corporation
David J. Malebranche, Emory University School of Medicine
Vickie M. Mays, University of California, Los Angeles
Patricia Robertson, University of California, San Francisco

Ronald Stall, University of Pittsburgh
Alan M. Zaslavsky, Harvard Medical School

Although the reviewers listed above have provided many constructive comments and suggestions, they were not asked to endorse the report's conclusions or recommendations, nor did they see the final draft of the report before its release. The review of this report was overseen by **Kristine M. Gebbie,** City University of New York, and **Bradford H. Gray,** The Urban Institute. Appointed by the National Research Council and the Institute of Medicine, they were responsible for making certain that an independent examination of this report was carried out in accordance with institutional procedures and that all review comments were carefully considered. Responsibility for the final content of this report rests entirely with the authoring committee and the institution.

Preface

In 1999 the Institute of Medicine (IOM) released the report *Lesbian Health*—the first IOM report that focused on the health of a sexual-minority population. In addition to presenting what was known about the health status of lesbians, the report highlighted the challenges inherent in conducting research on the health needs and risks of this population. The report created an awareness about the health of lesbians and the importance of research in improving their health.

Society has experienced many changes during the ensuing 12 years, yet much remains unknown about the health status of sexual and gender minorities. Moreover, many of the research challenges identified in *Lesbian Health* persist today. At the request of the National Institutes of Health (NIH), in 2010 the IOM convened a committee to assess the current state of knowledge about the health of lesbian, gay, bisexual, and transgender people, as well as to identify research gaps and formulate a research agenda that could guide NIH in enhancing and focusing its research in this area.

The task before the committee was broad and complex. In considering the health of sexual and gender minorities, the committee recognized that not only are lesbians, gay men, bisexual men and women, and transgender people all separate groups, but each of these groups encompasses subpopulations with their own unique health needs. This report presents a wealth of information that has, for the first time, been compiled and organized in a comprehensive fashion. It is the product of more than a year of information gathering, review, and deliberation. The committee benefited from three open meetings (two in Washington, DC, and one in San Francisco) where not only invited presenters but also members of the public generously gave of their time, shared their knowledge, and responded to questions from the committee. These sessions, along with materials submitted from various sources, were invaluable in furthering the committee's understanding of the topic.

On behalf of the committee, in addition to the presenters, reviewers, consultants, and members of the public who assisted in the creation of this report, I extend our deepest thanks to the project staff: Monica Feit, study director; Joshua Joseph, associate program officer; Jon Sanders, program associate; Karen Anderson, senior program officer; Sarah Isquick, Christine Mirzayan Science and Technology Policy Graduate Fellow, fall 2010; and Rick Erdtmann, board director. The committee could not have done its work without the outstanding support and guidance provided by these individuals.

It is the committee's hope that this report will not only assist NIH in its goal of promoting the nation's health through research, but also advance the public's understanding about the health of lesbian, gay, bisexual, and transgender people.

Robert Graham, *Chair*
Committee on Lesbian, Gay, Bisexual, and Transgender Health Issues and Research Gaps and Opportunities

Contents

Tables, Figures, and Boxes

TABLES

FIGURES

BOXES

Acronyms and Abbreviations

AAPOR	American Association for Public Opinion Research
ACASI	audio computer-assisted self-interview
AIDS	acquired immune deficiency syndrome
BMI	body mass index
BRFSS	Behavioral Risk Factor Surveillance System
CDC	Centers for Disease Control and Prevention
CHIS	California Health Interview Survey
DEBI	Diffusion of Effective Behavioral Interventions
DOMA	Defense of Marriage Act
DSM	*Diagnostic and Statistical Manual of Mental Disorders*
FBI	Federal Bureau of Investigation
FDA	U.S. Food and Drug Administration
GIDC	gender identity disorder of childhood
GLMA	Gay and Lesbian Medical Association
GnRH	gonadotropin-releasing hormone
GSI	General Severity Index
GSS	General Social Survey
GUTS	Growing Up Today Study
HIV	human immunodeficiency virus

HPV	human papillomavirus
HRT	hormone replacement therapy
IOM	Institute of Medicine
LGB	lesbian, gay, and bisexual
LGBT	lesbian, gay, bisexual, and transgender
MA BRFSS	Massachusetts Behavioral Risk Factor Surveillance System
MIDUS	Midlife Development in the United States
NAS	National Academy of Sciences
NCAVP	National Coalition of Anti-Violence Programs
NCS	National Comorbidity Survey
NESARC	National Epidemiologic Survey on Alcohol and Related Conditions
NHANES	National Health and Nutrition Examination Survey
NHBS	National HIV Behavioral Survey
NHIS	National Health Interview Survey
NHS	Nurses' Health Study
NHSDA	National Household Survey of Drug Abuse
NHSLS	National Health and Social Life Survey
NIH	National Institutes of Health
NLHCS	National Lesbian Health Care Survey
NNHS	National Nurses Health Survey
NORC	National Opinion Research Center
NSFG	National Survey of Family Growth
NSHAP	National Social Life, Health, and Aging Project
NSSHB	National Survey of Sexual Health and Behavior
NTDS	National Transgender Discrimination Survey
RCT	randomized controlled trial
STD	sexually transmitted disease
STI	sexually transmitted infection
THIS	Transgender Health Initiative Survey
VDH	Virginia Department of Health
WPATH	World Professional Association for Transgender Health

Summary

Lesbian, gay, bisexual, and transgender (LGBT) individuals experience unique health disparities. Although the acronym LGBT is used as an umbrella term, and the health needs of this community are often grouped together, each of these letters represents a distinct population with its own health concerns. Furthermore, among lesbians, gay men, bisexual men and women, and transgender people, there are subpopulations based on race, ethnicity, socioeconomic status, geographic location, age, and other factors. Although a modest body of knowledge on LGBT health has been developed, these populations, stigmatized as sexual and gender minorities, have been the subject of relatively little health research. As a result, a number of questions arise: What is currently known about the health status of LGBT populations? Where do gaps in the research exist? What are the priorities for a research agenda to address these gaps?

At the request of the National Institutes of Health (NIH), the Institute of Medicine convened a consensus committee to answer these questions. The 17-member Committee on Lesbian, Gay, Bisexual, and Transgender Health Issues and Research Gaps and Opportunities comprised experts in the fields of mental health, biostatistics, clinical medicine, adolescent health and development, aging, parenting, behavioral sciences, HIV research, demography, racial and ethnic disparities, and health services. The committee was asked to

- conduct a review and prepare a report assessing the state of the science on the health status of lesbian, gay, bisexual, and transgender populations; identify research gaps and opportunities; and outline a research agenda that will assist NIH in enhancing its research efforts in this area.

STUDY APPROACH

In conducting this study, the committee used a variety of sources: five formal committee meetings, including four public meetings with presentations from researchers, individuals, advocacy groups, and service providers; a literature review; commissioned papers; and consultants. The committee's work was guided by four conceptual frameworks:

- The *life-course framework* acknowledges that events at each stage of life influence subsequent stages and recognizes that experiences are shaped by one's age cohort and historical context.
- The *minority stress model* posits that sexual and gender minorities experience chronic stress as a result of their stigmatization.
- *Intersectionality* examines an individual's multiple identities and the ways in which they interact.
- The *social ecology perspective* emphasizes that individuals are surrounded by spheres of influence, including families, communities, and society.

These frameworks complement each other and structured and informed the committee's deliberations.

CONTEXT FOR UNDERSTANDING LGBT HEALTH

The committee believed that to examine the health of LGBT people, it was important to understand the contextual factors that influence their lives. Some of those factors include the history of LGBT people in the United States, the effects of stigma, laws and policies, demographic factors, and barriers to care. These factors are interrelated. For example, many historical events have contributed to the stigmatization of nonheterosexual and gender-variant individuals. The inclusion of homosexuality in the *Diagnostic and Statistical Manual of Mental Disorders* until 1973 shaped sexual-minority patients' interactions with the health care system. Likewise, the legal landscape affects aspects of people's lives that influence health. For instance, laws prohibiting marriage between same-sex individuals often affect the access of lesbians, gay men, and bisexual people to employer-sponsored health insurance. Other barriers to care include the limited availability of providers with adequate training to treat transgender patients in a culturally competent manner and LGBT patients' previous negative experiences with the health care system.

The HIV/AIDS epidemic resulted in the deaths of thousands of gay and bisexual men; at the same time, it created a resilient and more unified LGBT community. HIV/AIDS remains one of the most critical health issues faced by some subgroups within LGBT populations in the United States—

particularly gay and bisexual men, as well as transgender women. The epidemic serves as an example of some of this report's key themes: not only resilience, but also stigma, racial and ethnic disparities, and the importance of research funding.

CHALLENGES TO CONDUCTING RESEARCH ON LGBT POPULATIONS

A number of challenges are associated with conducting health research on LGBT populations. These include the following:

- Sexual orientation and gender nonconformity are multifaceted concepts, and defining them operationally can be challenging.
- Individuals may be reluctant to answer research questions about their same-sex sexual behavior or gender nonconformity.
- Because LGBT populations represent a relatively small proportion of the U.S. population, it is labor-intensive and costly to recruit a large enough sample in general population surveys for meaningful analysis of these populations and their subgroups.

Despite these challenges, many researchers currently conduct health research on LGBT populations. In so doing, as with research on any populations, researchers must choose a sampling strategy and a data collection method. While probability samples allow findings to be generalized to the study's target population, they are expensive and difficult to implement with LGBT populations given the research challenges listed above. However, the use of established statistical techniques makes it possible to improve the precision of estimates for small populations by combining two or more data sets.

Research on the health status of LGBT populations more commonly uses nonprobability samples. Even though the extent to which findings based on such samples accurately characterize these populations is unknown, these samples have yielded valuable information for expanding the field of LGBT research and identifying possible gaps in health services. In addition to providing general descriptive data for LGBT populations and their subgroups, nonprobability samples have served to reveal the existence of certain phenomena, to suggest relationships among variables, to identify possible differences among groups, and to generate hypotheses and formulate ideas that can be advanced for systematic study in the future. A variety of methods are used to generate nonprobability samples, including purposive, quota, and snowball sampling. While much of what is currently known about the health of LGBT populations comes from studies with nonprobability samples, the field of LGBT health would benefit if more data came from probability samples.

Best practices for research on the health status of LGBT populations include scientific rigor and respectful involvement of individuals who represent the target population. Scientific rigor includes incorporating and monitoring culturally competent study designs, such as the use of appropriate measures to identify participants and implementation processes adapted to the unique characteristics of the target population. Respectful involvement refers to the involvement of LGBT individuals and those who represent the larger LGBT community in the research process, from design through data collection to dissemination.

HEALTH STATUS OVER THE LIFE COURSE

Drawing on the life-course framework, the committee examined the health status of LGBT populations in three life stages: childhood and adolescence, early/middle adulthood, and later adulthood. Within these age blocks, the committee looked at mental health, physical health, risk and protective factors, health services, and contextual influences. Research on sexual- and gender-minority populations has been uneven. More research has focused on gay men and lesbians than on bisexual and transgender people. Research has not adequately examined subpopulations, particularly racial and ethnic groups. Most research has been conducted among adults; very few studies have focused on children, more on adolescents and young adults, and few again on LGBT elders. Some of the key findings of this study across the life course are summarized below.

Childhood/Adolescence

- The burden of HIV falls disproportionately on young men, particularly young black men, who have sex with men.
- LGB youth are at increased risk for suicidal ideation and attempts as well as depression. Small studies suggest the same may be true for transgender youth.
- Rates of smoking, alcohol consumption, and substance use may be higher among LGB than heterosexual youth. Almost no research has examined substance use among transgender youth.
- The homeless youth population comprises a disproportionate number of LGB youth. Some research suggests that young transgender women are also at significant risk for homelessness.
- LGBT youth report experiencing elevated levels of violence, victimization, and harassment compared with heterosexual and non-gender-variant youth.
- Families and schools appear to be two possible focal points for intervention research.

Early/Middle Adulthood

- As a group, LGB adults appear to experience more mood and anxiety disorders, more depression, and an elevated risk for suicidal ideation and attempts compared with heterosexual adults. Research based on smaller convenience samples suggests that elevated rates of suicidal ideation and attempts as well as depression exist among transgender adults; however, little research has examined the prevalence of mood and anxiety disorders in this population.
- Lesbians and bisexual women may use preventive health services less frequently than heterosexual women.
- Lesbians and bisexual women may be at greater risk of obesity and have higher rates of breast cancer than heterosexual women.
- HIV/AIDS continues to exact a severe toll on men who have sex with men, with black and Latino men being disproportionately affected.
- LGBT people are frequently the targets of stigma, discrimination, and violence because of their sexual- and gender-minority status.
- LGB adults may have higher rates of smoking, alcohol use, and substance use than heterosexual adults. Most research in this area has been conducted among women, with much less being known about gay and bisexual men. Limited research among transgender adults indicates that substance use is a concern for this population.
- Gay men and lesbians are less likely to be parents than their heterosexual peers, although children of gay and lesbian parents are well adjusted and developmentally similar to children of heterosexual parents.

Later Adulthood

- Limited research suggests that transgender elders may experience negative health outcomes as a result of long-term hormone use.
- HIV/AIDS impacts not only younger but also older LGBT individuals. However, few HIV prevention programs target older adults, a cohort that also has been deeply affected by the losses inflicted by AIDS.
- There is some evidence that LGBT elders exhibit crisis competence (a concept reflecting resilience and perceived hardiness within older LGBT populations).
- LGBT elders experience stigma, discrimination, and violence across the life course.
- LGBT elders are less likely to have children than heterosexual elders and are less likely to receive care from adult children.

RECOMMENDATIONS

The committee's primary recommendation is the implementation of a research agenda that will assist NIH in enhancing its research efforts in the area of LGBT health. The committee also recommends six additional actions to advance understanding of LGBT health.

Research Agenda

> **Recommendation 1. NIH should implement a research agenda designed to advance knowledge and understanding of LGBT health.**

The committee believes that building the evidence base on LGBT health issues will not only benefit LGBT individuals but also provide new research on topics that affect heterosexual and non-gender-variant individuals as well. Given the large number of areas in LGBT health in which research is needed, the committee formulated a research agenda that reflects those areas of highest priority. Within each of those areas, the conceptual frameworks identified above are evident as cross-cutting perspectives that should be considered. Figure S-1 illustrates the interactions between the priority research areas identified by the committee and these cross-cutting perspectives.

As noted above, although lesbians, gay men, bisexual men and women, and transgender people each are separate populations, they frequently are considered as a group. The primary driving force behind combining these populations is that they are nonheterosexual or gender nonconforming

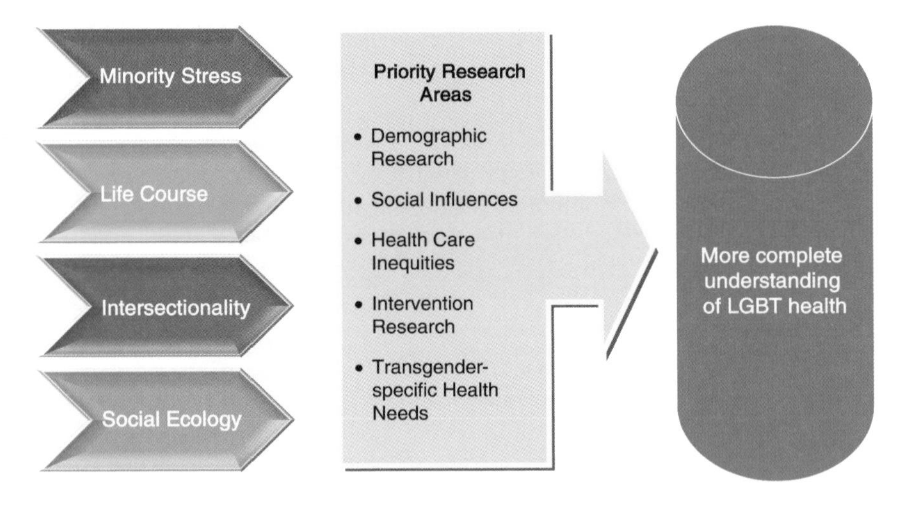

FIGURE S-1 Research agenda. A number of different conceptual perspectives can be applied to priority areas of research in order to further the evidence base for LGBT health issues.

and are frequently stigmatized as a consequence. These populations also are often combined in some way for research purposes. For example, researchers frequently merge lesbians, gay men, and bisexual people into a group labeled "nonheterosexual." Similarly, in some HIV research, study participants are combined in a single category that may include gay men, bisexual men, transgender women, and men who do not identify as any of the above but still have sex with other men. Combining these populations in this way obscures differences among them.

Given that lesbians, gay men, bisexual women and men, and transgender people are in fact separate populations, it is important to note that most of the research on these populations has focused on lesbians and gay men. Much less research has been conducted on bisexual and transgender people. The committee therefore recommends research that focuses on all of these populations.

Cross-Cutting Perspectives

The following perspectives should inform research on LGBT health:

- **A minority stress perspective**—Experiences of stigma shared by sexual and gender minorities and the impact of minority stress should be considered.
- **A life-course perspective**—Cohort and age differences influence health needs. Longitudinal studies and studies that analyze data with respect to different age groups are needed to gain a better understanding of LGBT health.
- **An intersectional perspective**—Sexual- or gender-minority status is only one of many factors that influence the lives and health of individuals. An examination of the health status of LGBT people in the context of racial, ethnic, socioeconomic, and geographic diversity will provide a more complete understanding.
- **A social ecological perspective**—An individual's health is affected by community and social circumstances. LGBT health research should consider both the individual and the various contexts, including interpersonal relationships, in which the individual lives.

Research Areas

Research in the following areas is essential for building a solid evidence base in LGBT health:

- **Demographic research**—More demographic data on lesbian, gay, bisexual, and transgender people across the life course are needed, as are data on LGBT subpopulations.

- **Social influences on the lives of LGBT people**—Social support plays an important part in mental health. The role of social structures—such as families, schools, workplaces, religious institutions, and community organizations—in the lives of LGBT people should be understood more fully.
- **Inequities in health care**—LGBT people face barriers to equitable health care that profoundly affect their overall well-being. Understanding outcome disparities, provider attitudes and education, ways in which the care environment can be improved, and the experiences of LGBT individuals seeking care would provide a base from which to address these inequities.
- **Intervention research**—Research is needed to develop and test the effectiveness of interventions designed to address health inequities and negative health outcomes experienced by LGBT people. Interventions that increase access to care or address the mental or physical conditions that lead to impaired health would assist in reducing these disparities. Interventions focused on subgroups are especially needed.
- **Transgender-specific health needs**—An evidence base for providing transgender-specific health care to address gender dysphoria should be created. Most such research is based on small, non-probability samples. A more rigorous research program is needed to understand the health implications of hormone use and other transgender-specific issues.

Research Gaps and Opportunities

In its statement of task, the committee was asked to identify research gaps and opportunities related to LGBT health. In the committee's view, one sets out to identify research gaps by reviewing a body of evidence that needs additional work in selected areas. However, this was not the committee's experience in reviewing the literature on LGBT health. Instead, the committee found that the existing body of evidence is sparse and that substantial research is needed. The positive view of this situation is that there are many research opportunities related to LGBT health.

The research agenda proposed by the committee was drawn from the many research opportunities that currently exist. All of the topics on this agenda represent multiple opportunities for research that extends across the life course. In some cases, the focus is on specific subpopulations or fields, while in others it is on types of research or particular contexts. While not representing an exhaustive list, some specific research opportunities are noted at the end of Chapters 2 through 6 and in Chapter 7 in Table 7-1.

Data Collection

Recommendation 2. Data on sexual orientation and gender identity should be collected in federally funded surveys administered by the Department of Health and Human Services and in other relevant federally funded surveys.

Similar to race and ethnicity data, data on sexual and gender minorities should be included in the battery of demographic information that is collected in federally funded surveys. These data would help those seeking to undertake the demographic research recommended as part of the research agenda proposed by the committee. For example, given the interactions between social and economic circumstances and health, data from social and economic surveys could provide valuable information on the context for health disparities experienced by LGBT people. Similarly, surveys on crime and victimization, housing, and families would provide data on variables that relate to the health of sexual and gender minorities. This data collection would be aided by the development of standardized measures for sexual orientation and gender identity (see Recommendation 4 below).

Recommendation 3. Data on sexual orientation and gender identity should be collected in electronic health records.

The Office of the National Coordinator for Health Information Technology within the Department of Health and Human Services should include the collection of data on sexual orientation and gender identity as part of its meaningful-use objectives for electronic health records. Collecting these detailed patient-level data, with adequate privacy and security protection as is needed for all data collected in electronic health records, could assist in identifying and addressing LGBT health disparities. At present, possible discomfort on the part of health care workers with asking questions about sexual orientation and gender identity, a lack of knowledge by providers of how to elicit this information, and some hesitancy on the part of patients to disclose this information may be barriers to the collection of meaningful data on sexual orientation and gender identity. Nonetheless, the committee encourages the Office of the National Coordinator to begin planning for the collection of these data as part of the required set of demographic data for electronic health records. Detailed patient-level data such as those found in electronic health records could provide a rich source of information about LGBT populations and subpopulations.

Methodological Research

Recommendation 4. NIH should support the development and standardization of sexual orientation and gender identity measures.

NIH should support the rigorous development of valid, reliable measures focused on sexual orientation and gender identity. The development and adoption of standardized measures in federally funded surveys would assist in synthesizing scientific knowledge about the health of sexual and gender minorities.

Recommendation 5. NIH should support methodological research that relates to LGBT health.

NIH should support research that will assist in addressing the methodological challenges associated with conducting research on LGBT health. Particularly helpful would be studies aimed at developing innovative ways to conduct research with small populations and determining the best ways to collect information on sexual and gender minorities in research, health care, and other settings.

Research Training

Recommendation 6. A comprehensive research training approach should be created to strengthen LGBT health research at NIH.

To encourage more research on LGBT health issues, NIH should expand its intramural and extramural training programs, focusing on three audiences: researchers who are working with or considering working with LGBT populations, researchers who may not be aware of LGBT health issues, and NIH staff. Training opportunities should be provided to postbaccalaureate, postdoctoral, graduate student, and career researchers.

Policy on Research Participation

Recommendation 7. NIH should encourage grant applicants to address explicitly the inclusion or exclusion of sexual and gender minorities in their samples.

Using the NIH policy on the inclusion of women and minorities in clinical research as a model, NIH should encourage grant applicants to address explicitly the extent to which their proposed sample includes or excludes sexual and gender minorities. Researchers would thereby be prompted to consider the scientific implications of including or excluding sexual and gender minorities and whether these groups will be included in sufficient numbers to permit meaningful analyses.

1

Introduction

At a time when lesbian, gay, bisexual, and transgender (LGBT) individuals are an increasingly open, acknowledged, and visible part of society, clinicians and researchers are faced with incomplete information about the health status of this community. Although a modest body of knowledge on LGBT health has been developed over the last two decades, much remains to be explored. What is currently known about LGBT health? Where do gaps in the research in this area exist? What are the priorities for a research agenda to address these gaps? This report aims to answer these questions.

THE LGBT COMMUNITY

The phrase "lesbian, gay, bisexual, and transgender community" (or "LGBT community") refers to a broad coalition of groups that are diverse with respect to gender, sexual orientation, race/ethnicity, and socioeconomic status. Thus while this report focuses on the community that is encapsulated by the acronym LGBT, the committee wishes to highlight the importance of recognizing that the various populations represented by "L," "G," "B," and "T" are distinct groups, each with its own special health-related concerns and needs. The committee believes it is essential to emphasize these differences at the outset of this report because in some contemporary scientific discourse, and in the popular media, these groups are routinely treated as a single population under umbrella terms such as LGBT. At the same time, as discussed further below, these groups have many experiences in common, key among them being the experience of stigmatization. (Differences *within* each of these groups related to, for example, race, ethnicity, socioeconomic status, geographic location, and age also are addressed later in the chapter.)

Lesbians, gay men, and bisexual men and women are defined according to their sexual orientation, which, as discussed in Chapter 2, is typically conceptualized in terms of sexual attraction, behavior, identity, or some combination of these dimensions. They share the fact that their sexual orientation is not exclusively heterosexual. Yet this grouping of "nonheterosexuals" includes men and women; homosexual and bisexual individuals; people who label themselves as gay, lesbian, or bisexual, among other terms; and people who do not adopt such labels but nevertheless experience same-sex attraction or engage in same-sex sexual behavior. As explained throughout the report, these differences have important health implications for each group.

In contrast to lesbians, gay men, and bisexual men and women, transgender people are defined according to their gender identity and presentation. This group encompasses individuals whose gender identity differs from the sex originally assigned to them at birth or whose gender expression varies significantly from what is traditionally associated with or typical for that sex (i.e., people identified as male at birth who subsequently identify as female, and people identified as female at birth who later identify as male), as well as other individuals who vary from or reject traditional cultural conceptualizations of gender in terms of the male–female dichotomy. The transgender population is diverse in gender identity, expression, and sexual orientation. Some transgender individuals have undergone medical interventions to alter their sexual anatomy and physiology, others wish to have such procedures in the future, and still others do not. Transgender people can be heterosexual, homosexual, or bisexual in their sexual orientation. Some lesbians, gay men, and bisexuals are transgender; most are not. Male-to-female transgender people are known as MtF, transgender females, or transwomen, while female-to-male transgender people are known as FtM, transgender males, or transmen. Some transgender people do not fit into either of these binary categories. As one might expect, there are health differences between transgender and nontransgender people, as well as between transgender females and transgender males.

Whereas "LGBT" is appropriate and useful for describing the combined populations of lesbian, gay, bisexual, and transgender people, it also can obscure the many differences that distinguish these sexual- and gender-minority groups. Combining lesbians and gay men under a single rubric, for example, obscures gender differences in the experiences of homosexual people. Likewise, collapsing together the experiences of bisexual women and men tends to obscure gender differences. Further, to the extent that lesbian, gay, and bisexual are understood as identity labels,

"LGB" leaves out people whose experience includes same-sex attractions or behaviors but who do not adopt a nonheterosexual identity. And the transgender population, which itself encompasses multiple groups, has needs and concerns that are distinct from those of lesbians, bisexual women and men, and gay men.

As noted above, despite these many differences among the populations that make up the LGBT community, there are important commonalities as well. The remainder of this section first describes these commonalities and then some key differences within these populations.

Commonalities Among LGBT Populations

What do lesbians, gay men, bisexual women and men, and transgender people have in common that makes them, as a combined population, an appropriate focus for this report? In the committee's view, the main commonality across these diverse groups is their members' historically marginalized social status relative to society's cultural norm of the exclusively heterosexual individual who conforms to traditional gender roles and expectations. Put another way, these groups share the common status of "other" because of their members' departures from heterosexuality and gender norms. Their "otherness" is the basis for stigma and its attendant prejudice, discrimination, and violence, which underlie society's general lack of attention to their health needs and many of the health disparities discussed in this report. For some, this "otherness" may be complicated by additional dimensions of inequality such as race, ethnicity, and socioeconomic status, resulting in stigma at multiple levels.

To better understand how sexuality- and gender-linked stigma are related to health, imagine a world in which gender nonconformity, same-sex attraction, and same-sex sexual behavior are universally understood and accepted as part of the normal spectrum of the human condition. In this world, membership in any of the groups encompassed by LGBT would carry no social stigma, engender no disgrace or personal shame, and result in no discrimination. In this world, a host of issues would threaten the health of LGBT individuals: major chronic diseases such as cancer and heart disease; communicable diseases; mental disorders; environmental hazards; the threat of violence and terrorism; and the many other factors that jeopardize human "physical, mental and social well-being."[1] By and large,

[1] This latter phrase carries quotation marks because it is drawn from the preamble to the Constitution of the World Health Organization (WHO, 1946), which defines health broadly, and appropriately, as a "state of complete physical, mental and social well-being and not merely the absence of disease or infirmity." For the purposes of this report, the committee defines "health" broadly in accordance with this definition. Therefore, health encompasses multiple dimensions including physical, emotional, and social well-being and quality of life.

however, these issues would be the same as those confronting the rest of humanity. Only a few factors would stand out for LGBT individuals specifically. There would be little reason for the Institute of Medicine (IOM) to issue a report on LGBT health issues.

We do not live in the idealized world described in this thought experiment, however. Historically, lesbians, gay men, bisexual individuals, and transgender people have not been understood and accepted as part of the normal spectrum of the human condition. Instead, they have been stereotyped as deviants. Although LGBT people share with the rest of society the full range of health risks, they also face a profound and poorly understood set of additional health risks due largely to social stigma.

While the experience of stigma can differ across sexual and gender minorities, stigmatization touches the lives of all these groups in important ways and thereby affects their health. In contrast to members of many other marginalized groups, LGBT individuals frequently are invisible to health care researchers and providers. As explained in later chapters, this invisibility often exacerbates the deleterious effects of stigma. Overcoming this invisibility in health care services and research settings is a critical goal if we hope to eliminate the health disparities discussed throughout this report.

It is important to note that, despite the common experience of stigma among members of sexual- and gender-minority groups, LGBT people have not been passive victims of discrimination and prejudice. The achievements of LGBT people over the past few decades in building a community infrastructure that addresses their health needs, as well as obtaining acknowledgment of their health concerns from scientific bodies and government entities, attest to their commitment to resisting stigma and working actively for equal treatment in all aspects of their lives, including having access to appropriate health care services and reducing health care disparities. Indeed, some of the research cited in this report demonstrates the impressive psychological resiliency displayed by members of these populations, often in the face of considerable stress.

As detailed throughout this report, the stigma directed at sexual and gender minorities in the contemporary United States creates a variety of challenges for researchers and health care providers. Fearing discrimination and prejudice, for example, many lesbian, gay, bisexual, and transgender people refrain from disclosing their sexual orientation or gender identity to researchers and health care providers. Regardless of their own sexual orientation or gender identity, moreover, researchers risk being marginalized or discredited simply because they have chosen to study LGBT issues (Kempner, 2008), and providers seldom receive training in specific issues related to the care of LGBT patients. In addition, research on LGBT health involves some specific methodological challenges, which are discussed in Chapter 3.

Differences Within LGBT Populations

Not only are lesbians, gay men, bisexual women and men, and transgender people distinct populations, but each of these groups is itself a diverse population whose members vary widely in age, race and ethnicity, geographic location, social background, religiosity, and other demographic characteristics. Since many of these variables are centrally related to health status, health concerns, and access to care, this report explicitly considers a few key subgroupings of the LGBT population in each chapter:

- **Age cohort**—One's age influences one's experiences and needs. Bisexual adolescents who are wrestling with coming out in a nonsupportive environment have different health needs than gay adult men who lack access to health insurance or older lesbians who are unable to find appropriate grief counseling services. In addition, development does not follow the same course for people of all ages. An older adult who comes out as gay in his 50s may not experience the developmental process in the same fashion as a self-identified "queer" youth who comes out during her teenage years. Similarly, as discussed further below, experiences across the life course differ according to the time period in which individuals are born. For example, an adolescent coming out in 2010 would do so in a different environment than an adolescent coming out in the 1960s. Moreover, some people experience changes in their sexual attractions and relationships over the course of their life. Some transgender people, for example, are visibly gender role nonconforming in childhood and come out at an early age, whereas others are able to conform and may not come out until much later in life.
- **Race and ethnicity**—Concepts of community, traditional roles, religiosity, and cultural influences associated with race and ethnicity shape an LGBT individual's experiences. The racial and ethnic communities to which one belongs affect self-identification, the process of coming out, available support, the extent to which one identifies with the LGBT community, affirmation of gender-variant expression, and other factors that ultimately influence health outcomes. Members of racial and ethnic minority groups may have profoundly different experiences than non-Hispanic white LGBT individuals.
- **Educational level and socioeconomic status**—An LGBT individual's experience in society varies depending on his or her educational level and socioeconomic status. As higher educational levels tend to be associated with higher income levels, members of the community who are more educated may live in better neighborhoods with

better access to health care and the ability to lead healthier lives because of safe walking spaces and grocery stores that stock fresh fruits and vegetables (although, as discussed in later chapters, evidence indicates that some LGBT people face economic discrimination regardless of their educational level). On the other hand, members of the LGBT community who do not finish school or who live in poorer neighborhoods may experience more barriers in access to care and more negative health outcomes.

- **Geographic location**—Geographic location has significant effects on mental and physical health outcomes for LGBT individuals. Those in rural areas or areas with fewer LGBT people may feel less comfortable coming out, have less support from families and friends, and lack access to an LGBT community. LGBT individuals in rural areas may have less access to providers who are comfortable with or knowledgeable about the treatment of LGBT patients. In contrast, LGBT people living in areas with larger LGBT populations may find more support services and have more access to health care providers who are experienced in treating LGBT individuals.

Although these areas represent critical dimensions of the experiences of LGBT individuals, the relationships of these variables to health care disparities and health status have not been extensively studied.

STATEMENT OF TASK AND STUDY SCOPE

In the context of the issues outlined above, the IOM was asked by the National Institutes of Health (NIH) to convene a Committee on Lesbian, Gay, Bisexual, and Transgender Health Issues and Research Gaps and Opportunities. The 17-member committee included experts from the fields of mental health, biostatistics, clinical medicine, adolescent health and development, aging, parenting, behavioral sciences, HIV research, demography, racial and ethnic disparities, and health services research. The committee's statement of task is shown in Box 1-1. The study was supported entirely by NIH.

Although intersexuality constitutes an additional type of "otherness" that is stigmatized and overlaps in some respects with LGBT identities and health issues, the committee decided it would not be appropriate to include intersexuality in the study scope. The majority of individuals affected by disorders of sex development do not face challenges related to sexual orientation and gender identity, although homosexuality, gender role nonconformity, and gender dysphoria (defined as discomfort with the gender assigned to one at birth [see Chapter 2]) are somewhat more prevalent among this population compared with the general population (Cohen-Kettenis and

BOX 1-1
Statement of Task

An IOM committee will conduct a review and prepare a report assessing the state of the science on the health status of lesbian, gay, bisexual, and transgender (LGBT) populations; identify research gaps and opportunities related to LGBT health; and outline a research agenda that will assist NIH in enhancing its research efforts in this area. Additionally, the committee will consider research training needs to foster the advancement of knowledge about LGBT health and identify impediments that hinder such advancement.

Areas of interest to the committee might include but are not limited to

- the state of knowledge regarding LGBT health, health risks and protective factors, health disparities, and access to and utilization of health care;
- the developmental process from childhood across the life course, in the context of family and social networks; the impact of family and social acceptance of sexual orientation, gender identity, and expression on health and well-being; and the experience of families with LGBT parents;
- the effects of age cohort, race, ethnicity, socioeconomic status, and geography (particularly urban vs. rural environments) on the health of LGBT persons;
- the effects of social determinants and cultural factors, including stigma, discrimination, and violence on the health and development of LGBT persons;
- the methodological challenges, including definitional and measurement issues, and study design issues involved in conducting research on the health of LGBT people, and identification of best practices for conducting research in these populations;
- research gaps, opportunities, and priorities for conducting research in the LGBT population; and
- research training to advance knowledge about LGBT health.

Pfafflin, 2003). The committee acknowledges that while very little research exists on the subject of intersexuality, it is a separate research topic encompassing critical issues, most of which are not related to LGBT issues, and hence is beyond the scope of this report.

In a similar vein, the committee decided not to address research and theory on the origins of sexual orientation. The committee's task was to review the state of science on the health status of LGBT populations, to identify gaps in knowledge, and to outline a research agenda in the area of LGBT health. The committee recognized that a thorough review of research and theory relevant to the factors that shape sexual orientation (including sexual orientation identity, sexual behavior, and sexual desire or attraction) would be a substantial task, one that would be largely distinct from the committee's main focus on LGBT health, and therefore beyond the scope of the committee's charge.

STUDY APPROACH

This study was informed by four public meetings that included 35 presentations (see Appendix A). Three of these meetings were held in Washington, DC, while the fourth took place in San Francisco. In addition, the committee conducted an extensive review of the literature using Medline, PsycInfo, and the Social Science Citation Index (see Appendix B for a list of search terms), as well as other resources. The committee's approach to the literature is described below, followed by a discussion of the various frameworks applied in this study. A brief note on the terminology used in this report is presented in Box 1-2.

Approach to the Literature

While acknowledging that peer-reviewed journals are the gold standard for the reporting of research results and making every effort to consult works published in major research journals, the committee chose to include in this study what it judged to be the best empirical literature available: journal articles, book chapters, empirical reports, and other data sources that had been critically reviewed by the committee members. Recognizing that academic journals differ in their publication criteria and the rigor of their peer-review process, the committee gave the greatest weight to papers published in the most authoritative journals. Given that chapters, academic books, and technical reports typically are not subjected to the same peer-review standards as journal articles, the committee gave the greatest credence to such sources that reported research employing rigorous methods, were authored by well-established researchers, and were generally consistent with scholarly consensus on the current state of knowledge.

With respect to articles describing current health issues in the LGBT community, the committee attempted to limit its review to these articles published since 1999. In the area of transgender populations, however, much of the most current research was conducted prior to 1999 and is

BOX 1-2
A Note on Terminology

As discussed, the committee adopted the commonly used shorthand LGBT to stand for lesbian, gay, bisexual, and transgender. In cases in which the literature refers only to lesbian, gay, and bisexual populations, the term LGB appears in the report without the T. Appendix C provides a glossary to assist the reader with any unfamiliar terminology.

cited throughout the report. Likewise, in the case of history and theory, the committee reviewed and cites older literature.

When evaluating quantitative and qualitative research, the committee considered factors affecting the generalizability of studies, including sample size, sample source, sample composition, recruitment methods, and response rate. The committee also considered the study design, saturation (the point at which new information ceases to emerge), and other relevant factors. In some cases, the committee decided that a study with sample limitations was important; in such cases, these limitations and limits on the extent to which the findings can be generalized are explicitly acknowledged. The inclusion of case studies was kept to a minimum given their limited generalizability.

Research on U.S. samples was given priority. In cases in which no U.S.-based data were available or the committee determined that it was important to include research on non-U.S. samples, however, this research is cited. This was frequently the case for research involving transgender people. Only English-language articles were considered.

The committee considered papers whose authors employed statistical methods for analyzing data, as well as qualitative research that did not include statistical analysis. For papers that included statistical analysis, the committee evaluated whether the analysis was appropriate and conducted properly. For papers reporting qualitative research, the committee evaluated whether the data were appropriately analyzed and interpreted. The committee does not present magnitudes of differences, which should be determined by consulting individual studies.

In some cases, the committee used secondary sources such as reports. However, it always referred back to the original citations to evaluate the evidence.

Conceptual Frameworks

In understanding the health of LGBT populations, multiple frameworks can be used to examine how multiple identities and structural arrangements intersect to influence health care access, health status, and health outcomes. This section provides an overview of each of the conceptual frameworks used for this study.

First, recognizing that there are a number of ways to present the information contained in this report, the committee found it helpful to apply a **life-course perspective**. A life-course perspective provides a useful framework for the above-noted varying health needs and experiences of an LGBT individual over the course of his or her life. Central to a life-course framework (Cohler and Hammack, 2007; Elder, 1998) is the notion that the experiences of individuals at every stage of their life inform subsequent experiences, as individuals are constantly revisiting issues encountered at earlier points in the life course. This interrelationship among experiences starts before birth and in fact, before conception. A life-course framework has four key dimensions:

- *Linked lives*—Lives are interdependent; social ties, including immediate family and other relationships, influence individuals' perspective on life.
- *Life events as part of an overall trajectory*—Significant experiences have a differential impact at various stages of the life course.
- *Personal decisions*—Individuals make choices influenced by the social contexts in which they live (e.g., family, peers, neighborhood, work setting).
- *Historical context*—A historical perspective provides a context for understanding the forces and factors that have shaped an individual's experiences; those born within the same historical period may experience events differently from those born earlier or later.

From the perspective of LGBT populations, these four dimensions have particular salience because together they provide a framework for considering a range of issues that shape these individuals' experiences and their health disparities. The committee relied on this framework and on recognized differences in age cohorts, such as those discussed earlier, in presenting information about the health status of LGBT populations.

Along with a life-course framework, the committee drew on the **minority stress model** (Brooks, 1981; Meyer, 1995, 2003a). While this model was originally developed by Brooks (1981) for lesbians, Meyer (1995) expanded it to include gay men and subsequently applied it to lesbians, gay men, and bisexuals (Meyer, 2003b). This model originates in the premise that sexual minorities, like other minority groups, experience chronic stress arising from their stigmatization. Within the context of an individual's environmental circumstances, Meyer conceptualizes distal and proximal stress processes. A distal process is an objective stressor that does not depend on an individual's perspective. In this model, *actual experiences of discrimination and violence* (also referred to as *enacted stigma*) are distal stress processes. Proximal, or subjective, stress processes depend on an individual's perception. They include *internalized homophobia* (a term referring to an individual's self-directed stigma, reflecting the adoption of society's negative attitudes about homosexuality and the application of them to oneself), *perceived stigma* (which relates to the expectation that one will be rejected and discriminated against and leads to a state of continuous vigilance that can require considerable energy to maintain; it is also referred to as *felt stigma*), and *concealment of one's sexual orientation or transgender identity*. Related to this taxonomy is the categorization of minority stress processes as both external (enacted stigma) and internal (felt stigma, self-stigma) (Herek, 2009; Scambler and Hopkins, 1986).

There is also supporting evidence for the validity of this model for transgender individuals. Some qualitative studies strongly suggest that stigma can negatively affect the mental health of transgender people (Bockting et al., 1998; Nemoto et al., 2003, 2006).

The minority stress model attributes the higher prevalence of anxiety, depression, and substance use found among LGB as compared with heterosexual populations to the additive stress resulting from nonconformity with prevailing sexual orientation and gender norms. The committee's use of this framework is reflected in the discussion of stigma as a common experience for LGBT populations and, in the context of this study, one that affects health.

In addition to the minority stress model, the committee believed it was important to consider the multiple social identities of LGBT individuals, including their identities as members of various racial/ethnic groups, and the intersections of these identities with dimensions of inequality such as poverty. An **intersectional perspective** is useful because it acknowledges simultaneous dimensions of inequality and focuses on understanding how they are interrelated and how they shape and influence one another. This framework also challenges one to look at the points of cohesion and fracture *within* racial/ethnic sexual- and gender-minority groups, as well as those *between* these groups and the dominant group culture (Brooks et al., 2009; Gamson and Moon, 2004).

Intersectionality encompasses a set of foundational claims and organizing principles for understanding social inequality and its relationship to individuals' marginalized status based on such dimensions as race, ethnicity, and social class (Dill and Zambrana, 2009; Weber, 2010). These include the following:

- Race is a social construct. The lived experiences of racial/ethnic groups can be understood only in the context of institutionalized patterns of unequal control over the distribution of a society's valued goods and resources.
- Understanding the racial and ethnic experiences of sexual- and gender-minority individuals requires taking into account the full range of historical and social experiences both within and between sexual- and gender-minority groups with respect to class, gender, race, ethnicity, and geographical location.
- The economic and social positioning of groups within society is associated with institutional practices and policies that contribute to unequal treatment.

- The importance of representation—the ways social groups and individuals are viewed and depicted in the society at large and the expectations associated with these depictions—must be acknowledged. These representations are integrally linked to social, structural, political, historical, and geographic factors.

Intersectional approaches are based on the premise that individual and group identities are complex—influenced and shaped not just by race, class, ethnicity, sexuality/sexual orientation, gender, physical disabilities, and national origin but also by the confluence of all of those characteristics. Nevertheless, in a hierarchically organized society, some statuses become more important than others at any given historical moment and in specific geographic locations. Race, ethnicity, class, and community context matter; they are all powerful determinants of access to social capital—the resources that improve educational, economic, and social position in society. Thus, this framework reflects the committee's belief that the health status of LGBT individuals cannot be examined in terms of a one-dimensional sexual- or gender-minority category, but must be seen as shaped by their multiple identities and the simultaneous intersection of many characteristics.

Finally, the **social ecology model** (McLeroy et al., 1988) draws on earlier work by Bronfenbrenner (1979), which recognizes that influences on individuals can be much broader than the immediate environment. This viewpoint is reflected in Healthy People 2020. In developing objectives to improve the health of all Americans, including LGBT individuals, Healthy People 2020 used an ecological approach that focused on both individual- and population-level determinants of health (HHS, 2000, 2011). With respect to LGBT health in particular, the social ecology model is helpful in conceptualizing that behavior both affects the social environment and, in turn, is affected by it. A social ecological model has multiple levels, each of which influences the individual; beyond the individual, these may include families, relationships, community, and society. It is worth noting that for LGBT people, stigma can and does take place at all of these levels. The committee found this framework useful in thinking about the effects of environment on an individual's health, as well as ways in which to structure health interventions.

Each of the above four frameworks provides conceptual tools that can help increase our understanding of health status, health needs, and health disparities in LGBT populations. Each complements the others to yield a more comprehensive approach to understanding lived experiences and their impact on LGBT health. The life-course perspective focuses on development between and within age cohorts, conceptualized within a historical context. Sexual minority stress theory examines individuals within a social and community context and emphasizes the impact of stigma on lived experiences. Intersectionality brings attention to the importance of multiple stigmatized identities (race, ethnicity, and low socioeconomic status) and to the ways in which these factors adversely affect health. The social ecology perspective emphasizes the influences on individuals' lives, including social ties and societal factors, and how these influences affect health. The chapters that follow draw on all these conceptualizations in an effort to provide a comprehensive overview of what is known, as well as to identify the knowledge gaps.

REPORT ORGANIZATION

This report is organized into seven chapters. Chapter 2 provides context for understanding LGBT health status by defining sexual orientation and gender identity, highlighting historical events that are pertinent to LGBT health, providing a demographic overview of LGBT people in the United States, examining barriers to their care, and using the example of HIV/AIDS to illustrate some important themes. Chapter 3 addresses the topic of conducting research on the health of LGBT people. Specifically, it reviews the major challenges associated with the conduct of research with LGBT populations, presents some commonly used research methods, provides information about available data sources, and comments on best practices for conducting research on the health of LGBT people.

As noted, in preparing this report, the committee found it helpful to discuss health issues within a life-course framework. Chapters 4, 5, and 6 review, respectively, what is known about the current health status of LGBT populations through the life course, divided into childhood/adolescence, early/middle adulthood, and later adulthood. Each of these chapters addresses the following by age cohort: the development of sexual orientation and gender identity, mental and physical health status, risk and protective factors, health services, and contextual influences affecting LGBT health. Chapter 7 reviews the gaps in research on LGBT health, outlines a research agenda, and offers recommendations based on the committee's findings.

REFERENCES

Bockting, W. O., B. E. Robinson, and B. R. Rosser. 1998. Transgender HIV prevention: A qualitative needs assessment. *AIDS Care* 10(4):505–525.

Bronfenbrenner, U. 1979. *The ecology of human development: Experiments by nature and design*. Cambridge, MA: Harvard University Press.

Brooks, K. D., L. Bowleg, and K. Quina. 2009. Minority sexual status among minorities. In *Sexualities and identities of minority women,* edited by S. Loue. New York: Springer Science. Pp. 41–63.

Brooks, V. R. 1981. The theory of minority stress. In *Minority stress and lesbian women,* edited by V. R. Brooks. Lexington, MA: Lexington Books. Pp. 71–90.

Cohen-Kettenis, P. T., and F. Pfafflin. 2003. *Transgenderism and intersexuality in childhood and adolescence: Making choices*. Thousand Oaks, CA: SAGE Publications.

Cohler, B. J., and P. L. Hammack. 2007. The psychological world of the gay teenager: Social change, narrative, and "normality." *Journal of Youth and Adolescence* 36(1):47–59.

Dill, T. B., and R. Zambrana. 2009. *Emerging intersections: Race, class and gender in theory, policy and practice*. New Brunswick, NJ: Rutgers University Press.

Elder, G. H. 1998. The life course as developmental theory. *Child Development* 69(1):1.

Gamson, J., and D. Moon. 2004. The sociology of sexualities: Queer and beyond. *Annual Review of Sociology* 30(1):47–64.

Herek, G. M. 2009. Sexual stigma and sexual prejudice in the United States: A conceptual framework. In *Contemporary perspectives on lesbian, gay, and bisexual identities*, edited by D. A. Hope. New York: Springer Science + Business Media. Pp. 65–111.

HHS (U.S. Department of Health and Human Services). 2000. *Healthy people 2010: Understanding and improving health*. Washington, DC: HHS.

HHS. 2011. *Lesbian, gay, bisexual, and transgender health*. http://www.healthypeople.gov/2020/topicsobjectives2020/overview.aspx?topicid=25 (accessed February 15, 2011).

Kempner, J. 2008. The chilling effect: How do researchers react to controversy? *PLoS Medicine/Public Library of Science* 5(11):e222.

McLeroy, K. R., D. Bibeau, A. Steckler, and K. Glanz. 1988. An ecological perspective on health promotion programs. *Health Education Quarterly* 15(4):351–377.

Meyer, I. H. 1995. Minority stress and mental health in gay men. *Journal of Health & Social Behavior* 36(1):38–56.

Meyer, I. H. 2003a. Minority stress and mental health in gay men. In *Psychological perspectives on lesbian, gay, and bisexual experiences*. 2nd ed., edited by L. D. Garnets and D. C. Kimmel. New York: Columbia University Press. Pp. 699–731.

Meyer, I. H. 2003b. Prejudice, social stress, and mental health in lesbian, gay, and bisexual populations: Conceptual issues and research evidence. *Psychological Bulletin* 129(5):674–697.

Nemoto, T., M. Iwamoto, and D. Operario. 2003. HIV risk behaviors among Asian and Pacific Islander male-to-female transgenders. *The Community Psychologist* 36:31–35.

Nemoto, T., L. A. Sausa, D. Operario, and J. Keatley. 2006. Need for HIV/AIDS education and intervention for MTF transgenders: Responding to the challenge. *Journal of Homosexuality* 51(1):183–202.

Scambler, G., and A. Hopkins. 1986. Being epileptic: Coming to terms with stigma. *Sociology of Health & Illness* 8:26–43.

Weber, L. 2010. *Understanding race, class, gender, and sexuality: A conceptual framework*. 2nd ed. New York: Oxford University Press.

WHO (World Health Organization). 1946. WHO definition of health. In *Preamble to the Constitution of the World Health Organization as adopted by the International Health Conference*. New York: WHO.

2

Context for LGBT Health Status in the United States

The current health status of lesbian, gay, bisexual, and transgender people of all races, ethnicities, ages, and social backgrounds can be understood only in cultural and historical context. To provide this context, this chapter reviews basic definitions and concepts concerning gender identity, gender expression, and sexual orientation; summarizes key historical events that have shaped contemporary LGBT culture and communities; describes the demography of LGBT people in the United States; and examines barriers to accessing health care for LGBT people. The chapter then presents a discussion of the case of HIV/AIDS as it relates to several important themes of this report. The final section summarizes key findings and research opportunities.

DEFINING GENDER IDENTITY, GENDER EXPRESSION, AND SEXUAL ORIENTATION

To discuss the context surrounding the health of LGBT populations, the committee has adopted working definitions for a number of key terms. *Sex* is understood here as a biological construct, referring to the genetic, hormonal, anatomical, and physiological characteristics on whose basis one is labeled at birth as either male or female. *Gender*, on the other hand, denotes the cultural meanings of patterns of behavior, experience, and personality that are labeled masculine or feminine.

Gender Identity and Expression

Gender identity refers to a person's basic sense of being a man or boy, a woman or girl, or another gender (e.g., transgender, bigender, or gender queer—a rejection of the traditional binary classification of gender). Gender identity can be congruent or incongruent with one's sex assigned at birth based on the appearance of the external genitalia. *Gender expression* denotes the manifestation of characteristics in one's personality, appearance, and behavior that are culturally defined as masculine or feminine. *Gender role conformity* refers to the extent to which an individual's gender expression adheres to the cultural norms prescribed for people of his or her sex.

Gender dysphoria refers to a discomfort with one's sex assigned at birth (Fisk, 1974). This dysphoria can manifest itself in a persistent unease with one's primary and secondary sex characteristics, a sense of inappropriateness in one's gender role, and a strong and persistent identification with and desire to live in the role of the other sex, which has been classified as gender identity disorder in the *Diagnostic and Statistical Manual of Mental Disorders*, Fourth Edition (DSM-IV) (American Psychiatric Association, 2000).

The term *transgender* has come to be widely used to refer to a diverse group of individuals who cross or transcend culturally defined categories of gender (Bockting, 1999); that is, they depart significantly from traditional gender norms. This group includes transsexuals (who desire or have had hormone therapy and/or surgery to feminize or masculinize their body and may live full time in the cross-gender role); cross-dressers or transvestites (who wear clothes and adopt a presentation associated with the other gender for emotional or sexual gratification, and may live part time in the cross-gender role); transgenderists (who live full time in the cross-gender role, may take hormones, but do not desire surgery); bigender persons (who identify as both man and woman, may take hormones, and may live part time in the cross-gender role); drag queens and kings (who dress in clothes associated with the other gender, adopt a hyperfeminine or hypermasculine presentation, and appear part time in the cross-gender role); and other identities, such as gender queer or two-spirit—a term used by some Native Americans for individuals who possess feminine and masculine qualities (who may or may not desire hormones or surgery, and may or may not live part or full time in the cross-gender role). Definitions of these categories vary and continue to evolve over time. The term *transgender* is increasingly used to encompass this family of gender-variant identities and expressions, but opinions on the term vary by geographic region and by individual. For example, some transsexual women differentiate themselves from those who self-identify as transgender to underscore that they are not gender variant or nonconforming, but instead identify unambiguously with the other gender. As explained in the previous chapter, a person whose gender identity differs from a male sex assignment at birth is often referred to as a *male-to-female* transgender woman. A person whose gender identity differs from a female sex assignment at birth is often referred to as a *female-to-male* transgender man. For research purposes, transsexuals are more often the focus of study than other transgender groups since they are more likely to seek clinical intervention, making data on this subgroup more accessible (Rosser et al., 2007).

Transgender people may be sexually oriented toward men, women, other transgender people, or any combination of these groups. There is no consensus in the research literature as to whether, when describing a transgender person's sexual orientation, sexual orientation labels should be based on the person's sex at birth or gender identity. However, transgender people themselves, especially those who live full time in the cross-gender role, more often than not anchor their sexual orientation on gender identity (e.g., a male-to-female transsexual woman who is attracted primarily to women is most likely to refer to herself as lesbian rather than heterosexual or straight) (Amercian Psychological Association, 2009a,b).

Sexual Orientation

The committee's working definition of *sexual orientation* incorporates three core ideas. First, sexual orientation is about intimate human relationships—sexual, romantic, or both. These relationships can be actualized through behavior or can remain simply an object of desire. Second, the focus of sexual orientation is the biological sex of a person's actual or potential relationship partners—that is, people of the same sex as the individual, people of the other sex, or people of either sex. Third, sexual orientation is about enduring patterns of experience and behavior. A single instance of sexual desire or a single sexual act generally is not regarded as defining an individual's sexual orientation.

Based on these considerations, the committee adopted the following working definition: *sexual orientation* refers to an enduring pattern of or disposition to experience sexual or romantic desires for, and relationships with, people of one's same sex, the other sex, or both sexes. As this definition makes clear, sexual orientation is inherently a relational construct. Whether a sexual act or romantic attraction is characterized as homosexual or heterosexual depends on the biological sex of the individuals involved, *relative to each other*. One's sexual orientation defines the population of individuals with whom one can potentially create satisfying and fulfilling sexual or romantic relationships. Such relationships help to meet basic human needs for love, attachment, and intimacy and are, for many people, an essential aspect of the self (Herek, 2006; Peplau and Garnets, 2000).

This working definition encompasses *attraction*, *behavior*, and *identity*. As explained in Chapter 3, most researchers studying sexual orientation have defined it operationally in terms of one or more of these three components. Defined in terms of *attraction* (or *desire*), sexual orientation is an enduring pattern of experiencing sexual or romantic feelings for men, women, transgender persons, or some combination of these groups. Defined in terms of *behavior*, sexual orientation refers to an enduring pattern of sexual or romantic activity with men, women, transgender persons, or some combination of these groups. Sexual orientation *identity* encompasses both *personal identity* and *social identity*. Defined in terms of *personal identity*, sexual orientation refers to a conception of the self based on one's enduring pattern of sexual and romantic attractions and behaviors toward men, women, or both sexes. Defined in terms of *social* (or *collective*) *identity*, it refers to a sense of membership in a social group based on a shared sexual orientation and a linkage of one's self-esteem to that group.

Although sexual attractions and behaviors are generally understood as ranging along a continuum from exclusively heterosexual to exclusively homosexual (Kinsey et al., 1948, 1953), sexual orientation is often discussed according to three main categories, especially when it is defined in terms of identity: (1) *heterosexuality* (for individuals who identify as, for example, "straight" or whose sexual or romantic attractions and behaviors focus exclusively or mainly on members of the other sex); (2) *homosexuality* (for individuals who identify as, for example, "gay," "lesbian," or "homosexual" or whose attractions and behaviors focus exclusively or mainly on members of the same sex); and (3) *bisexuality* (for individuals who identify as, for example, "bisexual" or whose sexual or romantic attractions and behaviors are directed at members of both sexes to a significant degree). Which of these categories is used in a particular study or health intervention will depend on the research or treatment goals. Individuals may also have a specific attraction toward transgender persons (Coan et al., 2005; Operario et al., 2008; Weinberg and Williams, 2010).

Some research suggests that within the subgroup of individuals identifying as bisexual, there exists considerable variability in self-identified orientation and identity groups. While some bisexual individuals exhibit approximately equal attraction to males and females, others exhibit varying levels of preference for one sex or another (Herek et al., 2010). Similarly, bisexual individuals may exhibit differing degrees of heterosexual, homosexual, or bisexual identity, identifying with all groups equally or more strongly with one than the others (Weinrich and Klein, 2002; Worthington and Reynolds, 2009).

Individuals vary in the extent to which their behavioral history and patterns of sexual attraction fit neatly within one of the three main sexual orientation categories. As explained in Chapter 3, most adults exhibit consistency across the three categories (e.g., they are exclusively heterosexual or homosexual in their attractions, sexual behavior, and self-labeled identity), but some do not. Moreover, the ways in which people use identity labels—such as gay and bisexual—often vary among cultural, racial, ethnic, socioeconomic, and age groups. They may also vary from one situation to another and change over time.

In addition, new labels and identities emerge over time in conjunction with societal changes. Since the 1960s, for example, "gay" has become a more widely used identity label than terms such as "homosexual" and "homophile." More recently, some individuals have adopted the term "queer"—long a derogatory epithet used for gay, lesbian, and bisexual individuals—as a positive self-label. In addition, adolescents and young adults have coined a variety of alternative labels, such as "boi-dyke" and "omnisexual." Nevertheless, the labels "gay," "lesbian," and "bisexual" remain widely used by both adolescents (Russell et al., 2009) and adults (Herek et al., 2010).

Variations in Sexual Orientation

Empirical research shows that men and women overlap considerably in their experiences of sexual desire and behavior. In some aspects of sexuality, however, the experiences of men and women may be more likely to differ, and these areas may have implications for health. Three examples are highlighted here.

First, on average, men tend to show greater interest in sex and express a desire to engage in sex more frequently than women; these patterns appear to occur in both heterosexual and homosexual populations (for a review, see Baumeister et al., 2001). In self-reports, for example, the frequency of solitary masturbation, which is a useful indicator of sexual interest insofar as it is not constrained by the availability of a partner, is generally higher among men than women (Oliver and Hyde, 1993), and this pattern appears among nonheterosexual as well as heterosexual individuals (Laumann et al., 1994a,b).

Second, on average, sexual-minority men and women may differ in their early experiences of their sexuality. Overall, lesbians appear to display greater variability than gay men in the age at which they recall reaching various developmental "milestones," such as awareness of same-sex attractions, experience of same-sex fantasies, and first pursuit of same-sex sexual contact (for a review, see Diamond, 2008). Data from a 2005 national probability sample reveal that gay men (n = 241) recalled recognizing their homosexual orientation at a significantly earlier average age than lesbians (n = 152) or bisexual women (n = 159), while the average age for bisexual men (n = 110) was between that of women and gay men (Herek et al., 2010).

Third, compared with that of men, women's sexuality may be more likely to be shaped and altered by cultural, social, and situational influences over time (Baumeister, 2000). As a group, women may exhibit greater fluidity in their sexuality than men; that is, they may be more likely to experience changes over the life span in their patterns of sexual attraction. As Diamond (2008, p. 3) notes, "This flexibility makes it possible for some women to experience desires for either men or women under certain circumstances, regardless of their overall sexual orientation . . . women of all orientations may experience variation in their erotic and affectional feelings as they encounter different situations, relationships, and life stages."

These examples of gender-linked patterns suggest that, on average, men and women may experience some aspects of their sexuality differently. As noted above, however, the sexes overlap considerably on these dimensions.

The extent to which patterns of same-sex sexual behavior differ across racial and ethnic groups is not clear. Using data from the General Social Survey, Turner and colleagues (2005) found that different racial groups did not differ in the extent to which they reported having engaged in same-sex sexual activity since age 18. Using data from the 2002 National Survey of Family Growth, however, Jeffries (2009) found that non-Mexican Latino men were significantly more likely than non-Latino white men to ever have had anal sex with a male partner and were significantly more likely than non-Latino black men to have had oral sex with a male partner. These relationships remained significant after controlling for age, education, and foreign birth. Chae and Ayala (2010) examined data from the National Latino and Asian American study, a national probability household sample of Latino and Asian adults over 18 years of age residing in the United States (n = 2,095 Asian and 2,554 Latino respondents, including 101 Asians and 111 Latinos reporting same-sex behavior during the previous 12 months). They found that 6.2 percent of Asian respondents reported any same-sex behavior during the previous 12 months, compared with 3.9 percent of Latino respondents. Because the authors reported no confidence intervals, however, comparison across the groups is difficult.

As highlighted by the concept of intersectionality, the experience of being a sexual minority is influenced by an individual's other identities. Thus, the experience of being lesbian, gay, or bisexual appears to vary according to the racial or ethnic group with which one identifies. Chae and Ayala (2010) compared Latino and Asian American respondents who were "LGB-identified" (i.e., self-labeled as homosexual, lesbian, gay, or bisexual) and "non-LGB-identified" (i.e., reporting same-sex behavior during the previous year but not self-labeling as homosexual, lesbian, gay, or bisexual). They found considerable heterogeneity between Asian and Latino respondents, with most participants identified as sexual minorities within the sample not self-identifying as LGB. Furthermore, they found an association between identifying as a sexual minority and psychological distress. There were variations within the two ethnic groups, with participants of

Chinese ancestry more likely than members of other Asian ethnic groups to identify as LGB, and participants of Mexican ancestry less likely than other Latino respondents to identify as LGB. In addition, socioeconomic status was associated with LGB identification: LGB-identified respondents of Asian ancestry were more likely to be employed than their non-LGB-identified counterparts, and non-LGB-identified Latinos had lower levels of education than LGB-identified Latinos (Chae and Ayala, 2010). Another study, conducted in Houston, Texas, with a nonprobability sample of 1,494 black, Latino, Asian, and white men and women, found that concordance rates between sexual behavior and identity varied across racial and ethnic groups (Ross et al., 2003).

Other data indicate that black men who have sex with men are less likely than white men who have sex with men to self-identify as gay (Chu et al., 1992; Doll et al., 1992; Goldbaum et al., 1998; Kramer et al., 1980; McKirnan et al., 1995, 2001; Montgomery et al., 2003; O'Leary et al., 2007; Torian et al., 2002) and are more likely to engage in sexual behavior with both males and females (Flores et al., 2009). Among adults who self-identify as lesbian, gay, or bisexual, self-identified bisexual men appear to be more likely than others to be black or Latino. A 2005 survey with a national probability sample of self-identified lesbian, gay, and bisexual adults found that only 43 percent of the bisexual men were non-Latino white, compared with more than 70 percent of the gay men, lesbians, and bisexual women. Whereas the racial and ethnic characteristics of the lesbian subsample generally corresponded to those of the U.S. adult population, the proportion of non-Latino whites was higher among self-labeled bisexual women than in the national population (Herek et al., 2010).

Consistent with this pattern, black lesbian, gay, and bisexual adults appear to be less likely than those of other races to disclose their sexual orientation in the workplace (Herek et al., 2010). Black men who have sex with men are less likely than other men who have sex with men to join gay-related organizations (Kennamer et al., 2000; Stokes and McKirnan, 1996). Black men who have sex with men also appear less likely than their counterparts of other races to disclose their same-sex behavior or sexual orientation identity to others (CDC, 2003; Kennamer et al., 2000; McKirnan et al., 1995; Stokes and McKirnan, 1996). Another study found that as education increased, white men who have sex with men were more likely to disclose their sexual identity, but black men who have sex with men were substantially less likely to do so (Kennamer et al., 2000). Research with black lesbian and bisexual women suggests that disclosure of sexual orientation varies according to several factors, including whether one's sexual orientation identity is considered more important than one's racial identity (Bowleg et al., 2008). In a convenience sample of New York City youths recruited from community organizations and local colleges (n = 156 youths aged 14–21), black participants reported less disclosure of their identity than white participants (Rosario et al., 1996).

A study examining gender identity affirmation among 571 male-to-female transgender persons focused on gender disclosure in six relationships—with parents, siblings, friends, fellow students, work colleagues, and sexual partners. The authors found that, compared with non-Latino whites, nonwhites had fewer relationships in which they were able to disclose their transgender identity, yet in the relationships available to them, they were more likely to disclose and to receive affirmation of their transgender identity (Nuttbrock et al., 2009).

HISTORICAL PERSPECTIVE

Contemporary health disparities based on sexual orientation and gender identity are rooted in and reflect the historical stigmatization of LGBT people. Most LGBT people encounter stigma from an early age, and this experience shapes how they perceive and interact with all aspects of society, including health-related institutions. Likewise, heterosexual people (including many health care professionals) have been socialized in a society that stigmatizes sexual and gender minorities, and this context inevitably affects their knowledge and perceptions of LGBT people. And institutions and systems that affect the health of LGBT people have evolved within a society that has historically stigmatized those populations, and this has important implications for their ability to address the needs of sexual and gender minorities.

Although an extensive discussion of the history of LGBT populations is beyond the scope of this report, this section highlights some key historical themes relevant to the current health status of LGBT individuals. Specifically, this section describes how LGBT individuals have been marginalized through the law and through psychiatric diagnoses, how they have been affected by the AIDS epidemic, and how their current legal status has evolved. In addition, this section notes some ways in which LGBT individuals' responses to their differential treatment and stigmatized status have implications for their health. Insofar as contemporary notions of sexual orientation and gender identity have their origins in the beginning of the twentieth century, this historical review focuses mainly on the past 100 years.

Lesbian, Gay, and Bisexual History

Inversion, Homosexuality, and the Origins of Contemporary Notions of Sexual Orientation

Although heterosexual and homosexual behaviors and attractions are ubiquitous across human societies, the idea that individuals can be meaningfully defined or categorized in terms of their patterns of sexual attraction and behavior emerged in science and medicine only in the nineteenth century. When this discourse emerged, its initial focus was on individuals who were perceived as deviating from cultural definitions of gender and sexual "normalcy."

The category of "the sexual invert" historically preceded that of "the homosexual" as a target for medical and scientific scrutiny. During the 1860s, Ulrichs proposed that male inverts, or "Urnings," should be understood as "individuals who are born with the sexual drive of women and who have male bodies" (Ulrichs, 1994b, vol. 1, p. 35). Hirschfeld supported this argument and later posited that inverts represented an intermediate sex, reflecting both male and female qualities (Hirschfeld, 2000). Sexual inversion originally described the individual in totality, with sexual conduct being only one of various aspects (Chauncey, 1982–1983). Male inverts were believed to possess "feminine" qualities, including passivity, weakness, and sexual attraction to "masculine" males. Female inverts were believed to manifest "masculine" qualities, including an active interest in sexuality—an abnormal quality in the eyes of a society that believed femininity was inherently passive (Chauncey, 1982–1983).

The modern notion of sexual orientation—defined in terms of whether one's sexual attractions and interest are directed toward men or women—is usually traced to Sigmund Freud (Freud, 1953). He introduced a distinction between the sexual aim (i.e., preferences for particular types of sexual activity) and the object toward which that aim is directed. Freud's theory and clinical practice focused on the sexual object, with "homosexuals" and "heterosexuals" being understood entirely in terms of their sexual object (respectively, a person of the same or the other sex). The construct of "the invert," which focused on the individual's sexual aim (passive sexuality among male inverts, active sexuality among females), fell into disuse (Chauncey, 1982–1983; Freud, 1953). However, the modern construct of "transgender" has similarities to the notion of sexual inversion insofar as both involve crossing socially defined boundaries of gender.[1]

Homosexual Conduct as a Crime, Homosexuality as a Diagnosis

Throughout much of the twentieth century, consensual same-sex sexual behavior was illegal, and homosexuality was considered a form of mental illness. This dual stigma historically attached to homosexual behaviors and persons has, as noted earlier, shaped the experiences of many people living today and has influenced many contemporary institutions that affect health.

[1] Personal communication, J. D'Emilio, University of Illinois, Chicago, October 22, 2010.

Long before Freud articulated his theory of sexuality, theological doctrine and secular law sought to regulate sexual behaviors and attached punishments to a variety of sex acts that were nonprocreative or occurred outside of marriage. Proscribed sexual behaviors were often referred to collectively as *sodomy*, a term that was not clearly defined in most religious and legal texts but included homosexual behavior as well as other nonprocreative and extramarital sexual acts (Jordan, 1997). U.S. sodomy laws, which existed in all of the states until 1961, when Illinois eliminated its statute, were the legacy of these prohibitions. Their language varied from state to state, and they outlawed various types of sexual behavior, including some forms of homosexual behavior. The main effect of sodomy laws was not prosecution for homosexual acts—such prosecutions were relatively infrequent. However, the laws were regularly used to justify differential treatment of sexual minorities in a variety of arenas, including employment, child custody, and immigration (Leslie, 2000).

The expansion of discourse about sexuality from the domains of law and theology into medicine, psychiatry, and psychology was considered a sign of progress by many at the time because it offered the hope of treatment and cure (rather than punishment) for phenomena that society generally regarded as problematic. Nevertheless, after Freud, the division of people into "heterosexuals" and "homosexuals" involved stigmatization of the latter. Many early physicians and sexologists regarded homosexuality as a pathology, in contrast to "normal" heterosexuality (e.g., Krafft-Ebing, 1900), although this view was not unanimous (e.g., Ellis, 1901; Ulrichs, 1994a). Freud himself believed that homosexuality represented a less than optimal outcome for psychosexual development, but did not believe it should be classified as an illness (Freud, 1951). In the 1940s, however, American psychoanalysts broke with Freud, and the view that homosexuality was an illness soon became the dominant position in American psychoanalysis and psychiatry (Bayer, 1987).

Thus by the beginning of World War II, sodomy laws continued to criminalize same-sex sexual behavior, even when it occurred in a private setting between consenting adults, while psychiatry and psychology generally regarded homosexuality as an illness. Around this time, the illness model became part of government personnel policies when the U.S. military incorporated psychiatric screening into its induction process and developed formal procedures for rejecting homosexual recruits. Whereas same-sex sexual *behavior* previously had been classified as a criminal offense under military regulations prohibiting sodomy, the armed services now sought to bar homosexual *persons* from their ranks (Berube, 1990). However, the screening process was often superficial, especially during the early years of the war when troops were desperately needed. Indeed, many lesbians and gay men served successfully in the military, often with the knowledge of their heterosexual comrades (e.g., Berube, 1990; Black et al., 2000; Menninger, 1948).

When the need for recruits diminished during the war's waning years, however, policies prohibiting homosexual personnel were more vigorously enforced, and many gay men and lesbians received undesirable discharges as sexual psychopaths (Berube, 1990). Such discharges had severely negative consequences. Denied benefits under the GI Bill of Rights and socially ostracized in civilian life, gay and lesbian veterans with undesirable discharges often could not secure employment. As Berube (1990, p. 229) notes, "Sometimes their lives became so unbearable as exposed homosexuals that they had to leave home or tried to kill themselves."

Ironically, the mass courts martial and discharges may have contributed to the development of modern lesbian and gay communities in U.S. urban centers. D'Emilio (1983) observed that, rather than returning to their hometowns after the war, many men and women chose to settle in major port cities and centers of war industry, such as Los Angeles, San Francisco, and New York. Still others later migrated to these cities to join the growing communities. Thus, large gay communities began to emerge in many American cities after World War II ended.

Although gay and lesbian civilians often found some degree of tolerance in the relative anonymity of these large cities, they nevertheless experienced negative consequences related to stigma. Because of the criminalization of homosexual acts and the stigmatization of homosexual identity, local police generally had the freedom to harass and pursue gay men and lesbians at will. Sexual minorities risked arrest when they gathered, even in private homes. Gay bars provided a venue for gay men and lesbians to socialize openly, but they also served as targets for harassment. Police raids were common, with bar patrons routinely being charged with offenses such as disorderly conduct, vagrancy, public lewdness, and solicitation (Boyd, 2003; Johnson, 2004). At the national level, a U.S. Senate committee issued a 1950 report concluding that homosexuals were not qualified for federal employment and that they represented a security risk because they could be blackmailed about their sexuality (Subcommittee on Investigations of the Senate Committee on Expenditures in the Executive Departments, 1950). In response to this report, President Eisenhower issued an executive order dismissing all homosexuals from federal employment, both civilian and military. Reporting on the government's campaigns against gay, lesbian, and bisexual employees by daily newspapers across the country reinforced the anxiety experienced by sexual minorities (D'Emilio, 1983).

In 1952, the newly created DSM listed homosexuality as a sociopathic personality disturbance, along with substance abuse and sexual disorders (American Psychiatric Association, 1952; Bayer, 1987). This classification of homosexuality was used as the basis for laws and regulations that denied homosexuals employment or prohibited them from being licensed in many occupations. Thousands lost their jobs (D'Emilio, 1983). Many states also passed sexual psychopath laws that applied to homosexuals as well as rapists, pedophiles, and sadomasochists. In an effort to prevent sex crimes, some psychiatrists encouraged the state to confine sexual nonconformists, including homosexuals, until they were declared "cured" (Chauncey, 1993).

During this time, many psychiatrists and psychologists attempted various "cures" (i.e., attempts to change homosexuals into heterosexuals), including psychotherapy, hormone treatments, aversive conditioning with nausea-inducing drugs, lobotomy, electroshock, and castration (e.g., American Psychological Association, 2009b; Feldman, 1966; Katz, 1976; Max, 1935; Thompson, 1949). These methods proved to be largely unsuccessful (American Psychological Association, 2009b; Friedman and Downey, 1998; Haldeman, 1994).

In summary, lesbians and gay men faced extensive stigma during the World War II era and the years immediately following. Although many of them served in the military during the war, substantial numbers were dishonorably discharged as the war concluded. Public disclosure of one's sexual orientation could lead not only to personal rejection and ostracism, but also to unemployment and even arrest, fostering a need for considerable secrecy in one's daily life. Gay men and lesbians were officially classified as mentally ill. Many were pressured to seek psychiatric treatment to become heterosexual, although interventions purporting to change sexual orientation were generally ineffective. At the same time, emerging gay and lesbian communities and enclaves in large urban centers offered their members the opportunity to meet others who shared their sexual orientation. These communities provided a basis for the development of organizational and individual challenges to the stigmatized status of homosexuality.

Creating Community and Change

In the post–World War II era, most gay men and lesbians accepted their stigmatized status as inevitable. However, some organized politically, forming groups that began quietly to endeavor to change societal attitudes and laws while also serving as safe havens for their members. Homophile organizations, such as the Mattachine Society and the Daughters of Bilitis, were, of necessity, highly secret groups whose initial goal was to provide social support and assistance. By the early 1960s, however, some of their members began to advocate for a strategy of publicly confronting antihomosexual discrimination.

Meanwhile, some scientific research challenged the illness model. In 1948 and 1953, Alfred Kinsey and his colleagues published their groundbreaking reports on human sexual behavior (Kinsey et al., 1948, 1953), demonstrating that same-sex attraction and behavior were common among American adults. Also around this time, Ford and Beach (1951) published an extensive review of cross-cultural and cross-species studies of sexual behavior, concluding that same-sex sexual behavior occurs in many animal species and that homosexual behavior of some sort was considered normal and socially acceptable in a majority of the societies for which detailed ethnographic data were available (Ford and Beach, 1951).

In a landmark study funded by the National Institute of Mental Health, psychologist Evelyn Hooker directly tested the assumption underlying homosexuality's inclusion in the DSM, namely, that homosexuality was inherently linked with psychopathology. Based on her data, Hooker (1957) concluded that homosexuality is not inherently associated with psychopathology and is not a clinical entity, a conclusion that received extensive support in subsequent empirical research (e.g., Gonsiorek, 1991) and eventually became the consensus view of mainstream mental health professionals in the United States (see below). The scholarship of Kinsey, Ford and Beach, and Hooker challenged widespread assumptions that homosexuality was a rare and pathological form of sexuality, practiced only by a small number of social misfits.

By the 1960s, homophile activists had begun to challenge publicly the idea that homosexuality was an illness and to seek an end to job discrimination and harassment. The Mattachine Society of Washington, DC, for example, began working to change Civil Service Commission policies regarding the employment of sexual minorities. In 1965, the group organized small demonstrations at locations such as the White House to protest discrimination against homosexuals in government employment (D'Emilio, 1983). And in 1966, the Washington Mattachine Society passed a resolution stating that "in the absence of valid evidence to the contrary, homosexuality is not a sickness, disturbance, or other pathology in any sense, but is merely a preference, orientation, or propensity, on par with, and not different in kind from, heterosexuality" (D'Emilio, 1983, p. 164). Although the homophile movement achieved some small success in its attempts to ensure civil rights for homosexual persons, its membership remained small until the end of the 1960s.

A watershed event occurred on June 27, 1969, in response to a routine police raid on the Stonewall Inn, a New York City gay bar. Such raids were a common occurrence, and police typically encountered little resistance. That night, however, the Stonewall patrons, along with neighborhood residents and passersby, resisted the police in a confrontation that escalated into a riot that continued for several nights. The Stonewall Rebellion, as it is now called, is widely considered to have marked the beginning of the contemporary movement for sexual-minority civil rights. In the wake of

Stonewall, the movement grew rapidly and inspired many sectors of society to reevaluate long-standing assumptions about homosexuality (Adam, 1995). Many lesbians and gay men "came out"—that is, they publicly revealed their sexual orientation—in the professions, academia, churches, and the military.

In the face of rapidly changing cultural views about homosexuality, and recognizing that empirical data to support the illness model were lacking, the American Psychiatric Association's board of directors voted in December 1973 to remove homosexuality as a diagnosis from the DSM (Bayer, 1987; Minton, 2002).[2] Their decision was affirmed by a subsequent vote of the Association's membership (Bayer, 1987). In 1975, the American Psychological Association strongly endorsed the psychiatrists' actions and urged its members to work to eradicate the stigma historically associated with a homosexual orientation (Conger, 1975).

The 1970s saw the growth of gay and lesbian communities across the United States. A wide variety of organizations, associations, businesses, and self-help groups formed. More than half of the states repealed their sodomy laws, and some municipalities passed legislation prohibiting discrimination on the basis of sexual orientation. Meanwhile, businesses and social organizations catering to a gay clientele proliferated, and lesbian and gay communities expanded significantly in major cities (Faderman, 1991; Levine, 1979). Nevertheless, gay people remained widely stigmatized. Many gay rights statutes that were passed in the early and mid-1970s were subsequently overturned by voters (Adam, 1987). By the beginning of the 1980s, candidates and organizations that opposed the gay community's modest gains were increasingly visible in national politics.

The AIDS Epidemic

The first cases of what would come to be known as AIDS were detected in gay men in 1981 (Gottlieb et al., 1981). AIDS has since claimed the lives of a significant portion of the generations of gay and bisexual men who came of age during and after the World War II era, and has dramatically altered the LGBT community in numerous ways. A detailed history of the impact of the AIDS epidemic on sexual and gender minorities is beyond the scope of this report and has been addressed elsewhere (see, e.g., various In-

[2] The diagnosis of homosexuality was replaced with a new, more restrictive diagnosis, "ego-dystonic homosexuality," indicated by a persistent lack of heterosexual arousal, which the patient experienced as interfering with initiation or maintenance of wanted heterosexual relationships, and persistent distress from a sustained pattern of unwanted homosexual arousal. This new diagnostic category, however, was widely criticized by mental health professionals and was eliminated in 1986. The revised DSM-III contained no diagnostic category for homosexuality (American Psychiatric Association, 1987; Bayer, 1987).

stitute of Medicine/National Research Council reports on AIDS, including IOM, 1991a,b,c, 2005; NRC, 1989, 1990, 1993, 1995; see also Epstein, 1996; Levine et al., 1997). Nor can the complete history of AIDS yet be written. HIV continues to spread throughout the world and in the United States, where newly diagnosed infections occur disproportionately among black and Latino men who have sex with men.

To better illuminate the historical context for understanding contemporary health disparities among sexual and gender minorities, this section highlights several long-term effects of AIDS. A detailed look at the AIDS epidemic is presented later in the chapter to illustrate a number of themes of particular relevance to the health of LGBT populations that pervade the discussion in the ensuing chapters.

First, AIDS was responsible for the deaths of thousands of gay and bisexual men in the United States. Apart from the individual tragedy represented by the loss of each of these lives, the cumulative loss inevitably affected the entire community. Several AIDS researchers (e.g., Levine, 1998; Martin et al., 1989) likened the epidemic to natural disasters such as floods and hurricanes, albeit without the physical destruction. Writing about AIDS, Levine (1989) noted that disasters can destroy a community's preexisting sociocultural order and foster both collective and individual trauma among survivors. Collective trauma refers to the loss of communality, that is, the network of relationships and shared meanings that provide intimacy, support, and a sense of self and that tie individuals to the social order. Individual trauma denotes the emotional response to death and devastation, that is, feelings of shock, disorientation, guilt, emotional depletion, and numbness (Levine, 1989; see generally Erikson, 1976).

In addition to individual and collective trauma, the LGBT community faced the challenge of how to respond to AIDS in a society they perceived as already hostile to them. Many sexual- and gender-minority individuals wondered whether they would all be targeted for increased ostracism, discrimination, and stigmatization as a result of AIDS (Bayer, 1989). Mandatory testing of the members of so-called "risk groups" (especially gay and bisexual men) was widely discussed in the larger society, and many LGB individuals feared that such testing could lead to the development of government lists of sexual-minority people for subsequent quarantine and discrimination (Bayer, 1989). Concern was also widespread that state sodomy laws, many of which had been repealed during the 1960s and 1970s, would be reinstated on the pretext of preventing AIDS. This concern received additional impetus when the U.S. Supreme Court upheld the constitutionality of state sodomy laws in 1986 (American Psychological Association and APHA, 1986). One argument made for retaining sodomy laws was that they would contain the spread of AIDS, although an amicus brief filed jointly by the American Public Health Association and the American

Psychological Association rebutted this argument (American Psychological Association and APHA, 1986).

Faced with the challenge of providing care and support to its members, the LGBT community responded by organizing self-help groups and community-based organizations that offered a variety of medical, psychological, and social services to people with AIDS. It also created and maintained community-based prevention programs that disseminated information about sexual risk reduction and promoted norms that encouraged the practice of "safer sex." Although organizations in major urban centers—including the San Francisco AIDS Foundation, AIDS Project Los Angeles, and the New York Gay Men's Health Crisis—achieved national prominence, the organizing extended into midsized cities, towns, and rural areas as well. Funded by community donations, private foundations, and government entities, these organizations grew in size and sophistication as the epidemic wore on. They helped create the infrastructure for the provision of health and social services that currently exists in the LGBT community (NRC, 1993).

At the same time, the epidemic fostered widespread activism to speed the testing and approval of new AIDS treatments and to increase government funding for research and prevention. Frustrated by the slow pace of much AIDS-related biomedical research, LGBT activists teamed with health care workers to organize community-based research studies to test promising AIDS drugs. These efforts fostered a new model for health care in which patients and advocates played a highly active role in identifying and implementing treatment strategies (Epstein, 1996). Coalitions also were formed between community activists and public health workers to devise strategies for monitoring HIV transmission that would be sensitive to community concerns about stigma and discrimination.

AIDS probably changed public perceptions of sexual minorities. Although the epidemic was often ignored by the mass media or portrayed in sensationalist ways during its early years (Shilts, 1987), later coverage presented the lives of gay men with AIDS as multilayered. It also showed that many of these men were rejected by their biological relatives and were cared for by same-sex partners and extended gay and lesbian families (Herek, 2009c). In addition, the epidemic provided the impetus for unprecedented numbers of gay, lesbian, and bisexual people to disclose their sexual orientation to family members, friends, neighbors, coworkers, and society at large. Many men who contracted AIDS were involuntarily "outed" by the disease, but many others chose to come out in an attempt to reduce sexual stigma and prejudice. Social psychological research indicated that heterosexuals who reported knowing one or more gay men and lesbians personally were indeed more likely than others to be accepting and supportive of sexual minorities generally (e.g., Herek and Capitanio, 1996; Pettigrew and

Tropp, 2006). Thus as a result of the epidemic, many heterosexuals began to think about gay men and lesbians in ways that went beyond sexuality: as family members and friends, coworkers, contributors to society, and members of a besieged community (Herek, 2009c). These changes in perceptions of sexual minorities may have contributed to decreases in negative attitudes toward homosexuality that were observed in public opinion polls during the 1990s (e.g., Sherrill and Yang, 2000; Herek, 2009d).

Coincident with the first years of the AIDS epidemic was increased public recognition of individuals who identify as bisexual. Although bisexual people began forming social and political groups in the 1970s (Udis-Kessler, 1995; Weinberg et al., 1994), an organized bisexual community did not emerge until the 1980s (Herdt, 2001; Paul, 1983; Rust, 1995; Udis-Kessler, 1995). By the early 1990s, the inclusion of bisexual individuals in the organized gay movement was reflected in the addition of "bisexual" to the names of lesbian and gay organizations and events. It was also in the late 1980s and early 1990s that bisexuals were recognized as a group at heightened risk for HIV infection (Doll et al., 1992).

In summary, although the AIDS epidemic continues to ravage sexual-minority communities today, some of its long-term consequences are already apparent. Many HIV-positive gay and bisexual men are surviving and thriving today thanks to the development of new HIV treatments. Nevertheless, most of them require ongoing medical care and must adhere to drug regimens that are extremely expensive and often have debilitating side effects. Many uninfected gay and bisexual men, especially those who came of age before the era of AIDS, have lost life partners as well as entire networks of male friends and acquaintances. The lives of many lesbians and bisexual women similarly have been altered by extensive experiences with loss. If the epidemic had never occurred, those networks would today be a source of social and emotional support as their members continued through their life course. Yet while the epidemic had considerable impact on individual lives, it also changed the LGBT community, creating an infrastructure of organizations dedicated to meeting the health and social needs of LGBT individuals.

The Last 20 Years: Laws and Policies

During the 1990s and 2000s, the visibility of the LGBT community increased dramatically in most facets of U.S. society. The last 20 years have seen various events that have affected the lives of sexual minorities, including the U.S. Supreme Court decision in *Lawrence v. Texas*[3] that struck down all sodomy laws. This section focuses on some of these events, as

[3] *Lawrence v. Texas*, 539 U.S. 558 (2003).

well as trends that are particularly relevant to the health concerns of the contemporary LGBT community, with particular emphasis on the development of laws and policies that continue to shape the experience of sexual minorities today. Although the extent of legal inequalities experienced by LGBT individuals has declined during recent decades, sexual and gender minorities still enjoy overall fewer legal rights, protections, and benefits than the non-gender-variant, heterosexual population. Inequalities in the law can affect fundamental aspects of the lives of LGBT people and can directly impact their ability to access quality health care.

While federal laws and policies govern some areas of import to LGBT populations (e.g., military personnel policy, U.S. Food and Drug Administration [FDA] policy banning men who have sex with men from donating blood), many issues are determined by the laws of the individual states and, at times, those of smaller jurisdictions within the states. Because states vary in their treatment of these issues, the effects of laws and policies on LGBT individuals often depend on where they live or travel.

Criminal victimization and harassment. As noted above, sexual and gender minorities have long been subjected to violence and harassment because of their sexual orientation and gender identity. As early as the 1960s, LGBT communities began to organize to respond collectively to such attacks. By the 1980s, many community-based antiviolence organizations around the United States were conducting community patrols, documenting violent incidents, providing victim services, working with local law enforcement agencies, and organizing violence prevention programs (e.g., Herek, 1992; Wertheimer, 1992). These programs were part of an emerging national movement against hate crimes—criminal actions that are motivated in whole or in part by bias against the victim's perceived race, religion, ethnicity, sexual orientation, or disability (Department of Justice, 2009; see generally Jenness and Grattet, 2001).

During the 1980s, some states passed laws mandating the collection of data to document the occurrence of hate crimes, including those based on the victim's sexual orientation. In 1990, Congress passed and President George H. W. Bush signed the Hate Crimes Statistics Act, which mandated the collection of such data on a national scale by the Federal Bureau of Investigation (FBI). Throughout the 1990s and 2000s, antiviolence projects based in sexual- and gender-minority communities continued to collect data and provide related services as more states enacted hate crime laws. In addition to mandating the local collection of data on the extent of hate crimes, many states imposed sentencing enhancement (i.e., a more severe penalty than would otherwise be imposed) for such crimes. The federal Hate Crimes Sentencing Enhancement Act of 1994 directed the U.S. Sentencing Commission to provide a sentencing enhancement for hate crimes, including those based on the victim's sexual orientation. This law's impact was limited because it applied only to existing federal crimes, which, in the case of sexual orientation, included only crimes committed on federal property or during the course of federally protected activities. The Matthew Shepard and James Byrd, Jr. Hate Crimes Prevention Act, enacted in 2009, expanded federal hate crime law to allow federal prosecution of crimes motivated by a victim's sexual orientation and gender identity. It also mandated the collection of data on crimes motivated by bias against a particular gender or gender identity (FBI, 2010).

Since 1991, the FBI has recorded a substantial number of hate crimes based on sexual orientation annually (FBI, 2010). Through 2009 (the most recent year for which data were available when this report went to press), approximately 17,500 incidents based on sexual orientation had been reported to the FBI. The FBI's hate crime reports underestimate the actual number of such incidents for several reasons, including that the reports rely on the voluntary cooperation of local law enforcement agencies, that many victims do not report the crime to the police, and that many hate crimes are not accurately classified as such (e.g., Herek and Sims, 2008). Data from the National Crime Victimization Survey, conducted annually by the U.S. Bureau of Justice Statistics with a sample of approximately 42,000 households, suggested an annual average of 210,430 hate crime victimizations in the United States in 190,840 separate incidents between July 2000 and December 2003. Hate crimes were more likely to occur in urban than in suburban or rural settings. More than 37,800 (17.9 percent) of these victimizations were motivated by the victim's sexual orientation. Approximately 42 percent of those crimes were reported to police authorities (Harlow, 2005).

In addition to hate crimes, other long-standing forms of harassment based on sexual orientation or gender identity or expression were the focus of community organizing and government response during the 1990s and 2000s. Such harassment emerged as a special concern for LGBT youth, who can face harassment and bullying in school because of their actual or perceived sexual orientation or gender identity (see Chapter 4).

An extensive national study released in late 2008 by the Gay, Lesbian, and Straight Education Network found that 86.2 percent of public school LGBT students reported being verbally harassed because of their sexual orientation, 44.1 percent reported being physically harassed, and 22.1 percent reported being physically assaulted. In addition, 32.7 percent of the LGBT students surveyed reported missing a day of school because of feeling unsafe, compared with only 4.5 percent of a national sample of secondary school students (Kosciw et al., 2008). The nonprobability sample of students (n = 6,219, age range = 13–21 in grades 6–12) was recruited through community-based LGBT youth groups and Internet listservs and websites. The majority of these students did not report the incidents to school officials, believing that little to no action would be taken or that the situation might even be exacerbated if reported.

Currently, federal law does not explicitly prohibit school-based harassment based on sexual orientation or gender identity or expression. A minority of states explicitly prohibit bullying and harassment in public K–12 schools on the basis of sexual orientation or gender identity (Biegel and Kuehl, 2010).

Marriage and relationships. Perhaps one of the most striking developments over the past two decades has been the prominence of debate in the United States and around the world concerning societal recognition of the family relationships of sexual- and gender-minority persons. People in same-sex couples have long sought ways to solemnize and formalize their relationship, including through legal recognition (e.g., Nardi, 1997). In the 1980s, some California municipalities enacted statutes to recognize same-sex relationships (in the form of "domestic partnerships") and provided the same-sex partners of city employees some of the benefits granted to married heterosexual couples. Throughout the 1990s, other jurisdictions enacted similar legislation, and debate about the issue of marriage equality for same-sex couples began to emerge on a national level (for historical background, see Chauncey, 2004; Lewin, 1998; Nardi, 1997).

A 1996 Hawaii Supreme Court decision[4] raised the prospect that marriage rights might eventually be granted to same-sex partners in that state. In response, Congress passed the Defense of Marriage Act (DOMA). DOMA defines marriage as a legal union between one man and one woman for the purposes of federal law, and exempts states from recognizing marriages performed in another state between two people of the same sex (Defense of Marriage Act, 1996). Most states subsequently passed their own versions of DOMA through statute or constitutional amendment (Peterson, 2004; Vestal, 2009).

In 1999, California became the first state to pass a statewide bill recognizing same-sex couples. Although that law bestowed only limited rights, subsequent legislation gave same-sex couples many of the rights of heterosexual married couples. In 2000, Vermont passed the nation's first civil unions bill, which gave registered same-sex couples all of the same benefits and responsibilities accorded by the state to heterosexual married couples. Other states, including New Jersey, Washington, Oregon, Illinois, and Nevada, subsequently enacted legislation recognizing civil unions or domestic partnerships. Civil unions entitle couples to most of the spousal rights and obligations accorded by the state to different-sex married couples, while

[4] *Baehr v. Miike*, 950 P.2d 1234 (1996).

the level of rights conveyed by domestic partnerships varies among states. In addition, some state and local government entities offer limited benefits for the same-sex partners of their employees (e.g., access to group health insurance plans), as do many private employers.

Late in 2003, the Massachusetts Supreme Court ordered that state to begin recognizing marriages between same-sex couples within 6 months.[5] Since then, six other states and the District of Columbia have allowed same-sex couples to marry, either through legislation (Maine; New Hampshire; Vermont; Washington, DC) or as a result of a state court ruling (California, Connecticut, Iowa). However, voters passed constitutional amendments that revoked the right to marry in California and prevented the Maine statute from going into effect.

Because same-sex couples are not legally recognized in most states, and because the legal recognitions extended by a handful of states are not recognized by the federal government, same-sex couples are denied a large number of the rights and benefits associated with marriage. At the federal level, DOMA denies same-sex couples access to more than 1,138 federal rights and obligations (GAO, 2004), ranging from spousal immigration rights to the spousal exemption under federal estate tax law.[6] In addition, because of DOMA, same-sex couples are ineligible for spousal or survivor benefits from social security, a federal benefit plan (Goldberg, 2009). Even in states where couples with same-sex partners can legally marry, state law cannot require employers to recognize same-sex married couples for the purposes of benefits administered under the Employee Retirement Income Security Act, which governs the health care and retirement benefit plans of many employers (Goldberg, 2009). In states that do not grant same-sex partners the right to marry or do not have civil unions or extend full recognition to domestic partnerships, same-sex couples also are denied a variety of benefits at the state level in such areas as income taxes; inheritance rights; community property; and state-funded benefit programs providing for basic needs, including health care.

The lack of recognition of marriage between two partners of the same sex has other health implications as well. A large body of research has shown that positive health outcomes are associated with marriage (Herdt and Kertzner, 2006; Herek, 2006). These positive effects are derived in part from the increased social support and relative stability associated with a legally recognized commitment (Herek, 2006). One recent study conducted with a nonprobability sample via the Internet (n = 2,677 lesbian, gay, and

---

[5] *Goodridge v. Dept. of Public Health*, 798 N.E. 2d 941 (Mass. 2003).

[6] Under federal law, a heterosexual spouse may transfer unlimited assets to a surviving spouse upon death without incurring estate tax liability. This exemption is not available to same-sex spouses (Steinberger, 2009).

bisexual adults) found that same-sex couples in legally recognized relationships experienced fewer depressive symptoms, lower levels of stress, and more meaning in their lives compared with participants in similar long-term relationships that lacked legal recognition (Riggle et al., 2010).

Denial of legal recognition of marriage between same-sex couples also has a direct impact on LGB individuals' interactions with the health care system. In many cases, employer-sponsored health insurance is not extended to same-sex partners, affecting their access to affordable health care. In addition, LGB individuals often are unable to take medical leave from work to care for an unmarried same-sex partner to the same extent as married couples. In 2010, the U.S. Department of Labor expanded the scope of the Family and Medical Leave Act to ensure that employees would be allowed unpaid leave to care for the children of unmarried same-sex partners; however, the act still does not extend this leave to care for unmarried same-sex partners themselves. Some states have extended medical leave to unmarried same-sex partners, but most have not. LGB people also have experienced the denial of hospital visitation rights for same-sex partners and disregard for advance directives[7] with respect to the care of same-sex partners. In 2010, President Obama issued a memorandum directing the U.S. Department of Health and Human Services to adopt regulations requiring all hospitals receiving Medicaid or Medicare dollars to permit visitation by a designated visitor without regard to sexual orientation or gender identity and requiring those hospitals to respect all patients' advance directives. If a visitor is not designated or an advance directive is not in place before a patient is incapacitated, however, same-sex partners may still be disregarded in terms of visitation or medical decision making.

Transgender people also face some uncertainty concerning access to marriage. No court has issued a published decision regarding the validity of a marriage in which one of the spouses undergoes sex reassignment after the marriage has taken place, although many state agencies, many public and private employers, and several federal agencies have held that such marriages are valid.[8] Few courts have ruled on the validity of a marriage in which one of the spouses undergoes sex reassignment before the marriage has taken place, although in practice, the great majority of couples in this situation do not encounter legal problems. One appellate court decision has

[7] Advance directives provide for the right of a competent individual to control the course of his or her medical care in all circumstances, as well as the right to designate another person to make these choices in the event of the individual's mental incapacity.

[8] *Kikue Liedigk v. Social Security Administration*, Office of Hearings and Appeals, December 1, 2003.

recognized the validity of such a marriage,[9] and a number of trial courts have done so.[10]

Parenting and children. Before the emergence of visible gay communities in the United States, many lesbians, gay men, and bisexual people married heterosexually for a variety of reasons, including social and family pressures, a desire to avoid stigma, and a perception that such marriages were the only available route to having children. Sometimes individuals have recognized their homosexuality or bisexuality only after marrying a person of the other sex (e.g., Higgins, 2006). Many lesbian, gay, and bisexual individuals became parents through such marriages. In more recent times, many lesbian, gay, and bisexual adults have conceived and reared children while in a same-sex relationship. Other same-sex couples and sexual-minority individuals have adopted children. In a 2005 Internet survey with a national probability sample of self-identified lesbian, gay, and bisexual adults, approximately 35 percent of lesbians and 8 percent of gay men reported having at least one child, as did 67 percent of bisexual women and 36 percent of bisexual men (Herek et al., 2010). These numbers may be higher among younger sexual-minority individuals. Data from the 2002 National Survey of Family Growth (NSFG) indicate that more than 35 percent of lesbians aged 18–44 had given birth and that 16 percent of gay men in that age group had a biological or adopted child (Gates et al., 2007). Fewer sexual-minority than heterosexual individuals are parents, but there are many lesbian mothers and gay fathers in the United States today (Patterson, 2000, 2009).

Thus, many children are currently being reared by one or more sexual-minority parents. The legal status of those parents and of their children varies from state to state. For example, states differ on whether they consider a parent's sexual orientation to be relevant to custody or visitation in divorce proceedings (Patterson, 2009). In recent years, some states have enacted laws or policies forbidding gay and lesbian individuals or couples from foster-parenting or adopting children; other states have considered laws banning same-sex couples, or all unmarried couples, from foster-parenting or adopting children (Gates et al., 2007; Joslin and Minter, 2009; Patterson, 2009). A long-standing ban on adoptions by lesbian or gay parents in Florida was overturned in 2010. As discussed in later chapters, this variability in legal status has implications for the health of sexual-minority parents and their children.

---

[9] See *M.T. v. J.T. 355 A.2d 204*, N.J. Sup. Ct., 1976.

[10] See, e.g., *Vecchione v. Vecchione*, CA Civ. No. 95D003769 [Orange County Sup. Ct., filed October 22, 1998]; *Carter v. Carter*, Nos. 139,251 Division C & 139,252 Division D [East Baton Rouge Parish La. Fam. Ct., filed January 16, 2002].

Transgender people also can face difficulty in court disputes over custody of their children. Many courts have denied or restricted custody or visitation for transgender parents, or even terminated their parental rights, solely because of their gender identity or expression. Only a few state courts have held that a parent's transgender status is irrelevant absent evidence of harm to the child. Transgender people who have no biological or adoptive relationship to the children they are raising with a partner face even more difficulties, as they must first convince the court that a person who has raised a child without formal legal or adoptive ties is nonetheless entitled to custody or visitation (Joslin and Minter, 2009).

Transgender History

As noted above, gender and sexuality were closely linked in early conceptualizations of sexual orientation. Over the past century, many transgender people have been a part of the larger gay and lesbian community. Transgender individuals played a key role in the Stonewall Rebellion, and they were instrumental in the organization of a more active gay and lesbian community in the 1970s (Bullough and Bullough, 1993). In many ways, however, the history of the transgender community is distinct from that of the LGB community.

Throughout history, gender variance has at times been both accepted and rejected as a part of many cultures and religions. By the end of the seventeenth century in England, gender crossing (or dressing as the other sex) was considered a crime, which created a foundation for similar laws in the United States (Bullough and Bullough, 1993). Since individuals who cross-dressed were forced to keep their identity a secret, historical data on discrimination and violence toward transgender individuals are scant. However, individual accounts detail many instances of harassment, humiliation, and violence, as well as the fear of being discovered and arrested or killed for their gender variance (Feinberg, 1996).

Hormone Therapy and Genital Reconstructive Surgery

Prior to the twentieth century, the term transsexual was not used to describe individuals with a gender-variant identity. Early sexologists Magnus Hirschfeld and Havelock Ellis defined the term "transvestism," or "eonism," as a category distinct from homosexuality that included cross-gender identification as well as cross-dressing (Ellis, 1933; Hirschfeld, 1991). However, the notion of changing one's sex through surgery or other means existed well before the term transsexual became commonly used. In the early twentieth century, European scientists began to experiment with "sex transformation," first with animals and then with humans. In Germany, doctors at Magnus

Hirschfield's Institute for Sexual Science started performing sex-change operations in the 1920s and 1930s (Meyerowitz, 2002).

It is not clear when the first complete "sex-change" operation was performed in the United States, but by the early 1920s, reports emerged of men and women who convinced physicians to perform castrations or hysterectomies as a means of changing their sex (Yawger, 1940). During the 1930s, endocrinologist Harry Benjamin became one of the first physicians in the United States to routinely administer hormone therapy to individuals desiring to change their sex (Benjamin, 1966; Drescher, 2010). During the next 20 years, a few American physicians privately performed sex reassignment surgery on nonintersex patients (Meyerowitz, 2002). However, it was not until the 1950s that the term *transsexual* became widely used to describe individuals who desired to change their sex.

Although he refused to endorse sex reassignment surgery for nonintersex patients, David Oliver Cauldwell coined the term *transsexual* in his 1949 essay "Psychopathia Transexualis" to describe individuals whose sex assigned at birth, based on the appearance of their external genitalia, did not match their gender identity (Cauldwell, 1949). Although transsexual individuals who met these criteria later gained access to sex reassignment, many psychiatrists remained critical of sex reassignment surgery as a legitimate form of treatment; they maintained that transsexual individuals were mentally disordered, and they objected to using hormones and surgery to treat these patients irreversibly (Drescher, 2010). Yet over time, understanding and acceptance grew, confirmed by a body of follow-up research (Green and Fleming, 1990; Pfäfflin and Junge, 1992). During this same period, stories of "sex changes" were publicized in sensationalist American magazines and newspapers. However, individuals seeking sex reassignment from physicians were routinely denied and informed that surgery was only for cases of intersexuality (Meyerowitz, 2002).

Much of the popular knowledge about sex reassignment surgery changed in 1952 when Christine Jorgensen, born George Jorgensen, emerged as a public figure in a front-page article of the *New York Daily News* (White, 1952). Jorgensen underwent sex reassignment surgery in Denmark and lived out the rest of her life as a woman. In the popular press, Jorgensen's story was unique because she was heralded as the first nonintersex individual to undergo such surgery (Meyerowitz, 2006). Extensive coverage of Jorgensen's transformation demonstrated to other transsexual people that sex reassignment surgery was feasible. Jorgensen's story also led to greater awareness of a concept that would later become known as gender identity, a term coined by Robert Stoller (1968) and popularized by John Money (1985, 1994) in his attempt to explain the sexual development of intersex and transsexual individuals (Drescher, 2010). In 1966, The Johns Hopkins University announced its program to perform and evaluate the efficacy of sex reassignment surgery, thus providing professional legitimacy for sex reassignment as a treatment for transsexualism (Meyerowitz, 2002). This was soon followed by similar programs at the University of Minnesota (Hastings, 1969; Hastings and Markland, 1978) and other university medical centers (Meyerowitz, 2002).

Psychiatric Classification

In 1979, an interdisciplinary group of physicians, therapists, and researchers created the Harry Benjamin International Gender Dysphoria Association, now known as the World Professional Association for Transgender Health (WPATH). *Gender dysphoria* was defined as serious discomfort with one's gender identity or gender role, thus acknowledging a spectrum of clinical presentations for which sex reassignment could be therapeutic and broadening the narrowly defined criteria originally used in the early sex reassignment programs (Laub and Fisk, 1974). The Benjamin Association defined standards of care to ensure and legitimize access to quality sex reassignment procedures. It also defined a number of eligibility criteria, including evaluation and recommendation by a mental health professional and, for surgery, a real life experience, referring to a set period of time in which to live full time in the gender role to which one is aspiring (WPATH, 1979).

Around the same time, a formal diagnosis of gender dysphoria was introduced in DSM-III (American Psychiatric Association, 1980), further legitimizing it as a psychiatric condition and providing guidance for treatment. DSM-III included two diagnoses: gender identity disorder of childhood (GIDC) and transsexualism (referring to gender dysphoria in adolescents and adults). In the 1987 revision of DSM-III, a third diagnosis was added: gender identity disorder of adolescence and adulthood, nontranssexual type. In 1994, the fourth edition of the DSM, DSM-IV, omitted this last diagnosis and consolidated GIDC and transsexualism under the diagnosis of gender identity disorder, with different criteria for children, adolescents, and adults (Zucker and Spitzer, 2005). In the last 15 years, however, these diagnoses have become increasingly controversial in the context of a transgender movement advocating for recognition of gender diversity and the depathologizing of gender variance (Bockting and Ehrbar, 2006; Bockting et al., 2009; Knudson et al., 2010).

Emergence of the Transgender Movement

As debate over the psychiatric classification and treatment of transsexualism and gender dysphoria continued for many years in the health field, transsexual and transgender people were frequently targets of stigma and discrimination from both the public at large and the police. The increasing number of medical centers willing to perform sex reassignment surgery raised the visibility of transsexual persons. By the 1960s, for example, the Tenderloin neighborhood in San Francisco had become a home for many gender- and sexual-variant people. With the changing dynamics of the neighborhood, tension had increased between residents and the police (Meyerowitz, 1998). In August 1966, that tension came to a head at Compton's Cafeteria, a 24-hour establishment where young male-to-females, cross-dressers, and gay men congregated. When the police attempted to raid the cafeteria and make arrests, the customers fought back, breaking windows and carrying the fighting into the street, including setting a nearby newsstand on fire (Stryker and Van Buskirk, 1996). A watershed event like the 1969 Stonewall Rebellion, the Compton's Cafeteria riot demonstrated an increasing collective consciousness among transsexual and transgender people. In 1969, a number of transsexual individuals in San Francisco formed the National Transsexual Counseling Unit from a number of smaller organizations (Meyerowitz, 2002).

As transsexual and transgender people fought for recognition and rights during the sexual revolution, they met with resistance from many sides. They were often excluded by gay men and lesbians from the gay liberation movement. However, they continued to advocate for their rights and equal treatment. In 1978, advocates in California successfully pushed for a state law that allowed transsexual individuals to change the name and sex designation on their birth certificate. Around this same time, the publication of Meyer and Reter's (1979) study claiming that sex reassignment surgery did not "confer [any] objective advantage in terms of social rehabilitation" led to the closing of the Hopkins Gender Identity Clinic, and a number of other, smaller clinics followed (Meyerowitz, 2002), although many critics of Meyer's study quickly came forward to defend the surgery (Fleming et al., 1980). A handful of university-based gender identity clinics survived, including clinics at Stanford University, the University of Texas, Case Western Reserve University, and the University of Minnesota. Their approach to care gradually changed as research and clinical experience evolved and as a generation of sex-reassigned transsexual individuals and other transgender individuals with various gender-variant identities and expressions continued to gain visibility (e.g., Kimberly, 1997; Stone, 1991; Warren, 1993).

These developments culminated in a paradigm shift away from changing sex toward facilitating a transgender coming-out process (Bockting, 1997, 2008; Bockting et al., 2009). Instead of viewing gender as binary and helping transgender and transsexual individuals conform, the transgender movement revealed a wide range of gender-variant identities and expressions, consistent with what had been documented in other cultures and throughout history (Coleman et al., 1992; Feinberg, 1996; Nanda, 1990; Roscoe, 1991; Williams, 1986). The focus of clinical management shifted to ameliorating the negative effects of stigma associated with gender variance and assisting transgender individuals in finding a gender expression that is comfortable and consistent with their gender identity (Bockting and Ehrbar, 2006). Psychotherapy now focuses on facilitating a transgender coming-out process that no longer emphasizes "transitioning" to become a "passing" member of the "opposite" sex, but instead emphasizes affirming a unique transgender identity. Hormone therapy and surgery continue to be options for feminizing or masculinizing the body to alleviate gender dysphoria. Instead of these interventions being viewed as two steps in a linear process toward sex reassignment, however, treatment now may use either hormones or surgery, both, or neither (Bockting, 2008). While research has clearly established the efficacy of sex reassignment that includes hormone therapy and a full-time gender role change followed by genital reconstructive surgery (Murad et al., 2010), virtually no studies have evaluated the contemporary approach to treatment whereby hormone therapy is not necessarily followed by surgery, and gender identity and expression do not conform to binary conceptualizations of sex and gender.

The 1990s saw the creation of many new organizations as transgender activists began to build a community identity, often facilitated by the Internet. In addition, transgender communities established lasting coalitions with gay, lesbian, and bisexual communities to support one another in similar struggles for increased awareness, acceptance, and human rights. In 1992, Minnesota became the first state in the nation to adopt human rights and antidiscrimination legislation that included not only gay men, lesbians, and bisexual men and women but also transgender people (Minnesota Department of Human Rights, 1993). Since then, a number of states and cities have followed suit (Bockting et al., 1999). Also during the 1990s, the National Gay and Lesbian Task Force began to include transgender people in its advocacy, and WPATH revised its standards of care and included transgender community representatives in its deliberations (Levine et al., 1998; Meyerowitz, 2002). Today, the existence of gender identity disorder and its inclusion in the DSM remains controversial and is the subject of intense debate, complicated by the potential implications of further depathologization and removal of the diagnosis for access to transgender-specific health care, particularly treatment of gender dysphoria and the medical interventions of hormone therapy and surgery that continue to be medically necessary for many (Drescher, 2010).

A DEMOGRAPHIC OVERVIEW OF LGBT POPULATIONS IN THE UNITED STATES

Among the first questions typically addressed by researchers who are studying a minority population are its size and its demographic and social characteristics. Demographic studies of LGBT populations can help make these often hidden groups of individuals visible in public policy discussions and pave the way for economic and public health studies to identify disparities (Gates and Ost, 2004a). However, it has been an ongoing challenge for researchers to collect reliable data from sufficiently large samples to assess the demographic characteristics of LGBT populations. Data from the U.S. census or large, national probability samples are usually required to examine the characteristics of a particular population. As explained in Chapter 3, few such surveys currently include data on sexual orientation and gender identity; some examples of the types of questions asked on these surveys are presented in that chapter. Even when data are derived from probability samples, racial and ethnic minorities and other subgroups of the population may not be represented in sufficient numbers to permit meaningful conclusions to be drawn about their demographic characteristics. With these caveats in mind, this section summarizes what is known from the limited available data about the demographic characteristics of LGBT populations in the United States.

Population Prevalence of Sexual Orientation Categories

Given that sexual orientation encompasses attraction, behavior, and identity and that an individual's enduring patterns of desires and behaviors can range along a continuum, estimating the number of people in the various sexual orientation categories in the population at any given time is a complex task. Before discussing current population estimates, it is illustrative to consider some examples of earlier attempts and the limitations associated with their findings.

Early Attempts to Estimate Sexual Orientation

Perhaps the most well-known example of an attempt to describe the sexual behavior of the U.S. population is the work of Alfred Kinsey and his colleagues (1948, 1953). In their pioneering descriptive study of the sexual feelings and experiences of thousands of U.S. adults, the Kinsey researchers did not categorize research participants according to sexual orientation categories but instead reported the extent to which their sexual histories included heterosexual and homosexual desires and behavior. For example, Kinsey and colleagues (1948) reported that 37 percent of the males in their sample had had at least some overt homosexual experience to the point of orgasm between adolescence and old age, and another 13 percent had reacted erotically to other males without having overt homosexual contacts after the onset of adolescence. Generalizations from the Kinsey group's findings to the entire U.S. population are problematic for several reasons, including the fact that the data were not obtained from a probability sample.[11] However, this research demonstrated the feasibility of studying sexuality in the general population. It also showed that human sexual behavior is highly diverse and that a large number of people acknowledged having engaged in sexual behaviors that previously had been considered rare.

Despite Kinsey and colleagues' eschewal of sexual orientation categories, others extrapolated from their findings to estimate the proportion of the U.S. population in each of the different categories. Based on such an extrapolation (Voeller, 1990), the belief that 90 percent of the U.S. population was heterosexual and 10 percent was gay or lesbian became widely accepted during the early years of the U.S. gay rights movement. Data were lacking, however, with which to gauge the accuracy of this estimate.

Recent Estimates

As noted, while the Kinsey report was important in pioneering the study of sexuality, sampling limitations make the generalizability of its findings uncertain. However, credible estimates of the size of different sexual orientation groups can be derived from the National Health and Social Life Survey (NHSLS), which was conducted by researchers at the National Opinion Research Center (NORC) at the University of Chicago in 1992. The NHSLS is widely regarded as the most authoritative national survey to date of adult sexuality in the United States. It included assessment of the number of people by sexual attraction, behavior, and sexual orientation identity in a large probability sample (n = 3,432) of U.S. adults.[12] As detailed in Chapter 3, sexual desire was assessed by asking respondents about who they were "sexually attracted to" (men, mostly men, both women and men, mostly women, only women). A separate question also asked about the appeal of having sex with someone of the same sex. Sexual behavior was assessed with questions about the respondents' sexual acts with males and with females during three time periods (the past 30 days, the past 12 months, and since adolescence). Identity was assessed by asking respondents whether they thought of themselves as heterosexual, homosexual, bisexual, or something else.

Among the NHSLS respondents, approximately 90 percent of men and 92 percent of women reported exclusively heterosexual attraction, behavior,

---

[11] For methodological and statistical critiques at the time the studies were first released, see Terman (1948), Cochran et al. (1953), and Wallis (1949). For more recent discussions, see Michaels (1996) and NRC (1989).

[12] The NHSLS was originally designed to collect data from a much larger sample. However, when the study's federal funding was withdrawn, a smaller study, supported by private foundations, was necessitated (Laumann et al., 1994b; Miller, 1995).

TABLE 2-1 Estimated Percentage of People by Sexual Orientation and Behavior from Selected Sample Surveys

		Percent Identifying as Homosexual, Gay, Lesbian, or Bisexual		Percent Reporting Same-Sex Partners		Percent Reporting Some Same-Sex Desire or Attraction	
Survey	Ages	Men	Women	Men	Women	Men	Women
National Survey of Sexual Health and Behavior, 2010	18+	6.8	4.5	—	—	—	—
General Social Survey, 2008	18+	2.9	4.6	—	—	—	—
General Social Survey, 2008	18–44	4.1	4.1	10.0	10.0	—	—
National Survey of Family Growth, 2002	18–44	4.1	4.1	6.2	11.5	7.1	13.4
National Health and Social Life Survey, 1992	18–59	2.8	1.4	7.1	3.8	7.7	7.5

NOTES: Estimates are based on small sample sizes, resulting in large confidence intervals around the estimates; see the text for details. Also, differences in estimates can occur because of sampling error (that is, the estimates in the table are based on probability samples) and nonsampling error, errors due to differential nonresponse and coverage, differences in the target population (the cohorts surveyed), differences in the survey questionnaires used, year of implementation, mode of administration, and the survey respondent.
SOURCES: Herbenick et al. (2010), Table 1, for results from the NSSHB; Gates (2010), Figures 1 and 7, for results from the GSS; Mosher et al. (2005), Tables 12 and 13, for results from the NSFG; Laumann et al. (1994a), Table 8.2, for results from the 1992 NHSLS.

and identity. About 2.8 percent of the men and 1.4 percent of the women labeled themselves homosexual or bisexual and reported same-sex desire.[13] Others reported having had same-sex partners or some degree of same-sex desire, attraction, or appeal (Laumann et al., 1994a). As shown in Table 2-1, approximately 4 percent of women and 7 percent of men reported having same-sex partners at some point since puberty. More than 7 percent of both men and women reported same-sex desire, attraction, or appeal.

Because the absolute number of both men and women reporting any nonheterosexual attraction, behavior, or identity was quite small (143 men, 150 women), the margin of error associated with these estimates is fairly

[13] All but three of the men and women in this group also reported having engaged in same-sex sexual behavior.

large, and any generalizations to the national population must be made with caution (Laumann et al., 1994a).

More recent data from the 2002 NSFG, conducted by the Centers for Disease Control and Prevention's National Center for Health Statistics, also provide estimates for sexual orientation identification, same-sex sexual behaviors, and same-sex attraction. These estimates are for a more recent and younger cohort (aged 18–44) than those from the NHSLS. In the NSFG, sexual orientation identification was assessed with the question: "Do you think of yourself as heterosexual, homosexual, bisexual, or something else?" Among men aged 18–44, 90.2 percent identified as heterosexual, 2.3 percent as homosexual, 1.8 percent as bisexual, and 3.9 percent as something else; 1.8 percent did not report their orientation. Among women in this age range, 90.3 percent identified as heterosexual, 1.3 percent as homosexual, 2.8 percent as bisexual, and 3.8 percent as something else; again, 1.8 percent did not report their orientation. In terms of behavior, 6.2 percent of men reported same-sex oral or anal sexual behavior, while 11.5 percent of women reported a "sexual experience" with another woman. As Mosher and colleagues (2005) point out, this relatively high number of women may be due to the broad wording used for the question. As for attraction, 7.1 percent of men and 13.4 percent of women acknowledged some degree of same-sex attraction.

Two more recent surveys based on national probability samples provide estimates of LGB identification. Gates (2010) reports that in the 2008 General Social Survey (GSS), a survey with a national probability sample conducted by NORC, 2.2 percent of men identified as gay and 0.7 percent as bisexual, while 2.7 percent of women identified as lesbian and 1.9 percent as bisexual (n = 1,773 for the sexual orientation questions). As in the NHSLS and NSFG, data from the GSS show that rates of same-sex sexual behavior—reported by approximately 10 percent of individuals aged 18–44—are higher than rates of LGB self-identification. Estimates of the number of people who self-identify as LGB also are found in data from the recent 2009 National Survey of Sexual Health and Behavior, collected by Knowledge Networks (Herbenick et al., 2010). As the authors describe, Knowledge Networks generates a national probability sample using random-digit dialing and address-based sampling. Internet access and the necessary hardware are provided to participants who lack them. In this sample, 6.8 percent of men and 4.5 percent of women self-identified as lesbian, gay, or bisexual.

Differences in the rates reported in Table 2-1 are no doubt due in part to the time periods during which the surveys were administered. Differences are also likely to have resulted from age differences across the samples, as younger cohorts are more likely than older adults to report LGB identification and same-sex sexual behavior. Differences across studies may result as well from variation in the survey instruments used, mode of administration, and methods used to draw the samples. Finally, as discussed above with respect to the NHSLS, there is substantial sampling variation, as the estimates are based on relatively small samples. Consequently, the margin of error associated with each estimate is likely to be fairly large.

Data from these and other national probability samples, as well as U.S. census data, reveal other demographic characteristics of LGBT populations. It should be noted that, because of data limitations, most of the demographic characteristics reported here refer only to gay men and lesbians; demographic information on bisexual and transgender individuals are extremely limited.

Size of the Transgender Population

Data on the proportion of transgender people in the U.S. population are sorely lacking. Rough estimates are available based on parental reports for children and the number of adults seeking hormone therapy or surgery at specialty clinics for the treatment of gender dysphoria. Based on ratings on the Child Behavior Check List (a parental report checklist used to measure behavior problems in children) for non-clinic-referred children (n = 398 boys and 398 girls) 1 percent of boys and 3.5 percent of girls reported "wishes to be of opposite sex" (Zucker et al., 1997). However, it should be noted that boys are referred more often than girls, reflecting, perhaps, greater societal intolerance of gender role nonconformity among boys than among girls (Zucker and Lawrence, 2009). With respect to adults, based on the number of transsexual adults at specialty clinics around the world for treatment of gender dysphoria, the estimated size of the population ranges from 1:2,900 (in Singapore) to 1:100,000 (in the United States) for transsexual women and 1:8,300 (in Singapore) to 1:400,000 (in the United States) for transsexual men. While the estimates for the United States are based on older data (Pauly, 1968), they are included here because they are the only data available from the United States. However, the number of adults seeking treatment appears to be increasing, and the ratio of transgender women to transgender men appears to be decreasing (Zucker and Lawrence, 2009).

Geographic Distribution

Lesbian and gay individuals can be found throughout the United States, being present in 99 percent of all U.S. counties (Gates and Ost, 2004b). U.S. census data on same-sex couples have been the most widely used in studying the geographic distribution of the lesbian and gay populations because the census is the largest and most geographically diverse data source available. As noted in Chapter 3, however, the data are limited in important respects, including the fact that they exclude LGBT individuals who are not cohabiting with a same-sex partner.

While lesbian and gay populations exist throughout the United States, their distribution is not uniform across all regions. Midwestern states appear to have a disproportionately small concentration of lesbian and gay individuals (Herek et al., 2010). Vermont, California, Washington, Massachusetts, and Oregon are the states with the highest percentage of gay and lesbian inhabitants (Gates and Ost, 2004b). Large metropolitan areas tend to have relatively high concentrations of these populations, among the highest being in San Francisco; Washington, DC; and Atlanta (Black et al., 2000). Moreover, many neighborhoods and communities have proportions of gay and lesbian residents that far exceed the national average. In addition, the gay and lesbian populations themselves differ in their patterns of location. The states with the highest concentration of same-sex male and same-sex female couples differ. Additionally, a larger proportion of gay male than lesbian couples tend to live in urban areas (Gates and Ost, 2004b).

In a study comparing transgender people recruited through online convenience sampling (n = 1,229) with existing U.S. census data, Rosser and colleagues (2007) found that respondents exhibited a wide geographic distribution across the United States. While the proportion of participants from the 15 most populous states generally mirrored the relative population size, some states (Colorado, Minnesota, Missouri, and Oregon) were overrepresented relative to the population size.

Household Composition

Several data sources yield estimates of the proportion of gay men and lesbians in same-sex relationships and the proportions cohabiting. Using data from the NHSLS, Black and colleagues (2000) found that, depending on whether sexual orientation was defined in terms of exclusively same-sex sexual behavior during the previous year or self-labeled identity, between 18.5 percent and 28.6 percent of gay men were partnered at the time they were surveyed; partnership rates among women during the same period were 41.6–43.8 percent. The study also found that 67.9 percent of behaviorally defined gay men and 93.8 percent of behaviorally defined lesbians had lived with a same-sex partner at some point in their lives (Black et al., 2000). However, as with other estimates discussed above, a large margin of error is associated with these estimates because they are based on small numbers of respondents (e.g., just 28 men and 16 women fit the criterion of exclusively same-sex sexual behavior during the previous year). In a more recent survey with a national probability sample, Herek and colleagues (2010) found that approximately 40 percent of self-identified gay men (n = 241) and 75 percent of lesbians (n = 152) reported they were currently in a same-sex relationship. Approximately one-fourth of the coupled men and four-fifths of the coupled women reported being in a legally recognized relationship (e.g., marriage, civil union) or living with their partner. Recent analysis of data from California by Carpenter and Gates (2008) indicates that 37–46 percent of gay men and 51–62 percent of lesbian women aged 18–59 are in cohabiting partnerships. Finally, the 2000 U.S. census yields an estimate of the absolute number of cohabiting sexual minorities: nearly 1,200,000 individuals indicated that they were cohabiting in same-sex relationships. Recent numbers from the American Community Survey indicate that this number is growing more rapidly than the overall U.S. population (Gates, 2006).

Some data are also available on the numbers of same-sex-couple households with children. In the 2000 census, about 27.5 percent of such households reported having children under the age of 18 (Gates and Ost, 2004b). The proportion of partnered lesbians with children in the home is significantly larger than the proportion of partnered gay males. In households with children under 18, an average of two children are present in both all households nationwide and same-sex-couple households (Gates and Ost, 2004b). Black and Latina women in same-sex couple households were more than twice as likely to be raising a child and black and Latino men in same-sex-couple households were four times more likely to be raising a child than their non-Hispanic white counterparts in same-sex couple households (Gates and Romero, 2009). U.S. census data do not yield a complete picture of gay and lesbian parenting as they do not include data on single gay or lesbian parents, and the data may be more representative of white than of nonwhite respondents, biasing comparisons. An analysis of combined GSS and NHSLS data, which include single gay men and lesbians (either self-identified or reporting that they have sex exclusively with persons of the same sex), indicated that approximately 14 percent of single gay men and 28 percent of single lesbians had children in the household (Black et al., 2000). In the 2005 survey by Herek and colleagues (published in 2010), approximately 8 percent of self-identified gay men and 35 percent of self-identified lesbians reported having one or more children, including adopted and step-children (Herek et al., 2010).

In a study comparing an online convenience sample of the U.S. transgender population (n = 1,229) with the 2000 U.S. census data, Rosser and colleagues (2007) found that transgender participants were more likely to be single, never married, or divorced and less likely to be currently married than the general population.

Income and Education

In many data sources, gay and lesbian individuals report higher average levels of education than their heterosexual counterparts. For example, Black and colleagues (2000) derived such a result from GSS and NHSLS data and for partnered individuals from the 1990 census. The authors caution, however, that this finding could be driven, at least in part, by well-educated people being disproportionately willing to identify as gay or lesbian in the GSS and NHSLS or being disproportionately likely to identify as same-sex partnered in the census.

On average, it appears that gay men have lower incomes than heterosexual men with similar education and occupations (Allegretto and Arthur, 2001; Badgett, 1995; Black et al., 2003; Carpenter, 2007). By contrast, some research has suggested that lesbian women have higher incomes than heterosexual women (e.g., Black et al., 2007), although other studies have not found this difference (e.g., Badgett, 2001; Klawitter and Flatt, 1998). Regardless, it is important to note that, because of differential treatment with respect to taxes and insurance, even lesbian or gay couples whose gross incomes are identical to those of heterosexual men and women may have less disposable income. These factors may contribute to the finding of Black and colleagues (2007) that lesbians and gay men are less likely than heterosexual men and women to own their own homes.

Little research has examined economic outcomes for bisexual individuals specifically. Carpenter (2005) presents evidence from California that bisexual people fare less well than comparable heterosexuals (and comparable gay and lesbian individuals) in the labor market.

Finally, in the study described above, Rosser and colleagues (2007) found that transgender participants were more educated but reported less household income.

Age

As is the case for heterosexual people, all age groups include lesbians and gay men. Similarly, all age groups include transgender individuals (Rosser et al., 2007). Nearly 20 percent of members of cohabiting same-sex couples are at least 55 years of age according to the 2000 census (Gates and Ost, 2004b). Self-identified gay men tend to be older, on average, than self-identified lesbians and bisexual men and women (Herek et al., 2010). Using GSS data collected between 1988 and 2002, Turner and colleagues (2005) found that the number of women who self-reported same-sex behavior was negatively correlated with birth cohort: younger women were significantly more likely to report such behavior. For example, 1.6 percent of women born before 1920 reported ever having had same-sex contact, compared with 6.9 percent of women born after 1969. The authors note that the increased prevalence of women reporting same-sex contact coincides with an increase in societal tolerance of same-sex sexual activity, although it is not clear whether the two phenomena are linked. A comparable pattern was not evident among men, although men's self-reports of same-sex behavior increased somewhat during the 1990s.

BARRIERS TO ACCESSING HEALTH CARE

Sexual and gender minorities face a number of barriers to accessing health care, many of which can be traced to stigma and its consequences. Multiple components of stigma influence the health and well-being of sexual and gender minorities. This section defines the components of stigma, reviews barriers to accessing health care for members of LGBT populations, and describes how the cross-cutting theme of stigma is associated with these barriers at both the personal and structural levels.

Stigma

As used in this report, the term *stigma* refers to the inferior status, negative regard, and relative powerlessness that society collectively assigns to individuals and groups that are associated with various conditions, statuses, and attributes (Goffman, 1963; Herek, 2009a; Link and Phelan, 2001). Social scientists have long recognized that stigma is not inherent in a particular trait or in membership in a particular group. Rather, society collectively identifies and assigns negative meaning and value to certain characteristics and groups, thereby "constructing" stigma. Thus, in perhaps the best known theoretical analysis of the concept, Erving Goffman (1963, p. 5) characterized stigma as "an undesired differentness." *Sexual stigma* refers specifically to the stigma attached to any nonheterosexual behavior, identity, relationship, or community (e.g., Herek, 2009a). *Transgender stigma* is used here to refer to the stigma attached to individuals who self-identify as transgender or transsexual or whose gender expression or comportment varies from societal gender norms.

Access and Barriers to Care

The Institute of Medicine (IOM) defines access to health care as the "timely use of personal health services to achieve the best possible outcomes" (IOM, 1993, p. 4). Drawing on the social ecology model, the committee categorized barriers to accessing high-quality care as both personal and structural. LGBT individuals face both types of barriers. Although many of these barriers can be traced to sexual and transgender stigma, many LGBT individuals also experience barriers to care related to their membership in other marginalized groups in society (e.g., racial/ethnic minorities, low-income groups, and those from certain geographic locations).

It is worth noting that while most of the literature on access to care focuses on adults, there are some issues specific to adolescents as well. In its report *Adolescent Health Services*, the IOM (2009) highlights the importance of providing all adolescents with health services that attract and engage them and give them opportunities to discuss sensitive health issues. Moreover, states the report, health services that are confidential are perceived as more accessible and are more likely to be utilized by adolescents, particularly for issues related to sexual behavior. For adolescents who are sexual or gender minorities, these factors may be more complex. LGBT adolescents may have access to providers, but if they are not given an opportunity to discuss such topics as sexual or gender orientation, they may not seek care or discuss confidential information. Similarly, if care is not confidential, LGBT adolescents may be less likely to access it.

Personal-Level Barriers

Personal-level barriers are created by the attitudes, beliefs, and behaviors of individuals within the health care system—both providers and patients. Individual expressions of sexual and transgender stigma create significant personal barriers for LGBT people attempting to access high-quality care. Three such expressions are discussed here: enacted stigma, felt stigma, and internalized stigma (Herek, 2009d).

Enacted stigma. *Enacted stigma* refers to explicit behaviors that express stigma. These behaviors can take the form of verbal epithets, shunning, overt discrimination, and even violence. Individuals are often targeted for enactments of sexual stigma because of their perceived gender nonconformity, and transgender individuals are often targeted because they are assumed to be homosexual. Thus, many stigma enactments against sexual and gender minorities alike are rooted in both sexual and transgender stigma.

Some LGBT individuals face discrimination in the health care system that can lead to an outright denial of care or to the delivery of inadequate care. There are many examples of manifestations of enacted stigma against LGBT individuals by health care providers. LGBT individuals have reported experiencing refusal of treatment by health care staff, verbal abuse, and disrespectful behavior, as well as many other forms of failure to provide adequate care (Eliason and Schope, 2001; Kenagy, 2005; Scherzer, 2000; Sears, 2009).

Felt stigma. Because any individual may be perceived to be gay, lesbian, or bisexual, virtually anyone—regardless of sexual orientation—can be the target of an enactment of sexual stigma. Most people, heterosexuals and nonheterosexuals alike, recognize this possibility, and that recognition often leads them to modify their own behavior to avoid such an experience. Heterosexuals and nonheterosexuals alike may modify or adapt their behavior in a variety of ways to avoid stigma; sexual-minority individuals may hide their sexual orientation from others, including health care providers. This awareness of the possibility that stigma will be enacted in particular situations is referred to as *felt stigma*. Felt stigma can be adaptive to the extent that it protects the individual from enacted stigma. At the same time, this adaptation has costs. Fear of stigmatization or previous negative experiences with the health care system may lead LGBT individuals to delay seeking care. Confidentiality also can be an issue, given that most health insurance is provided through an individual's place of employment. If he or she is not "out" as a sexual or gender minority in the workplace, and because there is no legal protection in many jurisdictions for sexual or gender minorities in the workplace, patients may fear loss of employment due to their sexual- or gender-minority status. Ponce and colleagues (2010) suggested this explanation after demonstrating significant disparities in health care access for gay men and lesbians compared with heterosexuals. In addition, many LGBT individuals do not disclose their sexual orientation because of fear of provider bias, although it should be noted that many patients, regardless of sexual orientation, are unwilling to disclose information about their sexual behaviors to a health care provider (Jillson, 2002). For example, in-depth qualitative interviews with LGBT individuals in a rural setting revealed that many would strategically remain silent to health care providers about their sexuality or gender status (Willging et al., 2006). Others may fail to complete advance directives and powers of attorney for partners as a way of concealing their sexual orientation.

Internalized stigma. A third way in which individuals manifest stigma is by accepting the legitimacy of society's negative regard for the stigmatized group. In non-gender-variant heterosexuals, this *internalized stigma* is expressed as prejudice against sexual minorities (commonly labeled *sexual prejudice* or *homophobia*) and transgender people (sometimes labeled *transphobia* and referred to here as *transgender prejudice*).

Sexual prejudice on the part of health care providers often underlies enactments of stigma. Although there has been little recent research investigating provider attitudes toward LGBT patients, earlier studies have shown that provider attitudes toward sexual-minority patients can be barriers to care (IOM, 1993; Jillson, 2002). From the available literature, it appears that many providers are uncomfortable with providing services to LGBT patients. In one study published during the 1980s, 40 percent of physicians surveyed reported being sometimes or often uncomfortable providing care to lesbian or gay patients (Mathews et al., 1986). In a survey conducted with a nonprobability sample of members of the Gay and Lesbian Medical Association (GLMA), 67 percent of respondents believed they had seen gay or lesbian patients receive substandard care because of their sexual orientation (Schatz and O'Hanlan, 1994). On the other hand, in a recent follow-up to the earlier Matthews and colleagues (1986) study, Smith and Mathews (2007) found that levels of sexual prejudice among health care providers had declined substantially.

Among sexual- and gender-minority individuals, internalized stigma leads to denigration of the self, termed *self-stigma* (this phenomenon has been labeled *internalized homophobia* in sexual-minority individuals). Self-stigma may cause sexual and gender minorities to feel that they do not deserve respect from their health care provider or the same access to health care as heterosexuals. As a result, they may not disclose key information to their provider, may avoid seeking treatment, or may refrain from challenging discrimination and other forms of enacted stigma.

Other personal barriers. As noted, in addition to stigma related to their sexual-minority status, LGBT individuals may face barriers to care due to other characteristics, such as their racial/ethnic minority status, education level, income level, geographic location, language, immigration status, knowledge, and cultural beliefs. The intersection of these dimensions with the stigma associated with sexual- and gender-minority status results in unique barriers and challenges to accessing high-quality care for many LGBT individuals.

Structural Barriers

Structural barriers relate to the health care system at the institutional level. These barriers operate regardless of the attitudes of individuals. Examples of such barriers include an employer-based health care system that limits LGBT individuals' access to marital benefits, including eligibility for health insurance; lack of training in LGBT health received by providers; and insurance practices that limit the types of care covered for LGBT individuals.

Structural stigma. *Structural stigma* (or *institutional stigma*) is the manifestation of stigma within the institutions of society (Corrigan et al., 2005). Structural stigma often perpetuates stigma-based differentials in status and power (Link and Phelan, 2001) and may operate even in the absence of prejudice on the part of individual members of an institution. For example, if a health maintenance organization provides care for members' different-sex spouses but not their same-sex partners, its sexual-minority members have a lower status than their heterosexual counterparts, regardless of whether individual staff members are personally prejudiced against sexual minorities. Just as institutional racism works "to the disadvantage of racial minority groups even in the absence of individual prejudice or discrimination" (Link and Phelan, 2001), structural sexual stigma disadvantages and restricts the opportunities of sexual and gender minorities by perpetuating their lower status and power relative to non-gender-variant heterosexuals (Herek, 2009b).

As discussed earlier, structural stigma occurs in the health care system as well in society at large (e.g., with respect to employment benefits for same-sex couples and government rules and regulations regarding marriage between same-sex couples). For example, a major structural barrier is the lack of legal recognition of partners, which has prevented many hospitals and health care providers from according partners and family members of LGBT individuals the same rights to visit and access information that are provided to heterosexual spouses. There have been cases of legal refusal to recognize the partner of a sexual-minority patient as a health care proxy even when so designated by the patient (IOM, 1999).

Provider knowledge and training. With respect to the health care provided to LGBT people, a number of structural barriers result from providers' lack of training in the health needs of LGBT patients. *Cultural competency*, referring to a set of skills that allows providers to give culturally appropriate high-quality care to individuals of cultures different from their own, is an important aspect of care (IOM, 1999). Patient–provider communication is important. In fact, studies suggest that poor patient–provider communication is strongly associated with adverse health behaviors such as decreased levels of adherence to physician advice; it is also associated with decreased rates of satisfaction (Cortes et al., 2009; Inui and Carter, 1989; Stewart, 1995). Yet many providers are not trained to provide care for LGBT individuals, and providers themselves report a lack of knowledge about the issues facing their sexual- and gender-minority patients. Particularly for transgender patients, access to providers who are knowledgeable about transgender health issues is critical. In fact, few physicians are knowledgeable about or sensitive to LGBT health risks or health needs (IOM, 1999, p. 43). Medical schools teach very little about sexuality in general and little or nothing about the unique aspects of lesbian, gay, and bisexual health (Makadon, 2006; Tesar and Rovi, 1998; Wallick et al., 1993), and it is rare for medical students to receive any training in transgender health (AAMC GSA and AAMC OSR, 2007).

While the Association of American Medical Colleges issued recommendations for institutional programs and educational activities to address the needs of LGBT patients in 2007, including training in communication skills regarding sexual orientation and gender identity, it is not evident that all medical schools have embraced these recommendations. The Lesbian, Gay, Bisexual, and Transgender Medical Education Research Group, a group of medical students at Stanford University, surveyed deans of medical education at 116 universities in the United States and Canada. They found variability in the content and quality of the LGBT-specific instruction medical students received, with HIV, sexual orientation, and gender identity being the most common LGBT topics included in the curricula. Fully 70 percent of the deans rated their school's curriculum in this area as "fair" or worse (Obedin-Maliver et al., 2010).

While many providers report high levels of discomfort with taking the sexual history of any patient, this lack of training exacerbates this discomfort when providers are dealing with LGBT patients. A qualitative study involving 13 HIV providers found that discomfort with asking questions was one of their greatest issues with respect to the treatment and care of transgender patients (Lurie, 2005). Likewise, a survey of 60 pediatricians in Washington, DC, that examined their approach to the health of LGB youth found that discussions of sex and sexual orientation were difficult even for those who were well intentioned (East and El Rayess, 1998).

Health insurance. Lack of health insurance is a major structural barrier to care, and LGBT people and their children are more likely to lack health insurance than heterosexual people and their children (Badgett, 1994; Cochran, 2001; Diamant et al., 2000; Ponce et al., 2010). This is due at least partially to the fact that LGBT families often lack access to employer-sponsored health insurance (Ash and Badgett, 2006; Heck et al., 2006). As was noted in the earlier discussion of laws and policies, unmarried same-sex partners of employees often are ineligible for employer-sponsored health insurance. While 57 percent of Fortune 500 companies now extend domestic partner benefits to their LGB employees (HRC, 2010), this practice is much less common for smaller companies. Ponce and colleagues (2010) examined disparities in health insurance coverage faced by same-sex couples and found significant disparities in access to care. Using population-based data from California, the authors found that partnered gay men were less than half as likely (42 percent) as married heterosexual men to receive employer-sponsored dependent coverage, and partnered lesbians were 28 percent less likely to receive such coverage than married heterosexual women. As a result, gay men and partnered lesbians are more than twice as likely to be uninsured as married heterosexuals (Ponce et al., 2010).

Even when LGBT people have access to health insurance, they often are still at a disadvantage in relation to their heterosexual peers. Unlike most heterosexual married couples, employees are required to pay federal taxes on employer-provided health insurance for a same-sex partner (Badgett, 2007). Moreover, health plans often fail to cover many services that impact LGBT individuals, including infertility treatment for lesbians. In some instances, access to reproductive and fertility services is denied on the basis of marital status or sexual orientation (Ethics Committee of the American Society for Reproductive Medicine, 2009).

High levels of joblessness and poverty among transgender populations, particularly those of color, make lack of health insurance a problem for these individuals (Xavier et al., 2005). In addition, both private and public health care plans severely limit transgender people's access to sex reassignment surgery or other treatments related to transgender status. Most private insurance plans, as well as Medicare, contain explicit exclusions for such treatments.

THE CASE OF HIV/AIDS

In the chapters that follow, this report addresses a variety of issues related to the health of LGBT populations. Several themes pervade this discussion, including stigma, the resilience of LGBT communities and individuals, the importance of research funding, and persistent health inequities among racial and ethnic minority LGBT individuals. This section returns to the HIV/AIDS epidemic, whose history and impact were briefly described above, to set the stage for the following chapters by illustrating how these themes continue to influence LGBT health today. The IOM has a long history of studying AIDS, having published more than 20 reports on the subject since 1986.

The HIV/AIDS epidemic remains one of the most critical health issues faced by some subgroups within the LGBT population in the United States, namely gay and bisexual men and transgender women. As discussed below, the epidemic is another example of how the intersection of multiple identities (e.g., racial, ethnic, socioeconomic, sexual, and gender) increases risks for some individuals.

Stigma

As noted earlier, the first cases of what would eventually be labeled AIDS were diagnosed in the United States in 1981 in several white gay men (Gottlieb, 2001). The public continued to regard AIDS mainly as a "gay disease" long after health professionals had abandoned this idea (Herek and Capitanio, 1999). The association of AIDS with homosexuality and its attendant stigma shaped and intensified societal responses to AIDS while hindering research and prevention efforts.

As a new, transmissible disease that was not understood by medical science and was perceived as inevitably fatal, AIDS probably would have evoked stigma regardless of whom it affected. But the fact that the public associated it with gay men—an already marginalized group, as explained earlier in this chapter—compounded the stigma experienced by those who were diagnosed with the disease (Herek, 1990). Public opinion surveys conducted in the United States during the epidemic's early years revealed widespread fear of AIDS, inaccurate beliefs about how it could be transmitted, and a willingness to restrict the civil liberties of people perceived to be at risk for contracting it (Blake and Arkin, 1988; Clendinen, 1983; Herek, 1990). Such beliefs and opinions tended to be strongest among respondents with negative attitudes toward gay men and lesbians. In numerous studies, respondents who expressed negative attitudes toward gay people were more likely than others to be poorly informed about AIDS, to overestimate the risks of HIV transmission through casual social contact, to endorse punitive and restrictive AIDS-related policies (e.g., mass quarantine), and to stigmatize people with the disease (D'Augelli, 1989; Goodwin and Roscoe, 1988; Herek and Glunt, 1991; Pleck et al., 1988; Price and Hsu, 1992; Pryor et al., 1989; Stipp and Kerr, 1989).

Negative attitudes toward AIDS and its perceived association with gay men found expression in a variety of ways. Men with AIDS faced ostracism and discrimination both because of their illness and because they were assumed to be gay. Many were fired from their jobs, evicted from their homes, and shunned by their relatives and friends (NRC, 1993). When public awareness about AIDS increased during the mid-1980s, groups that monitored antigay violence reported an increase in incidents, with many assailants making verbal references to AIDS during the attacks (Berrill, 1990). More than 7,200 incidents of antigay harassment and victimization were reported to the National Gay and Lesbian Task Force in 1988. Of these, 17 percent were AIDS-related. The percentages were similar in 1986 and 1987 (Berrill, 1992).

In its early stages, AIDS was perceived not as a national health problem but as a problem for homosexuals and intravenous drug users. Because of the marginal status of these groups, societal response to the epidemic was slow. It was not until there was widespread awareness that AIDS was affecting the "mainstream" population that the disease garnered significant attention. Indeed, it was Ryan White, an Indiana adolescent who contracted AIDS through treatment for hemophilia, who became the sympathetic face of AIDS to the nation (White and Cunningham, 1991).

The response of the federal government to the epidemic also was slow. Inadequate efforts were undertaken to intervene in the spread of HIV, especially compared with the response to other new diseases. Throughout most of the 1980s, the disease was seldom acknowledged by the federal government. President Ronald Reagan mentioned AIDS publicly for the first time only in 1987.

Furthermore, HIV/AIDS research and prevention efforts were hampered by the stigma associated with homosexual behavior. Researchers and public health officials were hindered from the outset of the epidemic by the relative lack of reliable scientific data on gay and bisexual men and the LGBT community. Early in the epidemic, researchers and public health officials attempting to respond to the epidemic had to base many of their predictions and much of their planning on population estimates derived from the Kinsey studies of the 1940s and 1950s. As noted above, the generalizability of these data was questionable. However, the funding and resources needed to collect data on homosexuality and bisexuality from high-quality probability samples had not been made available during the intervening years. In addition, scientists conducting research on sexual behavior among gay and bisexual men, men who have sex with other men but do not identify as gay or bisexual, and transgender people often came under political scrutiny.

Facing stigma related to both HIV/AIDS and homosexuality, many gay and bisexual men, as well as other men who have sex with men, have been reluctant to undergo HIV testing, to seek treatment for HIV, and to participate in scientific research (Chesney and Smith, 1999; Herek, 1999; Stall et al., 1996).

The marginalized status of transgender people similarly delayed government's responses to HIV/AIDS in the transgender community. As noted by Herbst and colleagues (2008), there was virtually no attention to infection rates in the transgender community until the mid-1990s, largely because transgender individuals were not included in federal surveillance efforts.

Although the cultural climate regarding HIV-positive individuals has become more inclusive since the early days of the AIDS epidemic, stigmatization continues to affect all LGBT people.

Resilience

As discussed earlier, AIDS was a devastating disease for LGBT people, yet they responded to this unprecedented challenge with resilience. Community-based organizations were created and provided a variety of medical, psychological, and social services to people with AIDS and disseminated information about sexual risk reduction and "safer sex." These organizations were visible in major urban centers, but these kinds of activities extended into smaller cities and towns as well.

It can be argued that the AIDS epidemic created a greater sense of community among LGBT people than had previously existed, with far-reaching effects. In the absence of an early political or cultural response to

AIDS, gay-based organizations were the first to respond, caring for those who were infected, advocating for increased attention, and raising funds to promote scientific research. The disease forged new and stronger bonds among LGBT people. For example, although political divides along gender lines were often evident in the LGB community during the 1970s, lesbians and bisexual women, who themselves were considerably less likely to be infected with HIV than gay and bisexual men, played prominent roles in the community's response to the epidemic.

Gerald (1989, p. 450) notes that "far from destroying the gay community, the concern over AIDS has strengthened it." A sense of community emerged that was able to confront the challenges posed by the disease. With the creation of this organized community, new models of care and support for members of the community were developed. In addition, LGBT organizations learned how to work with foundations and corporations in new ways to access funding to address the epidemic. The community built partnerships and coalitions with research and health institutions and with federal, state, and local policy makers. The mobilization of the LGBT community was a major positive response to the epidemic, and the structures created in response to the disease continue to exist today.

Importance of Research Funding

One of the major successes that emerged from the AIDS epidemic was the confirmation that funding for research can drive progress. "Beginning in 1981 with the allocation of several hundred thousand dollars for research, U.S. government spending on HIV/AIDS nearly doubled every year between FY1982 and FY1989. Since then, annual increases in Federal spending have been more gradual" (Funders Concerned About AIDS, 2003, p. 45).

While the initial response of the federal government was slow, a strong funding commitment since the late 1980s can be linked to impressive advances. After the discovery of HIV as a viral agent, the development of a blood test to diagnose HIV-infected patients and screen the blood supply followed rapidly. In 1987, the licensing of Zidovudine (AZT), the first clinically effective drug against HIV, appeared to offer great promise. As HIV quickly became resistant to AZT, however, the initial optimism dissipated (Fauci, 2008; Sepkowitz, 2001).

By 1990, 9 years after the epidemic emerged, researchers had achieved great progress in understanding the epidemiology, natural history, and pathogenesis of the disease (IOM, 1991a). In 1991, the discovery of two other pharmaceutical agents that could be used in combination with AZT to target the virus led to the development of highly active antiretroviral therapy. By the mid-1990s, protease inhibitors had reached the market and were used successfully in combination with existing therapies to improve the prognosis of many HIV-infected individuals. Within 2 years, the AIDS death rate in the United States dropped by more than two-thirds (Fauci, 2008).

Given that the most effective strategy against AIDS was to prevent infection in the first place and that HIV transmission occurs between people in social settings and involves individual behavior, the social and behavioral sciences clearly had an important role to play in the fight against AIDS (IOM, 1995). Much of the dramatic decline in AIDS cases observed among gay and bisexual men during the 1980s was attributable to large-scale behavior changes within the community, in which social and behavioral research played a key role (IOM, 2001).

AIDS prevention activities began in gay communities in the early 1980s in San Francisco and New York City (Shilts, 1987). Later efforts led by the Centers for Disease Control and Prevention expanded prevention activities to other populations. These early interventions focused mainly on increasing knowledge about HIV transmission, but over time, interventions were developed at the individual, small-group, and community levels that were aimed at changing behavior associated with HIV transmission (CDC, 2006).

Behavior change strategies for men who have sex with men utilized a variety of interventions, including problem solving, self-management, skills building, delivery of information, and fostering of heightened self-efficacy and intentions to reduce risk (NIH, 1997). Studies using a variety of evaluation designs (descriptive studies, nonrandomized and randomized studies) showed that risk reduction strategies for men who have sex with men had positive behavioral effects (NIH, 1997).

Figure 2-1 shows discretionary funding (including funding for research, prevention, and treatment) by the Department of Health and Human Services for HIV/AIDS from fiscal year 1981 to fiscal year 2008. It should be noted that much of the research that has been undertaken on LGBT health generally has been made possible through HIV funding.

Today, the budget for the National Institutes of Health's (NIH) AIDS research program totals more than $3 billion, representing approximately 10 percent of the total NIH budget. Funding priorities encompass not only etiology and pathogenesis, epidemiology, preventive measures, and treatment, but also the investigation of innovative means of prevention (NIH, 2010).

Health Inequities

The progress mentioned in the previous section has not translated into benefits for all members of the LGBT community. An estimated 28,720 new HIV cases occurred among men who have sex with men in 2006. Although black people made up only 12.8 percent of the U.S. population in 2006 (U.S. Census Bureau, 2006), 35 percent (10,130) of the estimated new HIV

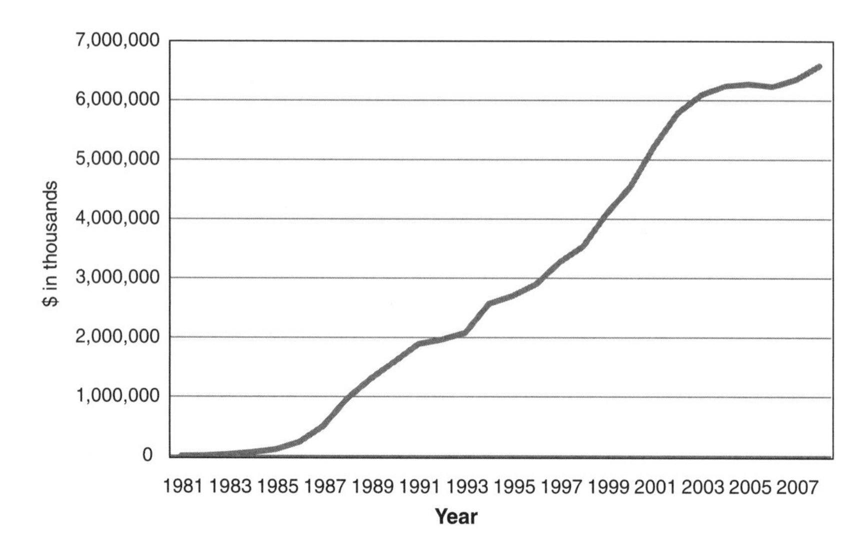

FIGURE 2-1 Discretionary funding for HIV/AIDS by the Department of Health and Human Services in thousands of dollars.
SOURCE: Adapted from a table prepared by the Congressional Research Services based on analysis from HHS Budget Office, March 20, 2008 (Johnson, 2008).

cases were among black men who have sex with men, while 46 percent (13,230) were among white men who have sex with men. Similarly, Latino people accounted for 14.8 percent of the U.S. population in 2006 (U.S. Census Bureau, 2006), but Latino men who have sex with men accounted for 18.6 percent (5,360) of new HIV cases (CDC, 2010). While HIV/AIDS diagnoses among American Indians and Alaska Natives represented less than 1 percent of all HIV/AIDS diagnoses in 2005, this group is ranked third among the U.S. population in rates of diagnosis (behind blacks and Latinos). Of the 1,447 American Indian/Alaska Native men with HIV/AIDS at the end of 2005, 74 percent had been infected through male-to-male sexual contact or male-to-male sexual contact combined with intravenous drug use (CDC, 2008).

The disproportionate impact of HIV/AIDS on nonwhite men who have sex with men may not be linked exclusively to individual risk behaviors. Social determinants, such as low education level, can be associated with a number of factors that have been understood to play a significant role in the spread of HIV/AIDS, although their effects have been largely understudied. These factors include a higher likelihood of unemployment or low-wage employment, less likelihood of having health care coverage, inferior quality of care, limited accessibility of treatment medications and interventions, community destabilization, and sexual networks composed of high-risk (more likely to have HIV infection) members (Peterson and Jones, 2009).

Black transgender individuals have a significantly higher infection rate than other racial or ethnic groups, with male-to-females being at a particularly high risk of infection. In their systematic review, Herbst and colleagues (2008) found that some of the risk factors that may contribute to the high infection rates among male-to-females include multiple sex partners who are male, casual sex, and sex while under the influence of drugs or alcohol. The authors also note that the studies considered in their meta-analysis included a high percentage of male-to-females who engage in sex work. Figure 2-2 presents a breakdown of new HIV infections in 2006, the most recent year for which data are available, by race/ethnicity among men who have sex with men. Note that the figure presents absolute numbers.

Members of racial and ethnic minority groups have typically been underrepresented in the mainstream LGBT movement. HIV in racial and ethnic minority communities, particularly the black community, is complicated by a range of issues, including, among others, a lower likelihood of getting tested, greater discomfort with the health care system and with medical institutions, lower levels of acceptance of same-sex and bisexual sexual behavior, and racism (Peterson and Jones, 2009).

Furthermore, a systematic review of HIV interventions notes the lack of interventions targeting black, Latino, or other racial and ethnic minority men who have sex with men (Lyles et al., 2007). Similarly, no evidence-based HIV prevention interventions have been identified as effective for members of the black transgender community (Herbst et al., 2008).

The health inequities illustrated by the HIV/AIDS example persist in

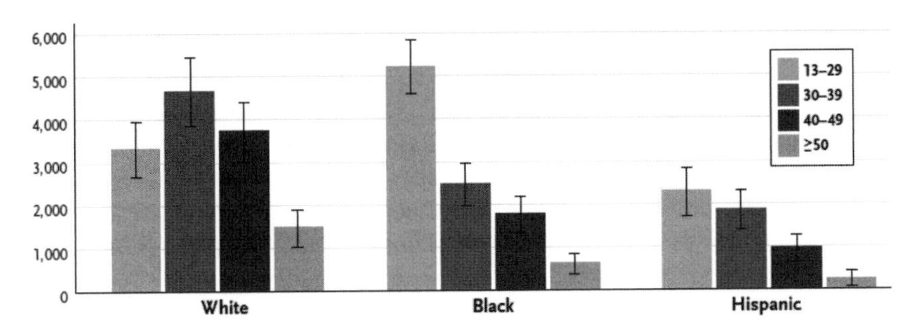

FIGURE 2-2 Estimated number of new HIV infections by race/ethnicity among men who have sex with men.
NOTES: Incidence estimates are adjusted for reporting delays and reclassification of cases reported without a known risk factor for HIV, but not for underreporting; non-Hispanic whites and non-Hispanic blacks are referred to as white and black, respectively. Persons of Hispanic ethnicity might be of any race; the "I" bars denote the data range for each confidence interval.
SOURCE: CDC, 2010.

many areas of LGBT health today. The challenges associated with understanding racial, ethnic, geographic, socioeconomic, and other LGBT subpopulations are discussed throughout the remainder of the report.

SUMMARY OF KEY FINDINGS AND RESEARCH OPPORTUNITIES

Findings

Operationally defining LGBT populations requires considerable care and attention to the focus of the research question. Basic demographic data, which are critical to understanding and meeting the needs of populations, are lacking for LGBT populations. From the data that are available, much more is known about lesbians and gay men than about bisexual and transgender people. Further complicating the situation is the fact that not only are lesbians, gay men, bisexual women, bisexual men, transgender women, and transgender men all discrete populations, but each group is further shaped by racial, ethnic, and other cultural influences. The available demographic data fail to adequately describe the variations within each LGBT population; however, existing research provides some pertinent findings:

- Self-identification as lesbian, gay, or bisexual and disclosure of this identity may vary by race, ethnicity, income level, or geographic location.
- If one examines the historical trajectory of LGBT populations in the United States, it is clear that stigma has exerted an enormous and continuing influence on the life and consequently the health status of LGBT individuals.
- LGBT individuals live in most geographic areas throughout the United States, but studies have shown higher proportions in urban areas on the East and West Coasts.
- On average, gay men appear to have lower incomes than heterosexual men with similar education and occupations. While some research has suggested that lesbian women have higher incomes than heterosexual women, other studies have not found this difference. In comparison with non-gender-variant heterosexual adults, bisexual and transgender people also appear to have lower incomes.
- As a result of differential treatment in such areas as taxes and insurance, even lesbian or gay individuals whose gross incomes are identical to those of heterosexual men and women can be expected to have less disposable income.
- While lesbians and gay men are less likely to be parents than their heterosexual peers, substantial numbers of lesbians and gay men have children.

- Lesbians, gay men, and bisexual and transgender people exist across all age groups.
- LGBT individuals face financial barriers, limitations on access to health insurance, insufficient provider knowledge, and negative provider attitudes that can be expected to have an effect on their access to health care.
- A lack of training for health care providers may lead to less than optimal care for LGBT adolescents and adults.
- LGBT individuals face barriers to care related to sexual and transgender stigma, and some are further marginalized by additional barriers such as racial/ethnic minority status, low income, immigrant status, and limited English proficiency.

Research Opportunities

Research on the influence of contextual factors (e.g., income, geographic location, race, ethnicity, stigma) on LGBT health status is lacking. Although limited data are available with which to assess how many individuals identify as lesbian, gay, bisexual, or transgender, as well as how many report same-sex sexual behavior, demographic data on LGBT populations from large-scale surveys are largely absent from the literature. There are many opportunities for future research:

- large-scale surveys examining the demographic and social characteristics of sexual and gender minorities;
- patterns of household composition within LGBT populations, specifically rates of partnership and children with gay, lesbian, bisexual, or transgender parents;
- income and education differences among both single and partnered sexual- and gender-minority individuals;
- impacts of barriers to care—particularly provider knowledge about and attitudes toward LGBT patients, limited access to health insurance, and discrimination within the health care system—on the health of LGBT individuals; and
- the extent to which LGBT individuals experience enactments of stigma and the impact of sexual and transgender stigma, at both the personal and structural levels, on LGBT health.

REFERENCES

AAMC GSA and AAMC OSR (Association of American Medical Colleges Group on Student Affairs and Association of American Medical Colleges Organization of Student Representatives). 2007. *Institutional programs and educational activities to address the needs of GLBT students and patients*. Washington, DC: AAMC GSA and AAMC OSR.

Adam, B. D. 1987. *The rise of a gay and lesbian movement*. New York: Twayne Publishers.
Adam, B. D. 1995. *The rise of a gay and lesbian movement* (revised edition). New York: Twayne Publishers.
Allegretto, S. A., and M. M. Arthur. 2001. An empirical analysis of homosexual/heterosexual male earnings differentials: Unmarried and unequal? *Industrial and Labor Relations Review* 54:631–646.
American Psychiatric Association. 1952. *Mental disorders: Diagnostic and statistical manual*. Washington, DC: American Psychiatric Association.
American Psychiatric Association. 1980. *Diagnostic and statistical manual of mental disorders*. 3rd ed. Washington, DC: American Psychiatric Association.
American Psychiatric Association. 1987. *Diagnostic and statistical manual of mental disorders*. 4th ed. Washington, DC: American Psychiatric Association.
American Psychiatric Association. 2000. *Diagnostic and statistical manual of mental disorders (DSM-IV-TR)*. 4th ed. Washington, DC: American Psychiatric Association.
American Psychological Association. 2009a. *Report of the APA task force on gender identity and gender variance*. Washington, DC: American Psychological Association.
American Psychological Association. 2009b. *Report of the task force on appropriate therapeutic responses to sexual orientation*. Washington, DC: American Psychological Association.
American Psychological Association and APHA (American Public Health Association). 1986. *Bowers v. Hardwick: Brief for amicus curiae, Supreme Court of the United States*. Washington, DC: American Psychological Association and APHA.
Ash, M. A., and M. V. L. Badgett. 2006. Separate and unequal: The effect of unequal access to employment-based health insurance on same-sex and unmarried different-sex couples. *Contemporary Economic Policy* 24(4):582–599.
Badgett, M. V. L. 1994. *Civil rights, civilized research: Constructing a sexual orientation anti-discrimination policy based on the evidence*. Paper presented at APPAM Research Conference, San Francisco, CA.
Badgett, M. V. L. 1995. The wage effects of sexual orientation discrimination. *Industrial and Labor Relations Review* 48(4):726–739.
Badgett, M. V. L. 2001. *Money, myths, and change: The economic lives of lesbians and gay men*. Chicago, IL: University of Chicago Press.
Badgett, M. V. L. 2007. Unequal taxes on equal benefits: The taxation of domestic partner benefits. *Echelon Magazine* 22–22.
Baumeister, R. F. 2000. Gender differences in erotic plasticity: The female sex drive as socially flexible and responsive. *Psychological Bulletin* 126(3):347–374; discussion 385–389.
Baumeister, R. F., K. R. Catanese, and K. D. Vohs. 2001. Is there a gender difference in strength of sex drive? Theoretical views, conceptual distinctions, and a review of relevant evidence. *Personality and Social Psychology Review* 5(3):242–273.
Bayer, R. 1987. *Homosexuality and American psychiatry: The politics of diagnosis* (revised edition). Princeton, NJ: Princeton University Press.
Bayer, R. 1989. *Private acts, social consequences: AIDS and the politics of public health*. New York: The Free Press.
Benjamin, H. 1966. *The transsexual phenomenon*. New York: Julian Press.
Berrill, K. T. 1990. Anti-gay violence and victimization in the United States. *Journal of Interpersonal Violence* 5(3):274-294.
Berrill, K. T. 1992. Anti-gay violence and victimization in the United States: An overview. In *Hate crimes: Confronting violence against lesbians and gay men*, edited by G. M. Herek and K. T. Berrill. Newbury Park, CA: SAGE Publications. Pp. 19–45.
Berube, A. 1990. *Coming out under fire: The history of gay men and women in World War Two*. New York: The Free Press.

Biegel, S., and S. J. Kuehl. 2010. *Safe at school: Addressing the school environment and LGBT safety through policy and legislation.* Los Angeles, CA: The Williams Institute, The Great Lakes Center for Education Research and Practice, and the National Education Policy Center.

Black, D., G. Gates, S. Sanders, and L. Taylor. 2000. Demographics of the gay and lesbian population in the United States: Evidence from available systematic data sources. *Demography* 37(2):139–154.

Black, D. A., H. R. Makar, S. G. Sanders, and L. J. Taylor. 2003. The earnings effects of sexual orientation. *Industrial and Labor Relations Review* 56:449–469.

Black, D. A., S. G. Sanders, and L. J. Taylor. 2007. The economics of lesbian and gay families. *The Journal of Economic Perspectives* 21:53–70.

Blake, S. M., and E. B. Arkin. 1988. *AIDS information monitor: A summary of national public opinion surveys on AIDS: 1983 through 1986.* Washington, DC: American Red Cross.

Bockting, W. O. 1997. Transgender coming out: Implications for the clinical management of gender dysphoria. In *Gender blending*, edited by B. Bullough, V. L. Bullough, and J. Elias. Amherst, NY: Prometheus Books. Pp. 48–52.

Bockting, W. O. 1999. From construction to context: Gender through the eyes of the transgendered. *SIECUS Report* 28(1):3–7.

Bockting, W. O. 2008. Psychotherapy and the real-life experience: From gender dichotomy to gender diversity. *Sexologies* 17(4):211–224.

Bockting, W. O., and R. Ehrbar. 2006. Commentary: Gender variance, dissonance, or identity disorder. *Journal of Psychology and Human Sexuality* 17(3/4):125–134.

Bockting, W. O., B. R. Rosser, and K. Scheltema. 1999. Transgender HIV prevention: Implementation and evaluation of a workshop. *Health Education Research* 14(2):177–183.

Bockting, W., A. Benner, and E. Coleman. 2009. Gay and bisexual identity development among female-to-male transsexuals in North America: Emergence of a transgender sexuality. *Archives of Sexual Behavior* 38(5):688–701.

Bowleg, L., G. Burkholder, M. Teti, and M. L. Craig. 2008. The complexities of outness: Psychosocial predictors of coming out to others among black lesbian and bisexual women. *Journal of LGBT Health Research* 4(4):153–166.

Boyd, N. A. 2003. *Wide-open town: A history of queer San Francisco to 1965.* Berkeley: University of California Press.

Bullough, V. L., and B. Bullough. 1993. *Crossdressing, sex, and gender.* Philadelphia, PA: University of Pennsylvania Press.

Carpenter, C. S. 2005. Self-reported sexual orientation and earnings: Evidence from California. *Industrial and Labor Relations Review* 58(2):258–273.

Carpenter, C. S. 2007. Revisiting the income penalty for behaviorally gay men: Evidence from NHANES III. *Labour Economics* 14(1):25–34.

Carpenter, C. S., and G. J. Gates. 2008. Gay and lesbian partnership: Evidence from California. *Demography* 45(3):573-590.

Cauldwell, D. O. 1949. Psychopathia transexualis. *Sexology* 16:139–152.

CDC (Centers for Disease Control and Prevention). 2003. *HIV/STD risks in young men who have sex with men who do not disclose their sexual orientation—six U.S. cities, 1994–2000.* Atlanta, GA: CDC.

CDC. 2006. Evolution of HIV/AIDS prevention programs—United States, 1981-2006. *Morbidity and Mortality Weekly Report* 55(21):597–603.

CDC. 2008. *HIV/AIDS among American Indians and Alaska natives.* Atlanta, GA: CDC.

CDC. 2010. *HIV and AIDS among gay and bisexual men.* Atlanta, GA: CDC.

Chae, D. H., and G. Ayala. 2010. Sexual orientation and sexual behavior among Latino and Asian Americans: Implications for unfair treatment and psychological distress. *Journal of Sex Research* 47(5):451–459.

Chauncey, G., Jr. 1982–1983. From sexual inversion to homosexuality: Medicine and the changing conceptualization of female deviance. *Salmagundi* 58–59:114–146.
Chauncey, G., Jr. 1993. The postwar sex crime panic. In *True stories from the American past*, edited by W. Graebner. New York: McGraw-Hill. Pp. 160–178.
Chauncey, G, Jr. 2004. *Why marriage? The history shaping today's debate over gay equality*. New York: Basic Books.
Chesney, M. A., and A. W. Smith. 1999. Critical delays in HIV testing and care. *American Behavioral Scientist* 42(7):1162–1174.
Chu, S. Y., T. A. Peterman, L. S. Doll, J. W. Buehler, and J. W. Curran. 1992. AIDS in bisexual men in the United States: Epidemiology and transmission to women. *American Journal of Public Health* 82(2):220–224.
Clendinen, D. 1983. AIDS spreads pain and fear among ill and healthy alike. *New York Times*, A1, B4.
Coan, D. L., W. Schrager, and T. Packer. 2005. The role of male sexual partners in HIV infection among male-to-female transgendered individuals. In *Transgender health and HIV prevention: Needs assessment studies from transgender communities across the United States*, edited by W. Bockting and E. Avery. New York: The Haworth Medical Press. Pp. 21–30.
Cochran, S. D. 2001. Emerging issues in research on lesbians' and gay men's mental health: Does sexual orientation really matter? *American Psychologist* 56(11):931–947.
Cochran, W. G., F. Mosteller, and J. W. Tukey. 1953. Statistical problems of the Kinsey Report. *Journal of the American Statistical Association* 48(264):673–716.
Coleman, E., P. Colgan, and L. Gooren. 1992. Male cross-gender behavior in Myanmar (Burma): A description of the acault. *Archives of Sexual Behavior* 21(3):313–321.
Conger, J. J. 1975. Proceedings of the American Psychological Association, Incorporated, for the year 1974: Minutes of the annual meeting of the Council of Representatives. *American Psychologist* 30:620–651.
Corrigan, P. W., A. C. Watson, M. L. Heyrman, A. Warpinski, G. Gracia, N. Slopen, and L. L. Hall. 2005. Structural stigma in state legislation. *Psychiatric Services* 56(5):557–563.
Cortes, D. E., N. Mulvaney-Day, L. Fortuna, S. Reinfeld, and M. Alegría. 2009. Patient-provider communication. *Health Education & Behavior* 36(1):138–154.
D'Augelli, A. R. 1989. Lesbians' and gay men's experiences of discrimination and harassment in a university community. *American Journal of Community Psychology* 17(3):317–321.
D'Emilio, J. 1983. *Sexual politics, sexual communities*. Chicago, IL: The University of Chicago Press.
Department of Justice. 2009. *2008 hate crime statistics: Incidents, offenses, victims, and known offenders by bias motivation*. http://www2.fbi.gov/ucr/hc2008/data/table_01.html (accessed November 4, 2010).
Diamant, A. L., C. Wold, K. Spritzer, and L. Gelberg. 2000. Health behaviors, health status, and access to and use of health care: A population-based study of lesbian, bisexual, and heterosexual women. *Archives of Family Medicine* 9(10):1043–1051.
Diamond, L. M. 2008. *Sexual fluidity: Understanding women's love and desire*. Cambridge, MA: Harvard University Press.
Doll, L. S., L. R. Petersen, C. R. White, E. S. Johnson, J. W. Ward, and The Blood Donor Study Group. 1992. Homosexually and nonhomosexually identified men who have sex with men: A behavioral comparison. *Journal of Sex Research* 29(1):1–14.
Drescher, J. 2010. Queer diagnoses: Parallels and contrasts in the history of homosexuality, gender variance, and the diagnostic and statistical manual. *Archives of Sexual Behavior* 39(2):427–460.
East, J. A., and F. El Rayess. 1998. Pediatricians' approach to the health care of lesbian, gay, and bisexual youth. *Journal of Adolescent Health* 23(4):191–193.

Eliason, M. J., and R. D. Schope. 2001. Does "don't ask don't tell" apply to health care? Lesbian, gay, and bisexual people's disclosure to health care providers. *Journal of the Gay and Lesbian Medical Association* 5(4):125–134.

Ellis, H. 1901. *Studies in the psychology of sex: Volume 2: Sexual inversion*. Philadelphia, PA: F.A. Davis.

Ellis, H. 1933. *Psychology of sex*. London: William Heinemann.

Epstein, S. 1996. *Impure science: AIDS, activism, and the politics of knowledge*. Berkeley, CA: University of California Press.

Erikson, K. T. 1976. *Everything in its path: Destruction of community in the Buffalo Creek flood*. New York: Simon and Schuster.

Ethics Committee of the American Society for Reproductive Medicine. 2009. Access to fertility treatment by gays, lesbians, and unmarried persons. *Fertility & Sterility* 92(4): 1190–1193.

Faderman, L. 1991. *Odd girls and twilight lovers: A history of lesbian life in twentieth-century America*. New York: Columbia University Press.

Fauci, A. S. 2008. 25 years of HIV. *Nature* 453(7193):289–290.

FBI (Federal Bureau of Investigation). 2010. *About hate crime statistics*. http://www2.fbi.gov/ucr/hc2009/abouthcs.html (accessed December 7, 2010).

Feinberg, L. 1996. *Transgender warriors*. Boston, MA: Beacon Press.

Feldman, M. P. 1966. Aversion therapy for sexual deviations: A critical review. *Psychological Bulletin* 65(2):65–79.

Fisk, N. M. 1974. Editorial: Gender dysphoria syndrome—the conceptualization that liberalizes indications for total gender reorientation and implies a broadly based multi-dimensional rehabilitative regimen. *Western Journal of Medicine* 120(5):386–391.

Fleming, M., C. Steinman, and G. Bocknek. 1980. Methodological problems in assessing sex-reassignment surgery: A reply to Meyer and Reter. *Archives of Sexual Behavior* 9(5):451–456.

Flores, S. A., R. Bakeman, G. A. Millett, and J. L. Peterson. 2009. HIV risk among bisexually and homosexually active racially diverse young men. *Sexually Transmitted Diseases* 36(5):325–329.

Ford, C. S., and F. Beach. 1951. *Patterns of sexual behavior*. New York: Harper and Row.

Freud, S. 1951. Letter from Freud. *American Journal of Psychiatry* 107(10):786-787.

Freud, S. 1953. Three essays on the theory of sexuality. In *The standard edition of the complete psychological works of Sigmund Freud*, Vol. 7, edited by J. Strachey. London: Hogarth Press. Original edition, original work published in 1905. Pp. 123–243.

Friedman, R. C., and J. I. Downey. 1998. Psychoanalysis and the model of homosexuality as psychopathology: A historical overview. *American Journal of Psychoanalysis* 58(3):249–270.

Funders Concerned About AIDS. 2003. *HIV/AIDS philanthropy: History and current parameters, 1981–2000*. New York: Funders Concerned About AIDS.

GAO (General Accounting Office). 2004. *Defense of marriage act: Update to prior report*. Washington, DC: GAO.

Gates, G. 2006. *Same-sex couples and the gay, lesbian, bisexual population: New estimates from the American Community Survey*. Los Angeles, CA: The Williams Institute on Sexual Orientation.

Gates, G. J. 2010. *Sexual minorities in the 2008 General Social Survey: Coming out and demographic characteristics*. Los Angeles, CA: The Williams Institute.

Gates, G., and J. Ost. 2004a. Estimating the size of the gay and lesbian population. In *The gay and lesbian atlas*, edited by G. Gates and J. Ost. Washington, DC: The Urban Institute Press. Pp. 17–21.

Gates, G., and J. Ost. 2004b. *The gay and lesbian atlas*. Washington, DC: The Urban Institute Press.

Gates, G., and A. P. Romero. 2009. *Parenting by gay men and lesbians: Beyond the current research*. In Marriage and family: Perspectives and complexities, edited by E. Peters and C. M. Kamp Dush. New York: Columbia University Press. Pp. 227–243.

Gates, G., M. V. L. Badgett, J. E. Macomber, and K. Chambers. 2007. *Adoption and foster care by gay and lesbian parents in the United States*. Los Angeles, CA: The Williams Institute.

Gerald, G. 1989. What can we learn from the gay community's response to the AIDS crisis? *Journal of the National Medical Association* 81(4):449–452.

Goffman, E. 1963. *Stigma: Notes on the management of spoiled identity*. New York: Simon and Schuster.

Goldbaum, G., T. Perdue, R. Wolitski, C. Rietmeijer, A. Hedrich, R. Wood, M. Fishbein, D. Cohn, N. Corby, A. Freeman, C. Guenther-Grey, J. Sheridan, and S. Tross. 1998. Differences in risk behavior and sources of AIDS information among gay, bisexual, and straight-identified men who have sex with men. *AIDS and Behavior* 2(1):13–21.

Goldberg, N. G. 2009. *The impact of inequality for same-sex partners in employer-sponsored retirement plans*. Los Angeles, CA: The Williams Institute.

Gonsiorek, J. C. 1991. The empirical basis for the demise of the illness model of homosexuality. In *Homosexuality: Research implications for public policy*, edited by J. C. Gonsiorek and J. D. Weinrich. Newbury Park, CA: SAGE Publications. Pp. 115–136.

Goodwin, M. P., and B. Roscoe. 1988. AIDS: Students' knowledge and attitudes at a Midwestern university. *Journal of American College Health* 36(4):214–222.

Gottlieb, M. S. 2001. AIDS—past and future. *New England Journal of Medicine* 344(23): 1788–1791.

Gottlieb, M. S., H. M. Schanker, P. T. Fan, A. Saxon, J. D. Weisman, and I. Pozalski. 1981. Pneumocystis pneumonia—Los Angeles. *Morbidity and Mortality Weekly Report* 30:250–252, http://www.cdc.gov/mmwr/preview/mmwrhtml/june_5.htm (accessed December 22, 2010).

Green, R., and D. T. Fleming. 1990. Transsexual surgery follow-up: Status in the 1990s. *Annual Review of Sex Research* 1:163–174.

Haldeman, D. C. 1994. The practice and ethics of sexual orientation conversion therapy. *Journal of Consulting & Clinical Psychology* 62(2):221–227.

Harlow, C. W. 2005. *Hate crime reported by victims and police*. Washington, DC: Department of Justice.

Hastings, D., and C. Markland. 1978. Post-surgical adjustment of twenty-five transsexuals (male-to-female) in the University of Minnesota Study. *Archives of Sexual Behavior* 7(4):327–336.

Hastings, D. W. 1969. Inauguration of a research project on transsexualism in a university medical center. In *Transsexualism and sex reassignment*, edited by R. Green and J. Money. Baltimore, MD: Johns Hopkins Press. Pp. 243–251.

Heck, J. E., R. L. Sell, and S. S. Gorin. 2006. Health care access among individuals involved in same-sex relationships. *American Journal of Public Health* 96(6):1111–1118.

Herbenick, D., M. Reece, V. Schick, S. A. Sanders, B. Dodge, and J. D. Fortenberry. 2010. Sexual behavior in the United States: Results from a national probability sample of men and women ages 14–94. *The Journal of Sexual Medicine* 7:255–265.

Herbst, J. H., E. D. Jacobs, T. J. Finlayson, V. S. McKleroy, M. S. Neumann, N. Crepaz, and HIV/AIDS Prevention Research Synthesis Team. 2008. Estimating HIV prevalence and risk behaviors of transgender persons in the United States: A systematic review. *AIDS & Behavior* 12(1):1–17.

Herdt, G. 2001. Social change, sexual diversity, and tolerance for bisexuality in the United States. In *Lesbian, gay, and bisexual identities and youth: Psychological perspectives*, edited by A. R. D'Augelli and C. J. Patterson. New York: Oxford University Press. Pp. 267–283.

Herdt, G., and R. Kertzner. 2006. I do, but I can't: The impact of marriage denial on the mental health and sexual citizenship of lesbians and gay men in the United States. *Sexuality Research and Social Policy* 3(1):33–49.

Herek, G. M. 1990. Illness, stigma, and AIDS. In *Psychological aspects of serious illness: Chronic conditions, fatal diseases, and clinical care*, edited by P. T. Costa, Jr., and G. R. VandenBos. Washington, DC: American Psychological Association. Pp. 103–150.

Herek, G. M. 1992. The community response to violence in San Francisco: An interview with Wenny Kusuma, Lester Olmstead-Rose, and Jill Tregor. In *Hate crimes: Confronting violence against lesbians and gay men,* edited by G. M. Herek and K. T. Berrill. Thousand Oaks, CA: SAGE Publications. Pp. 241–258.

Herek, G. M. 1999. AIDS and stigma. *American Behavioral Scientist* 42(7):1106–1116.

Herek, G. M. 2006. Legal recognition of same-sex relationships in the United States—a social science perspective. *American Psychologist* 61(6):607–621.

Herek, G. M. 2009a. Hate crimes and stigma-related experiences among sexual minority adults in the United States: Prevalence estimates from a national probability sample. *Journal of Interpersonal Violence* 24(1):54–74.

Herek, G. M. 2009b. Sexual prejudice. In *Handbook of prejudice, stereotyping, and discrimination*, edited by T. D. Nelson. New York: Psychology Press. Pp. 441–467.

Herek, G. M. 2009c. Sexual stigma and sexual prejudice in the United States: A conceptual framework. *Nebraska Symposium on Motivation* 54:65–111.

Herek, G. M. 2009d. Sexual stigma and sexual prejudice in the United States: A conceptual framework. In *Contemporary perspectives on lesbian, gay, and bisexual identities*, edited by D. A. Hope. New York: Springer Science + Business Media. Pp. 65–111.

Herek, G. M., and J. P. Capitanio. 1996. "Some of my best friends": Intergroup contact, concealable stigma, and heterosexuals' attitudes toward gay men and lesbians. *Personality & Social Psychology Bulletin* 22:412–424.

Herek, G. M., and J. P. Capitanio. 1999. Sex differences in how heterosexuals think about lesbians and gay men: Evidence from survey context effects. *Journal of Sex Research* 36(4):348–360.

Herek, G. M., and E. K. Glunt. 1991. AIDS-related attitudes in the United States: A preliminary conceptualization. *Journal of Sex Research* 28(1):99–123.

Herek, G. M., and C. Sims. 2008. Sexual orientation and violent victimization: Hate crimes and intimate partner violence among gay and bisexual males in the United States. In *Unequal opportunity: Health disparities among gay and bisexual men in the United States*, edited by R. J. Wolitski, R. Stall, and R. O. Valdiserri. New York: Oxford University Press. Pp. 35–71.

Herek, G. M., A. Norton, T. Allen, and C. Sims. 2010. Demographic, psychological, and social characteristics of self-identified lesbian, gay, and bisexual adults in a US probability sample. *Sexuality Research and Social Policy* 7(3):176–200.

Higgins, D. J. 2006. Same-sex attraction in heterosexually partnered men: Reasons, rationales and reflections. *Sexual and Relationship Therapy* 21(2):217–228.

Hirschfeld, M. 1991. *The transvestites: The erotic drive to cross-dress.* Translated by M. A. Lombardi-Nash. Buffalo, NY: Prometheus Books. Original edition, 1910.

Hirschfeld, M. 2000. *The homosexuality of men and women* (2nd edition). Translated by M. A. Lombardi-Nash. Buffalo, NY: Prometheus Books.

Hooker, E. 1957. The adjustment of the male overt homosexual. *Journal of Projective Techniques* 21(1):18–31.

HRC (Human Rights Campaign). 2010. *LGBT equality at the fortune 500.* http://www.hrc.org/issues/workplace/fortune500.htm (accessed February 9, 2011).

Inui, T. S., and W. B. Carter. 1989. Design issues in research on doctor-patient communication. In *Communicating with medical patients*, edited by M. Stewart and D. Roter. London: SAGE Publications.

IOM (Institute of Medicine). 1991a. *The AIDS Research Program of the National Institutes of Health*. Washington, DC: National Academy Press.

IOM. 1991b. *Expanding access to investigational therapies for HIV infection and AIDS*. Washington, DC: National Academy Press.

IOM. 1991c. *HIV screening of pregnant women and newborns*. Washington, DC: National Academy Press.

IOM. 1993. *Access to health care in America*. Washington, DC: National Academy Press.

IOM. 1995. *HIV and the blood supply: An analysis of crisis decision making*. Washington, DC: National Academy Press.

IOM. 1999. *Lesbian health: Current assessment and directions for the future*. Washington, DC: National Academy Press.

IOM. 2001. *No time to lose: Getting more from HIV prevention*. Washington, DC: National Academy Press.

IOM. 2005. *Public financing and delivery of HIV/AIDS care: Securing the legacy of Ryan White*. Washington, DC: The National Academies Press.

IOM. 2009. *Adolescent health services: Missing opportunities*. Washington, DC: The National Academies Press.

Jeffries, W. L. T. 2009. A comparative analysis of homosexual behaviors, sex role preferences, and anal sex proclivities in Latino and non-Latino men. *Archives of Sexual Behavior* 38(5):765–778.

Jenness, V., and R. Grattet. 2001. *Making hate a crime: From social movement to law enforcement*. New York: Russell Sage.

Jillson, I. A. 2002. Opening closed doors: Improving access to quality health services for LGBT populations. *Clinical Research and Regulatory Affairs* 19(2–3):153–190.

Johnson, D. K. 2004. *The lavender scare: The Cold War persecution of gays and lesbians in the federal government*. Chicago: University of Chicago Press.

Johnson, J. A. 2008. *AIDS funding for federal government programs: FY1981–FY2009*. Washington, DC: Congressional Research Service.

Jordan, M. D. 1997. *The invention of sodomy in Christian theology*. Chicago, IL: University of Chicago Press.

Joslin, C. G., and S. P. Minter. 2009. *Lesbian, gay, bisexual and transgender family law*. Eagan, MN: Thomson West.

Katz, J. N. 1976. *Gay American history: Lesbians and gay men in the U.S.A.* New York: Thomas Y. Crowell Company.

Kenagy, G. P. 2005. Transgender health: Findings from two needs assessment studies in Philadelphia. *Health & Social Work* 30(1):19–26.

Kennamer, J. D., J. Honnold, J. Bradford, and M. Hendricks. 2000. Differences in disclosure of sexuality among African American and white gay/bisexual men: Implications for HIV/AIDS prevention. *AIDS Education & Prevention* 12(6):519–531.

Kimberly, J. A. 1997. I am transsexual—hear me roar. *Minnesota Law and Politics* 21–49.

Kinsey, A. C., W. B. Pomeroy, and C. E. Martin. 1948. *Sexual behaviour in the human male*. Philadelphia, PA: W.B. Saunders.

Kinsey, A. C., W. B. Pomeroy, C. E. Martin, and P. H. Gebhard. 1953. *Sexual behavior in the human female*. Philadelphia, PA: W.B. Saunders.

Klawitter, M. M., and V. Flatt. 1998. The effects of state and local antidiscrimination policies on earnings for gays and lesbians. *Journal of Policy Analysis and Management* 17(4):658–686.

Knudson, G., G. DeCuypere, and W. Bockting. 2010. Recommendations for revision of the DSM diagnoses of gender identity disorders: Consensus Statement of the World Professional Association for Transgender Health. *International Journal of Transgenderism* 12(2):115–118.

Kosciw, J. G., A. Diaz, and E. A. Greytak. 2008. *2007 National School Climate Survey: The experiences of lesbian, gay, bisexual and transgender youth in our nation's schools*. New York: The Gay, Lesbian and Straight Education Network.

Krafft-Ebing, R. V. 1900. *Psychopathia sexualis with especial reference to antipathetic sexual instinct: A medico-forensic study*. Chicago, IL: W.T. Keener.

Kramer, M. A., S. O. Aral, and J. W. Curran. 1980. Self-reported behavior patterns of patients attending a sexually transmitted disease clinic. *American Journal of Public Health* 70(9):997–1000.

Laub, D. R., and N. Fisk. 1974. A rehabilitation program for gender dysphoria syndrome by surgical sex change. *Plastic and Reconstructive Surgery* 53(4):388–403.

Laumann, E. O., J. H. Gagnon, R. T. Michael, and S. Michaels. 1994a. Homosexuality. In *The social organization of sexuality: Sexual practices in the United States*, edited by E. O. Laumann, J. H. Gagnon, R. T. Michael, and S. Michaels. Chicago, IL: The University of Chicago Press. Pp. 283.

Laumann, E. O., R. T. Michael, and J. H. Gagnon. 1994b. A political history of the national sex survey of adults. *Family Planning Perspectives* 26(1):34–38.

Leslie, C. 2000. Creating criminals: The injuries inflicted by "unenforced" sodomy laws. *Harvard Civil Rights-Civil Liberties Law Review* 35(1):103–181.

Levine, M. P. 1979. Gay ghetto. *Journal of Homosexuality* 4(4):363–377.

Levine, M. P. 1989. *The impact of AIDS on the homosexual clone community in New York City*. Paper presented at V International Conference on AIDS, Montreal.

Levine, M. P. 1998. *Gay macho: The life and death of the homosexual clone*. New York: New York University Press.

Levine, M. P., P. M. Nardi, P. M., and G. H. Gagnon. 1997. *In changing times: Gay men and lesbians encounter HIV/AIDS*. Chicago, IL: University of Chicago Press.

Levine, S. B., G. Brown, E. Coleman, P. Cohen-Kettenis, J. J. Hage, J. Van Maasdam, M. Petersen, F. Pfafflin, and L. C. Schaefer. 1998. The standards of care for gender identity disorders. *International Journal of Transgenderism* 2(2).

Lewin, E. 1998. *Recognizing ourselves*. New York: Columbia University Press.

Link, B. G., and J. C. Phelan. 2001. Conceptualizing stigma. *Annual Review of Sociology* 27(1):363.

Lurie, S. 2005. Identifying training needs of health-care providers related to treatment and care of transgendered patients: A qualitative needs assessment conducted in New England. In *Transgender health and HIV prevention: Needs assessment studies from transgender communities across the United States*, edited by W. Bockting and E. Avery. New York: The Haworth Medical Press. Pp. 93–112.

Lyles, C. M., L. S. Kay, N. Crepaz, J. H. Herbst, W. F. Passin, A. S. Kim, S. M. Rama, S. Thadiparthi, J. B. DeLuca, M. M. Mullins, and HIV/AIDS Prevention Research Synthesis Team. 2007. Best-evidence interventions: Findings from a systematic review of HIV behavioral interventions for US populations at high risk, 2000–2004. *American Journal of Public Health* 97(1):133–143.

Makadon, H. J. 2006. Improving health care for the lesbian and gay communities. *New England Journal of Medicine* 354(9):895–897.

Martin, J. L., L. Dean, M. Garcia, and W. Hall. 1989. The impact of AIDS on a gay community: Changes in sexual behavior, substance use, and mental health. *American Journal of Community Psychology* 17:269–293.

Mathews, W. C., M. W. Booth, J. D. Turner, and L. Kessler. 1986. Physicians' attitudes toward homosexuality—survey of a California county medical society. *Western Journal of Medicine* 144(1):106–110.

Max, L. W. 1935. Breaking up a homosexual fixation by the conditioned reaction technique: A case study. *Psychological Bulletin* 32:734.

McKirnan, D. J., J. P. Stokes, L. Doll, and R. G. Burzette. 1995. Bisexually active men: Social characteristics and sexual behavior. *Journal of Sex Research* 32(1):65–76.

McKirnan, D. J., P. A. Vanable, D. G. Ostrow, and B. Hope. 2001. Expectancies of sexual "escape" and sexual risk among drug and alcohol-involved gay and bisexual men. *Journal of Substance Abuse* 13(1–2):137–154.

Menninger, W. C. 1948. *Psychiatry in a troubled world*. New York: Macmillan.

Meyer, J. K., and D. J. Reter. 1979. Sex reassignment: Follow-up. *Archives of General Psychiatry* 36(9):1010–1015.

Meyerowitz, J. 1998. Sex change and the popular press: Historical notes on transsexuality in the United States, 1930-1955. *GLQ: A Journal of Lesbian and Gay Studies* 4(2):159–187.

Meyerowitz, J. 2002. *How sex changed: A history of transsexuality in the United States*. Cambridge, MA: Harvard University Press.

Meyerowitz, J. 2006. Transforming sex: Christine Jorgensen in the postwar U.S. (cover story). *OAH Magazine of History* 20(2):16–20.

Michaels, S. 1996. The prevalence of homosexuality in the United States. In *Textbook of homosexuality and mental health*, edited by R. P. Cabaj and T. S. Stein. Washington, DC: American Psychiatric Press. Pp. 43–63.

Miller, P. V. 1995. They said it couldn't be done: The National Health and Social Life Survey. *Public Opinion Quarterly* 59(3):404–419.

Minnesota Department of Human Rights. 1993. *How Minnesota protects gender identity*. http://www.humanrights.state.mn.us/education/articles/rs06_4gender_protections.html (accessed December 31, 2010).

Minton, H. L. 2002. *Departing from deviance: A history of homosexual rights and emancipatory science in America*. Chicago, IL: University of Chicago Press.

Money, J. 1985. *The destroying angel: Sex, fitness & food in the legacy of degeneracy theory, graham crackers, Kellogg's corn flakes & American health history*. Buffalo, NY: Prometheus Books.

Money, J. 1994. The concept of gender identity disorder in childhood and adolescence after 39 years. *Journal of Sex & Marital Therapy* 20(3):163–177.

Montgomery, J. P., E. D. Mokotoff, A. C. Gentry, and J. M. Blair. 2003. The extent of bisexual behaviour in HIV-infected men and implications for transmission to their female sex partners. *AIDS Care* 15(6):829–837.

Mosher, W. D., A. Chandra, and J. Jones. 2005. Sexual behavior and selected health measures: Men and women 15-44 years of age, United States, 2002. *Advanced Data* (362):1–55.

Murad, M. H., M. B. Elamin, M. Z. Garcia, R. J. Mullan, A. Murad, P. J. Erwin, and V. M. Montori. 2010. Hormonal therapy and sex reassignment: A systematic review and meta-analysis of quality of life and psychosocial outcomes. *Clinical Endocrinology* 72(2):214–231.

Nanda, S. 1990. *Neither man nor woman: The Hijras of India*. Belmont, CA: Wadsworth Publishing Company.

Nardi, P. M. 1997. Friends, lovers, and families: The impact of AIDS on gay and lesbian relationships. In *In changing times: Gay men and lesbians encounter HIV/AIDS*, edited by M. P. Levine, P. M. Nardi, and J. H. Gagnon. Chicago, IL: University of Chicago Press. Pp. 55–82.

NIH (National Institutes of Health). 1997. *Interventions to prevent HIV risk behaviors*. Bethesda, MD: NIH.

NIH. 2010. *FY 2011 trans-NIH AIDS research by-pass budget estimate*. Bethesda, MD: NIH.

NRC (National Research Council). 1989. *AIDS: Sexual behavior and intravenous drug use*. Washington, DC: National Academy Press.

NRC. 1990. *AIDS: The second decade*. Washington, DC: National Academy Press.

NRC. 1993. *The social impact of AIDS in the United States*. Washington, DC: National Academy Press.

NRC. 1995. *Assessing the social and behavioral science base for HIV/AIDS prevention and intervention: Workshop summary*. Washington, DC: National Academy Press.

Nuttbrock, L., W. Bockting, S. Hwahng, A. Rosenblum, M. Mason, M. Marci, and J. Becker. 2009. Gender identity affirmation among male-to-female transgender persons: A life course analysis across types of relationships and cultural/lifestyle factors. *Sexual and Relationship Therapy* 24(2):108–125.

O'Leary, A., H. H. Fisher, D. W. Purcell, P. S. Spikes, and C. A. Gomez. 2007. Correlates of risk patterns and race/ethnicity among HIV-positive men who have sex with men. *AIDS & Behavior* 11(5):706-715.

Obedin-Maliver, J., M. R. Lunn, E. Goldsmith, L. Stewart, E. Tran, W. White, M. Wells, S. Brenman, and G. Garcia. 2010, November 5-10. *Lesbian, gay, bisexual, and transgender-related content in medical curricula*. Paper presented at 2010 Annual Meeting of the Association of American Medical Colleges, Washington, DC.

Oliver, M. B., and J. S. Hyde. 1993. Gender differences in sexuality: A meta-analysis. *Psychological Bulletin* 114(1):29.

Operario, D., J. Burton, K. Underhill, and J. Sevelius. 2008. Men who have sex with transgender women: Challenges to category-based HIV prevention. *AIDS & Behavior* 12(1):18–26.

Patterson, C. J. 2000. Family relationships of lesbians and gay men. *Journal of Marriage & the Family* 62(4):1052–1069.

Patterson, C. J. 2009. Children of lesbian and gay parents: Psychology, law, and policy. *American Psychologist* 64(8):727–736.

Paul, J. P. 1983. The bisexual identity: An idea without social recognition. *Journal of Homosexuality* 9(2/3):45–63.

Pauly, I. B. 1968. The current status of the change of sex operation. *The Journal of Nervous and Mental Disease* 147(5):460–471.

Peplau, L. A., and L. D. Garnets. 2000. A new paradigm for understanding women's sexuality and sexual orientation. *Journal of Social Issues* 56(2):329–350.

Peterson, K. 2004. *50-state rundown on gay marriage laws*. http://www.stateline.org/live/ViewPage.action?siteNodeId=136&languageId=1&contentId=15576 (accessed December 13, 2010).

Peterson, J. L., and K. T. Jones. 2009. HIV prevention for black men who have sex with men in the United States. *American Journal of Public Health* 99(6):976–980.

Pettigrew, T. F., and L. R. Tropp. 2006. A meta-analytic test of intergroup contact theory. *Journal of Personality and Social Psychology* 90:751–783.

Pfäfflin, F., and A. Junge. 1992. *Sex reassignment. Thirty years of international follow-up studies after sex reassignment surgery: A comprehensive review, 1961–1991*. http://web.archive.org/web/20070503090247/http://www.symposion.com/ijt/pfaefflin/1000.htm (accessed November 17, 2010).

Pleck, J. H., L. O'Donnell, C. O'Donnell, and J. Snarey. 1988. AIDS-phobia, contact with AIDS, and AIDS-related job stress in hospital workers. *Journal of Homosexuality* 15(3–4):41–54.

Ponce, N. A., S. D. Cochran, J. C. Pizer, and V. M. Mays. 2010. The effects of unequal access to health insurance for same-sex couples in California. *Health Affairs* hlthaff.2009.0583.

Price, V., and M. L. Hsu. 1992. Public opinion about AIDS policies. The role of misinformation and attitudes toward homosexuals. *Public Opinion Quarterly* 56(1):29–52.

Pryor, J. B., G. D. Reeder, R. Vinacco, and T. L. Kott. 1989. The instrumental and symbolic functions of attitudes toward persons with AIDS. *Journal of Applied Social Psychology* 19(5):377–404.

Riggle, E. D., S. S. Rostosky, and S. G. Horne. 2010. Psychological distress, well-being, and legal recognition in same-sex couple relationships. *Journal of Family Psychology* 24(1):82–86.

Rosario, M., H. F. L. Meyer-Bahlburg, J. Hunter, T. M. Exner, M. Gwadz, and A. M. Keller. 1996. The psychosexual development of urban lesbian, gay, and bisexual youths. *Journal of Sex Research* 33(2):113–126.

Roscoe, W. 1991. *The Zuni man-woman.* Albuquerque, NM: The University of New Mexico Press.

Ross, M. W., E. J. Essien, M. L. Williams, and M. E. Fernandez-Esquer. 2003. Concordance between sexual behavior and sexual identity in street outreach samples of four racial/ethnic groups. *Sexually Transmitted Diseases* 30(2):110–113.

Rosser, B. R. S., J. M. Oakes, W. Bockting, and M. Miner. 2007. Capturing the social demographics of hidden sexual minorities: An Internet study of the transgender population in the United States. *Sexuality Research and Social Policy* 4(2):50–64.

Russell, S. T., T. J. Clarke, and J. Clary. 2009. Are teens "post-gay"? Contemporary adolescents' sexual identity labels. *Journal of Youth and Adolescence* 38(7):884–890.

Rust, P. C. 1995. *Bisexuality and the challenge to lesbian politics: Sex, loyalty, and revolution.* New York: New York University Press.

Schatz, B., and K. O'Hanlan. 1994. *Anti-gay discrimination in medicine: Results of a national survey of lesbian, gay, and bisexual physicians.* San Francisco, CA: American Association of Physicians for Human Rights/Gay Lesbian Medical Association.

Scherzer, T. 2000. Negotiating health care: The experiences of young lesbian and bisexual women. *Culture, Health & Sexuality* 2(1):87–102.

Sears, B. 2009. *Delaware—sexual orientation and gender identity law and documentation of discrimination.* Los Angeles, CA: The Williams Institute.

Sepkowitz, K. A. 2001. AIDS—the first 20 years. *New England Journal of Medicine* 344(23):1764–1772.

Sherrill, K., and A. Yang. 2000. From outlaws to in-laws: Anti-gay attitudes thaw. *The Public Perspective* 11(1):20–23.

Shilts, R. 1987. *And the band played on: Politics, people, and the AIDS epidemic.* New York: St. Martin's Press.

Smith, D. M., and W. C. Mathews. 2007. Physicians' attitudes toward homosexuality and HIV: Survey of a California medical society-revisited (PATHH-II). *Journal of Homosexuality* 52(3-4):1–9.

Stall, R., C. Hoff, T. J. Coates, J. Paul, K. A. Phillips, M. Ekstrand, S. Kegeles, J. Catania, D. Daigle, and R. Diaz. 1996. Decisions to get HIV tested and to accept antiretroviral therapies among gay/bisexual men: Implications for secondary prevention efforts. *Journal of Acquired Immune Deficiency Syndromes and Human Retrovirology* 11(2):151–160.

Steinberger, M. D. 2009. *Federal estate tax disadvantages for same-sex couples.* Los Angeles, CA: The Williams Institute.

Stewart, M. A. 1995. Effective physician-patient communication and health outcomes: A review. *Canadian Medical Association Journal* 152(9):1423–1433.

Stipp, H., and D. Kerr. 1989. Determinants of public opinion about AIDS. *The Public Opinion Quarterly* 53(1):98–106.

Stokes, J. P., and D. J. McKirnan. 1996. Female partners of bisexual men. *Psychology of Women Quarterly* 20(2):267.

Stoller, R. 1968. *Sex and gender: On the development of masculinity and femininity.* New York: Science House.

Stone, S. 1991. The empire strikes back: A posttranssexual manifesto. In *Body guards: The cultural politics of gender ambiguity*, edited by J. Epstein and K. Straub. New York: Routledge. Pp. 280–304.

Stryker, S., and J. Van Buskirk, eds. 1996. *Gay by the bay: A history of queer culture in the San Francisco Bay area.* San Francisco, CA: Chronicle Books.

Subcommittee on Investigations of the Senate Committee on Expenditures in the Executive Departments. 1950. *Interim report: Employment of homosexuals and other sex perverts in government.* Washington, DC: U.S. Senate, 81st Congress, 2nd Session.

Terman, L. M. 1948. Kinsey's sexual behavior in the human male; some comments and criticisms. *Psychological Bulletin* 45(5):443–459.

Tesar, C. M., and S. L. Rovi. 1998. Survey of curriculum on homosexuality/bisexuality in departments of family medicine. *Family Medicine* 30(4):283–287.

Thompson, G. N. 1949. Electroshock and other therapeutic considerations in sexual psychopathy. *Journal of Nervous and Mental Disease* 109(6):531–539.

Torian, L. V., H. A. Makki, I. B. Menzies, C. S. Murrill, and I. B. Weisfuse. 2002. HIV infection in men who have sex with men, New York City Department of Health sexually transmitted disease clinics, 1990-1999: A decade of serosurveillance finds that racial disparities and associations between HIV and gonorrhea persist. *Sexually Transmitted Diseases* 29(2):73–78.

Turner, C. F., M. A. Villarroel, J. R. Chromy, E. Eggleston, and S. M. Rogers. 2005. Same-gender sex among U.S. adults. *Public Opinion Quarterly* 69(3):439–462.

U.S. Census Bureau. 2006. *General demographic characteristics, 2006 population estimates, United States.* http://factfinder.census.gov/servlet/QTTable?-ds_name=PEP_2006_EST&-qr_name=PEP_2006_EST_DP1&-geo_id=01000US (accessed January 14, 2011).

Udis-Kessler, A. 1995. Identity/politics: A history of the bisexual movement. In *Bisexual politics: Theories, queries, and visions*, edited by N. Tucker. New York: Haworth Press.

Ulrichs, K. H. 1994a. *The riddle of "man-manly" love: The pioneering work on male homosexuality, Vol. 2.* Translated by M. A. Lombardi-Nash. Buffalo, NY: Prometheus Books.

Ulrichs, K. H. 1994b. *The riddle of man-manly love: The pioneering work on male homosexuality, Vol. 1.* Translated by M. A. Lombardi-Nash. Buffalo, NY: Prometheus Books.

Vestal, C. 2009. *Gay marriage legal in six states.* http://www.stateline.org/live/details/story?contentId=347390 (accessed December 13, 2010).

Voeller, B. 1990. Some uses and abuses of the Kinsey scale. In *Homosexuality/heterosexuality: Concepts of sexual orientation,* edited by D. P. McWhirter, S. A. Sanders, and J. M. Reinisch. New York: Oxford University Press. Pp. 32–38.

Wallick, M. M., K. M. Cambre, and M. H. Townsend. 1993. Freshman students' attitudes toward homosexuality. *Academic Medicine* 68(5):357–358.

Wallis, W. A. 1949. Statistics of the Kinsey Report. *Journal of the American Statistical Association* 44(248):463–484.

Warren, B. 1993. Transexuality, identity, and empowerment: A view from the front lines. *SIECUS Report* 14–16.

Weinberg, M. S., and C. J. Williams. 2010. Men sexually interested in transwomen (MSTW): Gendered embodiment and the construction of sexual desire. *Journal of Sex Research* 47(4):374–383.

Weinberg, M. S., C. J. Williams, and D. W. Pryor. 1994. *Dual attraction: Understanding bisexuality.* New York: Oxford University Press.

Weinrich, J. D., and F. Klein. 2002. Bi-gay, bi-straight, and bi-bi: Three bisexual subgroups identified using cluster analysis of the Klein sexual orientation grid. *Journal of Bisexuality* 2(4):109–139.

Wertheimer, D. M. 1992. Treatment and service interventions for lesbian and gay male crime victims. In *Hate crimes: Confronting violence against lesbians and gay men,* edited by G. M. Herek and K. T. Berrill. Newbury Park, CA: SAGE Publications. Pp. 227–240.

White, B. 1952. Ex-GI becomes blonde beauty: Operations transform Bronx youth. *New York Daily News*, December 1, 1952.

White, R., and A. M. Cunningham. 1991. *Ryan White, my own story*. New York: Dial Books.

Willging, C. E., M. Salvador, and M. Kano. 2006. Pragmatic help seeking: How sexual and gender minority groups access mental health care in a rural state. *Psychiatric Services* 57(6):871–874.

Williams, W. 1986. *The spirit and the flesh: Sexual diversity in American Indian culture*. Boston, MA: Beacon Press.

Worthington, R. L., and A. L. Reynolds. 2009. Within-group differences in sexual orientation and identity. *Journal of Counseling Psychology* 56(1):44–55.

WPATH (World Professional Association for Transgender Health). 1979. *Standards of care for gender identity disorders*. http://www.wpath.org/publications_standards.cfm (accessed February 23, 2011).

Xavier, J. M., M. Bobbin, B. Singer, and E. Budd. 2005. A needs assessment of transgendered people of color living in Washington, DC. *International Journal of Transgenderism* 8(2/3):31–47.

Yawger, N. S. 1940. Transvestism and other cross-sex manifestations. *The Journal of Nervous and Mental Disease* 92(1):41–48.

Zucker, K. J., and A. A. Lawrence. 2009. Epidemiology of gender identity disorder: Recommendations for the standards of care of the world professional association for transgender health. *International Journal of Transgenderism* 11(1):8–18.

Zucker, K. J., and R. L. Spitzer. 2005. Was the gender identity disorder of childhood diagnosis introduced into DSM-III as a backdoor maneuver to replace homosexuality? A historical note. *Journal of Sex & Marital Therapy* 31(1):31–42.

Zucker, K. J., S. J. Bradley, and M. Sanikhani. 1997. Sex differences in referral rates of children with gender identity disorder: Some hypotheses. *Journal of Abnormal Child Psychology* 25(3):217.

3

Conducting Research on the Health Status of LGBT Populations

As background for the review of existing research on sexual- and gender-minority health in Chapters 4, 5, and 6, the present chapter reviews research challenges associated with the study of LGBT populations, the research methods and data sources used in studying these populations, and best-practice principles for conducting research on the health of LGBT people. The final section presents a summary of key findings and research opportunities.

RESEARCH CHALLENGES

Three important challenges confront researchers attempting to gather valid and reliable data for describing LGBT populations and assessing their health: (1) operationally defining and measuring sexual orientation and gender identity, (2) overcoming the reluctance of some LGBT individuals to identify themselves to researchers, and (3) obtaining high-quality samples of relatively small populations. In addition, as emphasized in Chapter 1, although the acronym "LGBT" is applied to lesbians, gay men, bisexual men and women, and transgender people, these groups are distinct, and they also comprise subgroups based on race, ethnicity, geographic location, socioeconomic status, age, and other factors. These variations have implications for health research, including the need to obtain sample sizes that are large enough to understand differences among subgroups.

Operationally Defining and Measuring Sexual Orientation and Gender Identity

Many social, cultural, and behavioral phenomena pose measurement challenges to researchers. For example, multiple operational definitions have been used to assess education (Smith, 1995), political ideology (Knight, 1999), religiosity and religious fundamentalism (Hall et al., 2008; Kellstedt and Smidt, 1996), and race and ethnicity (NRC, 2004; Stephan and Stephan, 2000). Similarly, researchers who study LGBT populations face the challenges of defining sexual orientation and gender identity and developing procedures for operationalizing these constructs.

As explained in Chapter 2, sexual orientation is typically defined and measured in terms of three dimensions—behavior, attraction, and identity. Ideally, which of these dimensions is used in research is informed by a particular study's research goals. For example, a study of HIV risk in gay men would appropriately focus on sexual behavior, whereas a study of experiences with hate crimes or housing discrimination might focus on sexual orientation identity (Herek et al., 2010). Although most adults exhibit consistency across the three dimensions (e.g., they are exclusively heterosexual or homosexual in their sexual behavior, attractions, and self-labeled identity), some do not. Whether a particular study categorizes the latter individuals as lesbian, gay, homosexual, bisexual, heterosexual, or something else will depend on which specific dimension of sexual orientation is measured in that study. In a study that measures sexual orientation in terms of same-sex attraction or sexual behavior with a same-sex partner, for example, the sample may include some participants who do not label themselves as lesbian, gay, or bisexual.

Not only do studies vary in which facet of sexual orientation they measure, but they also can differ in how they define each of the three dimensions operationally. The current lack of standardized measures contributes to the variability of population estimates and can make comparisons across studies difficult. For example, if two studies defined sexual orientation operationally in terms of sexual behavior but used different time frames for screening participants (e.g., if one study used the criterion of any same-sex sexual behavior during the past 12 months, whereas the other used any same-sex sexual behavior since age 18), they might reach different conclusions about the target population. Moreover, the samples obtained for both studies would exclude individuals who were not sexually active during the specified time period even if they experienced same-sex attractions or self-identified as lesbian, gay, or bisexual. This variability in the criteria for operationally defining sexual orientation may produce what appear to be inconsistent findings across studies. Although it may appear obvious, it is important to make the point that researchers should carefully evaluate the appropriateness of their operational definition(s) of sexual orientation in light of the research question their study addresses and clearly explain their measurement procedures when reporting their results.

Similar definitional and measurement variability can be observed across studies of transgender populations. No uniformly accepted best measures of gender variance and gender nonconformity currently exist. One common approach is simply to ask participants whether they are transgender (e.g., Almeida et al., 2009), and, in some studies, whether they further self-identify as female-to-male or male-to-female. This question often follows immediately a question about sexual orientation. However, Buchting and colleagues (2008) have proposed combining the two questions by asking respondents: "Do you consider yourself to be one or more of the following: (a) Straight, (b) Gay or Lesbian, (c) Bisexual, (d) Transgender."

Because some gender-variant people do not use "transgender" to identify themselves, and some nontransgender individuals may not fully understand the term, simply asking individuals whether they are transgender may lead to underreporting and false positives (SMART, 2009). To address these concerns, some studies have provided respondents with a definition of "transgender" to increase the validity of responses (e.g., Massachusetts Department of Public Health, 2007). Conron and colleagues (2008) report the results of cognitive interviewing with a small nonprobability sample (n = 30) that included transgender youth. Using a question that combined biological sex and gender—asking respondents whether they were "female," "male," "transgender, female-to-male," "transgender, male-to-female," or "transgender (not exclusively male or female)"—they found that most transgender youth were able to choose a response option they felt was appropriate. However, the authors recommend further testing with slight modifications to the question (Conron et al., 2008). In addition, questions about gender transitioning have been included in several studies (Grant et al., 2010; Nemoto et al., 2005; Xavier et al., 2007).

Measuring the sexual orientation of transgender people poses special challenges because some respondents may answer questions about sexual orientation in terms of birth sex (their own or their partner's), whereas others may respond in terms of gender identity, and still others may find it difficult to answer in terms of a male–female dichotomy (e.g., Austin et al., 2007; Garofalo et al., 2006). Some HIV studies have included questions about the respondent's sexual behavior with males, females, transgender men, and transgender women.

While a number of effective measures of sexual orientation and gender identity have been developed, there remains a need for methodological research to determine the best ways to identify lesbian, gay, bisexual, and transgender people in health research. And while the most appropriate measures of sexual orientation and gender identity vary according to a particular study's research goals, standardization of measures in federally funded surveys would help improve knowledge about LGBT health because it would allow for the comparison and combination of data across studies.

Overcoming the Reluctance to Identify as LGBT to Researchers

Researchers studying sensitive topics must deal routinely with the reluctance of some participants to disclose accurate information about themselves. A topic may be sensitive because respondents perceive it as intruding on their privacy, because it raises concerns about the possible repercussions of disclosure to others, or because it triggers social desirability concerns (i.e., the desire to "look good" to others). Examples of sensitive topics include income, illegal activities, sexual practices, and membership in a stigmatized group. When confronted with a question about a sensitive topic, respondents may decline to answer or may intentionally give an inaccurate response. In some cases, respondents may decide not to participate in the study at all, thereby reducing the overall response rate and possibly making the sample less representative of the larger population. All of these outcomes have important implications for data quality (Lee, 1993; Tourangeau and Yan, 2007; Tourangeau et al., 2000).

Because they wish to avoid stigma and discrimination and are concerned about their privacy, some individuals are reluctant to disclose their membership in a sexual- or gender-minority group. McFarland and Caceres (2001), for example, describing the factors that lead to underestimation of HIV infection and risk among men who have sex with men, note that stigma and discrimination result in marginalization of these men, which in turn engenders suspicion toward government institutions, researchers, and service providers. Consequently, they argue, many men who have sex with men are unwilling or reluctant to participate in research studies.

As with research on other sensitive topics, challenges include nonparticipation and item nonresponse (which occurs when a respondent provides some of the requested information, but certain questions are left unanswered, or certain responses are inadequate for use). Nonparticipation and nonresponse threaten the generalizability of research data to the extent that those who do not disclose their sexual orientation or transgender identity accurately, or decline to participate altogether, differ in relevant ways from those who do disclose and participate.

A primary strategy to foster disclosure and reduce nonresponse is for researchers to establish a bond of trust with members of the target population. As with other populations, sexual and gender minorities are more likely to entrust researchers with sensitive information about themselves to the extent that they perceive the researchers to be professional, competent, and sensitive to their concerns about privacy (see, generally, Dillman et al., 2009). In addition, sexual- and gender-minority participants are more likely to trust researchers who evidence knowledge and sensitivity about their community and culture, characteristics commonly understood to be components of cultural competence.

As an adjunct to cultural competence, a number of techniques have been used to improve response rates to questions relating to sensitive topics. Modes of data collection that foster participants' sense of confidentiality or anonymity may yield higher rates of disclosure. For example, research participants may be more willing to disclose same-sex behavior or attractions when they provide their responses via computer rather than in a face-to-face interview (Villarroel et al., 2006; for a review, see Gribble et al., 1999). Collecting data in a private setting and taking steps to establish rapport before asking questions about sensitive topics may also increase respondents' willingness to disclose sensitive information. Variations in the wording and format of questions, as well as use of terminology that is familiar to the participant, have shown some success in eliciting responses (Catania et al., 1996).

Respondents may be more willing to disclose sensitive information about themselves when their participation is anonymous. If anonymity is not possible, understanding that their responses are confidential may increase the extent of participants' self-disclosure. Although it would not be required, a certificate of confidentiality from the National Institutes of Health (NIH) could be helpful in this regard (NIH, 2011).

Obtaining High-Quality Samples of Relatively Small Populations

As documented below and in subsequent chapters, numerous studies of sexual and gender minorities that have relied on nonprobability samples have yielded important information about and insights into LGBT life and health. If the goal of a study is to provide estimates that can be generalized with confidence to the entire LGBT population, however, the use of probability-based methods is necessary. Obtaining a probability sample of a relatively small population, such as a racial, ethnic, religious, sexual, or gender minority, requires considerably more resources than are required for sampling the population as a whole. This is the case because a large number of potential participants must be screened to obtain a sample of minority group members large enough for statistical analysis. Still more resources are required to collect samples that permit study of subpopulations within these groups, such as socioeconomic, age, and geographic groupings, and comparisons of respondents according to health-related characteristics.

Lacking such resources, relatively few studies designed specifically to examine LGBT individuals have been able to utilize large probability samples. There are, however, some exceptions. In the Urban Men's Health

Study, Catania and colleagues (2001) used a complex, two-stage sampling procedure in New York, Los Angeles, San Francisco, and Chicago to obtain a probability sample of men who have sex with men (n = 2,881) (see also Blair, 1999). Herek and colleagues used the Knowledge Networks panel to obtain a national probability sample of self-identified lesbian, gay, and bisexual adults (n = 662) (Herek, 2009; Herek et al., 2010). Knowledge Networks creates a panel using random-digit dialing to generate a national probability sample and administers an online survey to the panel. Internet access and the appropriate equipment are provided for those panel members who lack them.

Other researchers have conducted secondary analyses of health data collected from surveys of large national samples that included at least one question about respondents' sexual behavior (e.g., Cochran and Mays, 2000), sexual attraction (e.g., Consolacion et al., 2004), or sexual orientation identity (e.g., Cochran et al., 2003, 2007; Hatzenbuehler et al., 2009, 2010; Mays and Cochran, 2001; McLaughlin et al., 2010). The findings from many of these studies are discussed in later chapters of this report.

In addition to the data sets used in these secondary analyses, numerous other government and academic surveys routinely use large national probability samples to collect extensive data on the health of Americans. However, relatively few of these surveys have included measures of variables related to sexual orientation or gender identity. Consequently, many of the data sources widely used by health researchers do not yield insights into LGBT populations. As discussed later in this chapter, this situation can be remedied by routinely including measures of sexual orientation and gender identity in these surveys.

U.S. census data have also been used to obtain information about the LGBT population (Black et al., 2000; Gates, 2007; Rosenfeld, 2010), but the available information is limited. Since 1990, the census has reported data for same-sex partners who live in the same household, provided that one of them is designated the householder and both report their gender and relationship status on the household roster. However, an unknown number of same-sex partners who do not meet these conditions are not identified. Moreover, because census respondents' sexual orientation is not ascertained, lesbians, gay men, and bisexual adults who are not cohabiting in a same-sex relationship remain invisible in the data. Nor can transgender people be identified in census data. It should be noted that adding content to the census requires the approval of the U.S. Office of Management and Budget and, ultimately, the Congress.

A third approach to obtaining a national probability sample with a sufficient number of sexual- and gender-minority respondents involves combining data across studies. For ongoing studies that recruit new probability samples on a regular basis, it can be possible to combine sexual- and gender-minority respondents across years to produce a sample that is sufficiently large for analysis, provided that the studies all include comparable measures of key variables. Combining data from eight waves of the General Social Survey with data from the National Health and Social Life Survey (NHSLS) and the Chicago Health and Social Life Survey, for example, Wienke and Hill (2009) compared the well-being of partnered gay men and lesbians (n = 282) with that of single gay men and lesbians (n = 59) and married, cohabiting, dating, and single heterosexuals (sample sizes ranged from 614 to 6,734).

Combining data from multiple samples can be helpful in researching groups (like sexual and gender minorities) that represent a small domain in part of a larger survey. Because the numbers of these small groups often are not sufficiently large for analysis, combining data from multiple samples allows researchers to generate more accurate estimates. However, this method poses a variety of analytical challenges, and statistical methods for improving the estimation and analysis of small domains continue to be developed (Rao, 2003). These methods usually require assumptions about the statistical models employed and additional information related to the estimates the researcher wants to produce. For application to LGBT health research, these measures require the implementation and use of consistent measures to identify LGBT populations.

Raghunathan and colleagues (2007) provide an example that, although not involving LGBT populations, combines information from two data sets to improve the efficiency of county-level estimates. The authors use a statistical modeling approach—combining data from the Behavioral Risk Factor Surveillance System (BRFSS), a telephone survey conducted by state agencies, and the National Health Interview Survey (NHIS), an area probability sample surveyed through face-to-face interviews—to improve county-level prevalence rates of cancer risk factors that were developed from one survey alone. In a case study using data from the NHIS and the National Nursing Home Survey, Schenker and colleagues (2002) provide an example that illustrates the benefits of combining estimates from complementary surveys and discuss the analytic issues involved in doing so. Schenker and Raghunathan (2007) review four studies conducted by the National Center for Health Statistics that combine information from multiple surveys to improve various measures of health. In another example, Elliott and colleagues (2009) recognized that estimates of health care disparities in small racial/ethnic groups are often lacking in precision because of the small sample sizes involved. They developed an application of the Kalman filter (a recursive algorithm originally used in engineering applications; see Kalman, 1960) to use the available data more efficiently. By applying the Kalman filter to 8 years of data from the NHIS, they demonstrated how estimates for small populations could be improved by combining estimates from multiple years. In many cases, this method improved precision to an extent that would be similar to what would be achieved by doubling the sample size of the yearly data. When this method is used, the LGBT populations in the data sets that are statistically combined must be identified.

RESEARCH METHODS

In all empirical research, each component of the study design must be based on consideration of specific characteristics of the population being studied if effective methods for data gathering are to be developed. For LGBT studies, researchers must identify and select the most effective methods to compensate for the unique research challenges discussed above. This section reviews sampling issues, including the utility of probability and nonprobability sampling for generating study populations for LGBT health research, and describes quantitative and qualitative analytic methods used in LGBT research.

Research studies are designed to describe population characteristics, explore unanswered questions, or test hypotheses in order to validate previous findings or investigate areas that have not been fully explored. The applicability of research findings is directly related to the study design and the ability of the research team to identify an adequate sample for analysis. The manner in which the data collection methodology, the measurement design, and sample selection methods and subject recruitment are assembled into a coherent study design determines the relevance and generalizability of the findings.

Internal and external validity are important considerations for evaluating the relevance of LGBT research findings. Internal validity means that the measures of all variables are reliable, there is justification for linkages of relationships between independent and dependent variables, and other extraneous variables that are not logically associated are ruled out. External validity denotes the generalizability of study results beyond the specific study setting. These issues are discussed throughout the chapter.

Sampling Challenges

Careful sampling requires a precise definition of the target population of the study. The target population is the set of elements about which information is wanted and parameter estimates are required (OMB, 2001). For example, the target population could be all LGBT persons in the United States or in a state, community, or other geographic area. If members of the target population are selected into the sample by a random, unbiased mechanism such that every person in the target population has a known chance of being selected into the study, the resultant study sample can be used to draw inferences and generalize about the target population, and the sample thus generated is "representative" of the target population. After the desired target population for a study has been specified, selection of a sample requires identifying or developing a sampling frame or list of elements in the target population. The completeness of the sampling frame relative to the target population and the methods by which individual units are selected or identified for the study sample determine the limits of statistical inference and generalizability for the study results. Typically, researchers obtain study samples by selecting participants from a geographically defined population or a list of individuals who share a common characteristic, such as inclusion in a membership list of professionals. As discussed above, a variety of factors create challenges for generating samples that are representative of LGBT populations.

Recently, alternative models have been developed to identify a target population by starting with the community of interest and identifying samples that mirror characteristics of that community. A probability-based mechanism may or may not be used for selecting the study sample. For LGBT studies, both probability and nonprobability sampling methods have been used.

Probability Sampling

Probability sampling identifies a well-defined target population and sampling frame and uses a probabilistic method of selection to obtain a sample that is representative of the target population (Kalton, 2009). Although probability sampling can be expensive and the statistical methods employed can be complicated, the ensuing data lead to findings that can be generalized to the target population. If the target population were the nation's LGBT populations, the sampling frame had characteristics such that it was possible to identify all LGBT people, and a probability mechanism were defined that gave everyone in the sampling frame an equal chance of being selected, then the findings could be generalized to LGBT populations in the United States—within the scope of the study measures and subject to limitations of sampling and nonsampling error. Probability-based sampling methods rely on the assumption that a list of all eligible units of the target population can be constructed and that all units will have a known probability of selection.

Many approaches to obtaining a probability-based sample of a population ensure that valid inferences can be drawn. Kalton (2009) describes a number of such approaches for obtaining valid samples for subpopulations. When an existing sampling frame can identify whether an individual is a member of a subpopulation, drawing a sample of a specified size can be accomplished in a straightforward way. On the other hand, in many applications, individuals cannot be identified prior to selection of the sample. In such cases, major challenges exist within the probability-based framework. The approaches Kalton describes can be costly, as several require extensive screening to identify the subpopulation(s) of interest or can rely on a number of assumptions to permit valid inferences.

A common practice is to draw a large sample of the general population and then screen potential participants for inclusion in the study based on criteria that define the study's target population. With populations such as LGBT individuals, ineligible participants must be identified and eliminated from the study during the data collection process. This process is often implemented with a series of screening questions administered at the time the interviewer first contacts the household person. For example, the previously mentioned Urban Men's Health Study used telephone screening, along with other techniques, to obtain a probability sample of men who were gay or bisexual or reported having sex with men and who resided in New York, Chicago, Los Angeles, and San Francisco (Blair, 1999; Catania et al., 2001). To compare the yield of population-based methods for health needs assessments, Meyer and colleagues (2002) and Bowen and colleagues (2004) conducted paired surveys in Jamaica Plain, Massachusetts, using random-digit dialing and household area probability sampling in the same census tracts. Percentages of women who identified as sexual minorities were similar across the two sampling methods.

Another method, known as disproportionate stratification, can be effective for identifying small study populations. This method identifies areas where the target population is more highly concentrated and then samples a higher fraction of units within those areas. Disproportionate sampling may be an effective screening strategy for LGBT populations while ensuring that population estimates are possible. For example:

- Boehmer and colleagues (2010) used disproportionate sampling to select geographic units in census areas with a higher prevalence of lesbians and bisexual women.
- The 2003 California LGBT Tobacco Survey used disproportionate stratification in its random-digit dialing sampling design. The survey used areas identified by the 2000 decennial census as having a high proportion of unmarried same-sex partners and applied a weighting scheme to make the sample representative of the lesbian and gay population of California (Carpenter and Gates, 2008).
- Sampling using multiple sampling frames takes advantage of more than one partial listing of the target population to create a probability sample; care must be taken to remove duplicate listings of individuals when using this method. Aaron and colleagues (2003) used capture recapture methods with multiple lists and elimina-

tion of duplicates to estimate the lesbian population in Allegheny County, Pennsylvania.
- Network or multiplicity sampling uses sampled persons as proxy respondents for persons who are "linked" to them in a specific way, for example, as a family member (Sirken, 2004). An assumption required for this method is that all members of the linkage must know or be willing to report the rare population status of those linked to them (Kalton, 2009).

Probability sampling has seen limited use in the study of LGBT health. As explained above, the relatively small size of LGBT populations, the lack of research funding, and the sensitivity of questions relating to sexual behavior and gender expression have been barriers to effective probability sampling. Despite these challenges, some researchers have used probability samples for LGBT research. In addition to the examples cited earlier (Catania et al., 2001; Herek et al., 2010), the NHSLS, described in the previous chapter (Laumann et al., 1994), used multistage sampling to create a probability sample of U.S. households. Although sexual and gender minorities were not specifically targeted for the study, questions about sexual orientation were included in the survey instrument. Similarly, the federally sponsored National Survey of Family Growth (NSFG) does not specifically target LGBT people but does include questions about sexual orientation identity, behavior, and attraction (Mosher et al., 2005). A further example is the National Survey of Sexual Health and Behavior (Herbenick et al., 2010), which was based on data from an online survey using a cross-sectional sample of U.S. adolescents and adults participating in a Knowledge Networks panel and reported data on the sexual orientation and behavior of participants. Another study using a probability sample of self-identified lesbian, gay, and bisexual participants in the Knowledge Networks panel reported extensive data on demographic, psychological, and social commonalities and differences across sexual orientation subgroups (Herek et al., 2010). Illustrative examples of the study designs and sexual orientation measures used in some of these studies are shown in Box 3-1.

Sexual orientation and gender identity measures have also been included in state-level health surveys of probability-based samples, allowing some comparisons with heterosexual counterparts. The Massachusetts Department of Public Health has incorporated these measures into its Behavioral Risk Factor Surveillance System surveys since 2001 (transgender identity question added in 2010). Conron and colleagues (2010) aggregated 2001–2008 data from the Massachusetts Behavioral Risk Factor Surveillance System surveys to examine patterns in self-reported health by sexual orientation identity. The California Health Interview Survey (CHIS), conducted every 2 years, is a population-based random-digit dialing telephone

BOX 3-1
Examples of Probability Sample Studies with Sexual Orientation Measures

National Survey of Family Growth (NSFG)

Personal interviews were conducted with the civilian noninstitutionalized population to collect data on factors influencing pregnancy and women's health in the United States. Sexual orientation questions were asked and answered by audio computer-assisted self-interview.*

A national sample of adult men and women aged 15-44 was interviewed. In 2002, 12,751 interviews were completed (4,928 men and 7,643 women).

Asked of women and men:

Do you think of yourself as: Heterosexual, Homosexual, Bisexual, or something else?

Men were asked about oral and anal sex with another man; women were asked whether they had ever had any sexual experience of any kind with another female.

Men and women were asked whether they were sexually attracted to males, females, or both.

National Health and Social Life Survey (NHSLS)

The NHSLS was designed to be a representative and current survey of adult sexual behavior in the United States. The goals of the study were to describe the distribution of sexual practices in the general population and to examine the changes in these practices under current conditions. Multistage household sampling was used to develop an area probability sample of households; 3,432 adult respondents were included.

Identity Question: Do you think of yourself as . . . (1) heterosexual (2) homosexual (3) bisexual (4) or something else? (Specify) [Volunteered responses: (5) normal/straight (6) don't know]

Key Behavior Questions: Now thinking about the time since your 18th birthday and during the time before you started living with [(S)pouse/(C)ohabitant], how many people, including men and women, did you begin having sex with, even if only one time? (If one) Was this partner a male or female? (If two or more) How many of these partners were...(a) male? (b) female?

Now I would like to ask you some questions about sexual experiences with (SAME SEX AS R[espondent]; males/females) after you were 12 or 13, that is, after puberty. How old were you the first time that you had sex with a [male/female]?

Have your sex partners in the last {12 months/5 years} been . . . exclusively male; both male and female; female?

Now thinking about the time since your 18th birthday (including the recent past you've already told us about) how many {female/male} partners have you had sex with?

Attraction Questions: On a scale of 1 to 4, where 1 is very appealing and 4 is not at all appealing, how would you rate each of these activities: . . . (b) having sex with someone of the same sex.

FEMALE ONLY: In general, you are sexually attracted to (1) only men (2) mostly men (3) both men and women (4) mostly women (5) only women.

MALE ONLY: In general, you are sexually attracted to (1) only women (2) mostly women (3) both women and men (4) mostly men (5) only men.

---

* Audio computer-assisted self-interview allows participants to view a survey on a computer and hear a recorded voice stating the questions. Participants enter their answers on the computer.

survey of a sample of more than 42,000 California adults. In 2001 and 2003, the CHIS included questions about sexual orientation identity and gender (male/female) of recent sex partners. Data from the CHIS have been used to examine LGBT health issues, including obesity and body weight (Carpenter, 2003; Deputy and Boehmer, 2010) and smoking (Tang et al., 2004). The California Quality of Life Survey, a population-based health survey of adult Californians conducted in 2004–2005 (n = 2,272 adults), employed a sampling frame that was created from a subset of adults first interviewed in the 2003 CHIS and included an oversample of sexual-minority adults. These data have been used to examine physical health status, psychological distress, and mental health status in different sexual orientation groups (Cochran and Mays, 2007, 2009). These studies and others make use of survey vehicles designed for the general population to capture information about sexual and gender minorities that has localized relevance for priority setting at the state and substate levels. Illustrative examples of the study designs and sexual orientation measures of state-level probability-based studies are shown in Box 3-2.

The ability of researchers to draw valid inferences with probability samples hinges on three key elements: proper item design (i.e., questions that elicit the desired information from respondents), acceptably high completion rates,[1] and sufficiently large samples. Thus, for example, the NHSLS was carefully designed to elicit information on sensitive issues, and the

---

[1] Response rates for survey research in the United States have generally declined in recent decades. At the same time, some research suggests that, compared with studies with higher response rates, the data from studies with lower response rates are not necessarily of lower quality. Thus, in noting the desirability of a high response rate, the committee recognizes that the association between response rate and data quality is complex (see, e.g., Holbrook et al., 2008; Keeter et al., 2000).

BOX 3-2
Examples of State-Level Probability Sample Studies with LGBT Measures

Massachusetts Behavioral Risk Factor Surveillance System (MA BRFSS)

The Centers for Disease Control and Prevention's (CDC) Behavioral Risk Factor Surveillance System requires all states to implement annual random-digit dialing surveys of community-residing adults to gather information about a wide range of health-related behaviors. The primary focus has been on behaviors that are linked with the leading causes of death—heart disease, cancer, stroke, diabetes, and injury—and other important health issues. These behaviors include (1) not getting enough physical activity; (2) being overweight; (3) not using seatbelts; (4) using tobacco and alcohol; and (5) not getting preventive medical care that can save lives, such as flu shots, mammograms, Pap smears, and colorectal cancer screening tests. Although the inclusion of questions about sexual orientation and gender conformity is not required, six states and two urban areas have added such questions. Massachusetts has included sexual orientation measures since 2000 and began to include a transgender question in 2010.

Questions in 2009 MA BRFSS

Do you consider yourself to be: heterosexual or straight, homosexual or (if respondent is male read "gay"; else if female, read "lesbian"), bisexual or other?

Do you consider yourself to be transgender?

During the past 12 months, have you had sex with only males, only females, or with both males and females?

The last time you had sex, was your partner male or female?

California Health Interview Survey (CHIS)

The CHIS is the nation's largest state health survey. A random-digit dialing telephone survey conducted every 2 years on a wide range of health topics, the CHIS yields a detailed picture of the health and health care needs of California's large and diverse population. More than 50,000 Californians—including adults, teenagers, and children—are surveyed by the CHIS. Participants in the CHIS are chosen at random, and the sample is extensive enough to be statistically representative of California's diverse population. The CHIS is especially known for its difficult-to-find data on ethnic subgroups. CHIS telephone surveys are conducted in all 58 counties of California. The CHIS may also conduct oversampling and small-area estimates of certain counties, such as Los Angeles and San Diego. The CHIS is conducted by the University of California, Los Angeles (UCLA) Center for Health Policy Research in collaboration with the California Department of Public Health and Department of Health Care Services.

Questions in 2001

This next question is about your sexual orientation and I want to remind you again that your answers are completely confidential. Are you gay, (lesbian), or bisexual?

Questions in 2003

In the past 12 months, have your sexual partners been male, female, or both male and female?

Do you think of yourself as straight or heterosexual, as gay (lesbian) or homosexual, or bisexual (IF NEEDED SAY: "Straight or Heterosexual people have sex with, or are primarily attracted to people of the opposite sex, Gay (and Lesbian) people have sex with or are primarily attracted to people of the same sex, and Bisexuals have sex with or are attracted to people of both sexes.")

completion rate was close to 80 percent. The design team initially hoped to sample 20,000 individuals for the study, but, as noted in the previous chapter, received funding sufficient to complete a sample of only 3,432. The total number of women who reported nonheterosexual behavior, attraction, or identity was 150 (8.6 percent of the total), and the comparable number for men was 143 (10.1 percent). The consequence is that estimates for these key subpopulations are not precise; that is, they have relatively large margins of error. Thus, the sample is useful, but far from ideal, for the purpose of studying LGB populations, and it does not permit meaningful analysis of subgroups defined by race/ethnicity, age, and other sociodemographic characteristics. The study included no measure of gender identity.

Other studies have also examined subsets of sexual and gender minorities in LGBT populations using probability samples that were not designed to study those individuals. An example is the study of same-sex couples in the U.S. census. Questions were not designed for the purpose of learning about same-sex couples, but the data have well-known properties. The 2000 U.S. census long form (received by approximately one in every six households) is very large. Thus, inferences drawn have high internal validity for very specific population parameters and have high external validity for more general population parameters. See Box 3-3 for an example of an inference that can be drawn from U.S. census data.

Respondent-driven sampling. Respondent-driven sampling, a chain-referral method, attempts to create a sample based on the social networks of participants. It has been used to obtain samples of rare populations and is being used more frequently in LGBT research. Respondent-driven sampling is similar to snowball sampling, defined later in the chapter, in that a sample is developed by using referrals from initial recruiters (seeds) and existing participants, from which estimates can be made about the social patterns of the study population. Those estimates are then used in

BOX 3-3
Drawing an Inference from Census Data

Using data from the 2000 U.S. census, Black and colleagues (2007) were able to report on home ownership among cohabitating same-sex couples. They report that 60.4 percent of cohabiting male couples and 61.7 percent of cohabiting female couples owned their home (or were paying a mortgage). By comparison, 75.0 percent of heterosexual couples owned their home or were paying a mortgage. These data appear to be consistent with those from other sources (Herek et al., 2010).

conjunction with data generated by the study to draw inferences about the population as a whole.

Respondent-driven sampling is limited in that it relies on a number of assumptions to enable those generalizable inferences (Kalton, 2009). For example, a theory of respondent-driven sampling developed by Volz and Heckathorn (2008) assumes that respondents accurately report the number of people linked to them in their social network, that they recruit others at random, and that they have reciprocal relationships with those they recruit. Most probability sampling methods do not require such assumptions. As a result, respondent-driven sampling is applicable mainly in examining small domains where clear social networks exist (Kalton, 2009).

Reisner and colleagues (2010) examined data generated by 74 original seeds from four Massachusetts studies conducted between 2006 and 2008 that used respondent-driven sampling to reach high-risk men who have sex with men. Thirty-four percent of seeds generated two or more subsequent participants. Analysis of the data indicated that the size of a participant's social network was not significantly associated with generating additional participants. Social network size is frequently considered in developing a respondent-driven sample of men who have sex with men, but this study suggests that social network size alone is insufficient to identify participants who will recruit other participants. Factors such as the strength of social network ties and the frequency of a study-specific health behavior may be important as well.

Time-location sampling. This sampling approach uses multiple stages of data collection to increase the likelihood of developing a representative sample of the target study population, focusing on key social and behavioral characteristics. With community involvement, personal interviews with community leaders and gatekeepers and focus groups are included in an ethnographic assessment to generate an exhaustive list of sites where members of the target population congregate. A sample of the sites is drawn randomly for data collection, and specific time intervals are established when attendees are recruited for study participation. This method, described as *venue-based, time-space sampling*, has been used for studies of gay men and is one of the two methods employed by geographic sites within Centers for Disease Control and Prevention's (CDC's) National HIV Behavioral Surveillance program (Gallagher et al., 2007).

The strengths of this method include community participation that may result in a more comprehensive roster of potential sites than might otherwise be obtained and reduce suspicion among the study population. Its effectiveness depends on how well the ethnographic assessment is conducted, as well as the comprehensiveness and stability of sites in the initial roster (sampling frame). If probability-based methods are used at each stage of implementation, inferences about the target population are possible. The Community Intervention Trial for Youth relied on this method to evaluate the effects of a multicomponent, community-level intervention to promote safer sexual behavior among men aged 15–25 who reported having sex with other men. The researchers identified locations or venues attended by the target population and at what times (days and time periods). They selected venues and time periods randomly and then systematically sampled members of the target population at those venues during those time periods. The collection of data from these participants allowed the researchers to draw inferences about the target population (Muhib et al., 2001).

Nonprobability Sampling

For a variety of reasons, including a historical lack of the resources needed to obtain probability samples of sexual and gender minorities, the majority of studies addressing topics relevant to LGBT health have been conducted using nonprobability samples (Herek et al., 2010). A nonprobability sample is one in which all elements of the target population do not have a known, nonzero chance of being included. Consequently, in contrast to probability samples, the sampling error associated with population estimates derived from nonprobability samples cannot be computed, and the extent to which the sample represents the population from which it was drawn cannot be known. In the worst cases, nonprobability samples based on extremely biased assumptions about the population can lead to highly inaccurate conclusions, as when findings from studies of sexual minorities in prison and clinical samples were used during the early twentieth century to depict homosexuality as a pathological condition (Herek, 2010; Meyer and Wilson, 2009). In recent years, however, investigators have used increasingly sophisticated methods for obtaining large and diverse community-based nonprobability samples that have provided numerous insights into the health of sexual and gender minorities (Binson et al., 2007; Herek et al., 2010; Meyer and Wilson, 2009).

An array of strategies can be used to create nonprobability samples, the choice of which depends on the study's research question, data collection methods, and available resources. For example, venues such as bars and clubs, community events and organizations, Internet listservs, and social networks have often been used to recruit LGBT study participants (Herek et al., 2010; Meyer and Wilson, 2009). The samples drawn from such venues are often referred to as *convenience samples*, although Meyer and Wilson (2009) observe that "for most nonprobability sampling procedures, 'convenience' is a misnomer; nonprobability sampling requires very careful consideration, design, and execution" (p. 26). Whereas some researchers distinguish convenience samples from other types of nonprobability samples, the term often is used to refer generally to any type of nonprobability sample (Binson et al., 2007). Throughout this report, the committee attempts to characterize each study's sample using the terminology employed by the authors, with the consequence that *convenience sample* is used to refer to nonprobability samples obtained through a variety of techniques. Similarly, the terms *community sample* and *community-based study* are used in this report to refer to nonprobability samples that are obtained from a specific locale, such as a city or neighborhood. The various techniques for collecting nonprobability samples of LGBT populations, each of which can be understood as incorporating "some level of systematic exclusion and inclusion criteria" into the task of obtaining participants (Binson et al., 2007, p. 406), include *purposive sampling*, *quota sampling*, and *snowball sampling*.

Purposive sampling involves selecting specific sample elements because the researcher has reason to believe they are likely to provide the most useful information about the topic to be researched. For example, a study may select HIV-infected individuals to study behaviors that can lead to an increased risk of infection. Or researchers conducting a school-based study of LGBT adolescent health may include a particular high school in the sample because they believe it will yield especially valuable information. Diamond (1998), for example, recruited 89 nonheterosexual women aged 16–23 to participate in a longitudinal study of sexual identity development among young women. Participants were recruited at lesbian, gay, and bisexual community events; at classes on gender and sexuality issues at a large private university; and from lesbian, gay, and bisexual student groups at various universities. Of the 89 original participants, 79 participated in successive follow-up interviews over a period of 10 years. Two-thirds of those participants changed their sexual identity labels, and half did so two or more times (Diamond, 2008). This study made an important contribution to the discussion of sexual fluidity among women.

Quota sampling involves selecting a set number of participants to fill preestablished categories as a means of increasing the sample's variability or diversity (Binson et al., 2007). The researcher may begin by identifying the target number of sample elements in each of several categories (based on, for example, demographic groupings such as gender, race, and ethnicity). The goal may be to have a final sample in which the proportions of various key groups resemble the population from which the elements were drawn or to oversample relatively uncommon groups. Participants are then recruited to fill the various "quotas." Kennamer and colleagues (2000) used quota sampling to develop a sample of more than 700 Caucasian and African American men who have sex with men in order to conduct a statewide survey of HIV-related knowledge, behaviors, and attitudes in Virginia. The purpose of this study was to provide information for public health planning with respect to the HIV risks of men who have sex with men. As men who have sex with men were largely hidden, no population data were available from which to sample. Using population estimates from statewide and regional census information, the research team created target sizes for regional-level samples and used community and venue recruitment to identify participants. Additional efforts were made to recruit African American men who have sex with men, who tend to be underrepresented in surveys. The results assisted public health planners in determining regional allocations for HIV education and prevention programs. Although the study data would not be applicable to another state or geographic area, information about the methodology could be helpful to others considering such a study.

Snowball sampling relies on an initial core group of participants to recruit others into the study through their social networks; those individuals, in turn, may be asked to recruit additional participants from their networks, and so on (Binson et al., 2007; Meyer and Wilson, 2009). Sample development begins when members of the target population are identified and selected as seeds who will distribute surveys to or identify others who meet the study's inclusion criteria. This method was used prominently in early studies of sexual and gender minorities and continues to be applied when previously unstudied population groups are engaged in research. Like respondent-driven sampling (discussed earlier in this chapter), snowball sampling is a chain-referral method. Unlike respondent-driven sampling, however, it does not involve the use of probabilistic procedures for sample selection.

Many studies of sexual and gender minorities with large nonprobability samples have used a combination of the above and related methods (e.g., Bell and Weinberg, 1978; Herek et al., 1999; Kennamer et al., 2000; Martin and Dean, 1990; Meyer et al., 2008; Morris and Rothblum, 1999). The National Lesbian Health Care Survey (NLHCS), for example, conducted in 1984–1985, developed a national study of self-identified lesbians across the United States (Solarz, 1999). A community effort throughout, the NLHCS used snowball sampling strategies by organizing groups of women across the country to distribute questionnaires to other lesbians. Notices about the survey were posted across the country in bookstores and other locations frequented by lesbians, and a study phone number was provided for those with questions or concerns. Women who self-identified as lesbians were eligible to participate (Bradford et al., 1993). Each questionnaire was numbered and coded to enable identification of the initial and secondary distributors, such that the researchers could track them from the original distribution location through a second and sometimes third handler. NLHCS data were the earliest to suggest that lesbians experienced higher-than-expected rates of sexual abuse and stress-related behaviors, such as alcohol use and mental health support. The extent to which lesbians were open about their sexual orientation was associated with greater availability of mental health services (Bradford et al., 1993). At a time when lesbians were largely hidden, the study results provided a base of information from which successive studies employing more rigorous sampling methods could be developed.

Another creative use of sampling methods is demonstrated by studies that have recruited sexual- and gender-minority participants through various nonprobability methods and then asked sample members to recruit other participants who meet specific criteria. For example, Rothblum and Factor (2001) placed advertisements in local and national periodicals to recruit lesbians with at least one female sibling. Eligible women who responded to the ad were sent two copies of a questionnaire, one for them to complete and the other for their sister (the questionnaires did not indicate that the study focused on lesbians). Although the representativeness of the sample could not be known, the researchers were able to compare lesbians with heterosexual "controls" from highly similar backgrounds on multiple health variables. Similar sibling-control studies have been conducted with gay men and bisexuals (Rothblum et al., 2004) and with same-sex couples (Balsam et al., 2008).

The National Transgender Discrimination Survey (NTDS), conducted by the National Center for Transgender Equality and the National Gay and Lesbian Task Force, distributed online links to the survey site through a network of more than 800 transgender-serving and transgender-led advocacy and service organizations, support groups, listservs, and online social networks; 2,000 paper surveys were distributed to difficult-to-reach transgender and gender-nonconforming respondents, resulting in a total sample of 6,450 (Grant et al., 2010). Characteristics of this sample closely resembled a convergence of findings from a growing number of convenience studies conducted across the country, primarily in urban centers or at the state level. NTDS results pointed to critical concerns regarding unemployment and economic insecurity; employment challenges; and barriers to health care, such as a lack of health insurance and culturally competent providers (Grant et al., 2010).

Well-designed nonprobability studies have been useful for local and state-level health access initiatives. In 2004–2005, the Virginia Department of Health's HIV Prevention Community Planning Group drew on findings from existing nonprobability transgender health surveys to develop the Virginia Transgender Health Initiative Survey (THIS). This policy-oriented health assessment study used focus groups to determine constructs for a statewide survey of transgender people and to gather information about regional differences that could affect survey distribution methods. A questionnaire was developed and distributed through community outreach efforts at local and regional locations, including health care providers' offices, LGBT events, and balls and house parties. It was also made available on a protected website. At a time when few transgender studies had been conducted, and none at the state level, it was critical for community representatives, experienced scientists, and public health officials to craft an approach that would be useful and accepted in the context within which they were working (Xavier et al., 2005, 2007). Study results were used to increase awareness of transgender health needs, resulting in expanded services throughout the public health system.

Even though the extent to which their findings accurately characterize the entire LGBT population is unknown, studies based on nonprobability samples have yielded valuable information for expanding the field of LGBT research and addressing health service gaps (see Box 3-4). In addition to providing general descriptive data for LGBT populations and subgroups, they have served to demonstrate the existence of phenomena; to test experimentally the effectiveness of various behavioral and medical interventions; to assess relationships among study variables; to identify differences among groups; and in general, to provide insights into the health-related challenges faced by LGBT populations.

In addition, in the absence of data from probability samples, researchers often develop approximations of population patterns when the findings from multiple methodologically rigorous studies with different nonprobability samples converge. During the 1990s and 2000s, for example, multiple studies using nonprobability samples suggested that lesbians were considerably more likely than gay men to report that they were in a committed relationship at the time of data collection (e.g., Kurdek, 2004). Data from the U.S. census and a national probability sample confirmed this pattern (Gates, 2009; Herek et al., 2010).

Data Collection: Quantitative and Qualitative Methods

In addition to selecting an appropriate sampling frame, a major methodological concern is choosing quantitative or qualitative data collection methods.

Quantitative Data Collection Methods

Quantitative data collection methods include traditional survey research, Internet/online surveys, randomized controlled trials (RCTs), longitudinal cohort studies, and use of patient-level data.

Survey research. Survey methods are commonly used in LGBT health studies and are particularly valuable for determining population demographic

BOX 3-4
Examples of the Use of Nonprobability Sample Surveys to Address Transgender Health

National Transgender Discrimination Survey (NTDS)

The NTDS gathered data from self-identified transgender or gender-nonconforming individuals in the first national effort to document discrimination found in previous small sample studies and anecdotal reports. A 6-month data collection effort online and with paper surveys generated a total sample of 6,450, distributed across the United States in a pattern that closely replicated that of same-sex households in the 1990 and 2000 census data. Whites and persons of color were represented in proportions similar to those in the 2007 American Community Survey (ACS): whites made up 75.1 percent of the ACS sample and 76 percent of the NTDS sample; 24.9 percent of the ACS sample and 24 percent of the NTDS sample, respectively, were people of color (combined racial and ethnic categories).

Consistent with results of numerous earlier studies, 26 percent of respondents reported having lost their job because they were transgender or gender-nonconforming. Black (32 percent) and multiracial (37 percent) respondents were particularly hard hit. Harassment or mistreatment on the job was reported by 97 percent of respondents. Compared with the general population, 62 percent of whom had access to employer-based insurance, this was the case for only 40 percent of NTDS respondents. Other prominent concerns related to transgender status included poverty and housing instability.

Describing transgender identification:

"Transgender/gender non-conforming" describes people whose gender identity or expression is different, at least part of the time, from the sex assigned to them at birth.

1. Do you consider yourself to be transgender/gender non-conforming in any way? (Yes, No) **(If no, do NOT continue).**
2. What sex were you assigned at birth, on your original birth certificate? (Male, Female)
3. What is your primary gender identity today? (Male/Man; Female/Woman; Part time as one gender, part time as another; A gender not listed here, please specify________)
4. For each term listed, please select to what degree it applies to you. (Terms including transgender, transsexual, FTM [female to male], MTF [male to female], intersex, genderqueer, and others; degree measured as not at all, somewhat, strongly).

Virginia Transgender Health Initiative Survey

Focus groups were conducted to determine constructs for a statewide survey and to gather information about regional differences that could affect survey distribution methods. After considering various methods, including respondent-driven sampling, the statewide team decided on a mixed-method approach. A quantitative survey was available on a protected website and in paper-and-pencil form at local and regional locations, including health care providers' offices, LGBT events, balls and house parties, community outreach venues, and transgender listservs. A $15 incentive was provided for completed surveys, using blank money orders sent to a name and location stated by the respondent. A total of 367 self-identified transgender individuals completed the survey.

Across the state, 61 percent responded online, while 39 percent completed paper surveys. Characteristics of the subsamples differed by race/ethnicity, type of community (urban, suburban, rural), living alone or with others, home ownership, health insurance, and disclosure of gender nonconformity to primary care provider. If either method had been used alone, a distorted description of the target population would have resulted.

Describing transgender identification:

For the purposes of this study, we consider you to be transgender if you:

- Have lived or want to live full-time in a gender opposite your birth or physical sex;
- Have or want to physically modify your body to match who you feel you really are inside;
- Have or want to wear the clothing of the opposite sex, in order to express an inner, cross-gender identity.
- Using the above definition, answer each of the following questions:
- Do you consider yourself to be a transgender person?
- Are you 18 years old or older?
- Do you live in, or attend school in Virginia?

If you answered yes to all three of these questions, please continue.

and sociocultural characteristics, assessing knowledge and opinions, assessing behavior and behavioral intentions, and gathering data to describe the distribution of health conditions among populations and subpopulations. When a survey is used to gather information about a target population, it is important to assess the quality of the survey data to determine how useful the data are for drawing inferences about that population. Defined sources of error can and do affect all studies involving data collection, and researchers must strive to minimize their impact on the study results. A classification of error sources in data collection systems provides a framework with which analysts can evaluate the limitations of their data.

Survey data are subject to (1) the error inherent in examining a portion of the population (as opposed to surveying every individual of that population) and (2) errors that occur as a result of data collection procedures. Theoretically, the quality of survey data can be assessed in terms of total survey error, which is a combination of those two general sources of error, known as sampling error (when probability sampling methods are used) and nonsampling error (Biemer, 2010).

When a probability-based sample is used, sampling error refers to the error that occurs when the researcher draws a sample of a population using a probability-based mechanism rather than surveying every member of that population (Biemer, 2010; OMB, 2001). The sampling error associated with an estimate is a measure of the estimate's precision. Sampling error occurs by chance and is based on the random selection scheme used. The amount of expected variance due to sampling decreases as the size of the sample increases.

Nonsampling error refers to error that originates in the limitations of the data collection methods and procedures used in a study. This type of error may occur through a number of data collection mechanisms and is not easily quantified. Nonsampling error can be divided into four major categories: *coverage error*, *nonresponse error*, *measurement error*, and *processing error* (Biemer, 2010; OMB, 2001). See Table 3-1 for examples of these sources of error.

Coverage error occurs when members of the target population are excluded from the frame population, when members outside of the target

TABLE 3-1 Sources of Nonsampling Error in Survey Research

Coverage Error	Associated with differences between the target population (a set of characteristics defining the population to be studied) and the sampling frame population. Example: In a random-digit dialing survey that sampled only land lines, lesbians with cell phones but not land lines would be excluded.
Nonresponse Error	Occurs when study participants fail to answer survey questions, either completely or in part. Example: Questions relating to sexual behavior or gender nonconformity are at risk for nonresponse because of participants' reluctance to reveal information about such private behavior.
Measurement Error	Relates to the logistics of data collection—the influence of how and in what settings questions are asked—and comes from four major sources: the questionnaire, the data collection method, the interviewer (if used), and the respondent. Because of the unpredictable nature of these factors, measurement error has the most potential to reduce data quality. Example: When sensitive questions are included, a private setting can facilitate accurate reporting.
Processing Error	Occurs in the handling and use of information generated through the data collection process. Example: Quality control measures are not routinely carried out, or not all errors that are found are corrected.

population are included in the frame population, and when members of the target population are included in the sampling frame more than once (OMB, 2001). In the case of random-digit dialing telephone surveys, for example, low-income individuals and those living in rural areas may be disproportionately excluded as they are more likely to live in a household without a telephone line (Galesic et al., 2006). More recently, the exclusion of households without a land-line telephone has exacerbated the coverage error of random-digit dialing surveys and resulted in the need to include a cell phone sampling frame in addition to the land-line telephone sampling frame.

Nonresponse error takes two forms. *Unit nonresponse* refers to cases in which a particular sampling unit (e.g., household, person, business) fails to respond to all parts of a questionnaire. *Item nonresponse* occurs when a respondent provides some of the requested information but leaves certain questions unanswered or provides responses that are inadequate for use. Nonresponse errors can result in biased survey estimates if there are relevant differences between those who respond to a questionnaire (or a particular question) and those who do not. Item nonresponse can be a significant factor for questions that are sensitive in nature.

Measurement error relates to the processes involved in data collection. These processes include the questionnaire design, important for receiving an accurate response; question wording or survey instructions, which if ambiguous lead to incorrect responses; and the way the questionnaire is formatted. Data collection methods have been shown to influence responses; for example, in-person interviews may generate more accurate information than telephone interviews, while reporting on sensitive topics may be improved when the interview takes place over the telephone because of the anonymity of the interviewee. Interviewers vary in how they ask questions and administer the interview, affecting respondents' answers. Respondents can also be a source of error: they may differ in their comprehension of questions and in their memory of past events; they also may provide incorrect responses to questions, intentionally or unintentionally.

Processing error stems from inconsistencies or oversight during the handling and use of data generated through the data collection process (OMB, 2001). Such errors may take place when survey-generated data are transformed into published statistical results; when responses to survey questions are recorded incorrectly; and during data entry, when collected data are transferred to an electronic medium. More complicated errors can arise in applying mathematical algorithms to survey data in order to account for other sources of error; imputation, for example, is sometimes used for generating values to replace missing or erroneous data to facilitate analysis (Brick and Kalton, 1996; Kalton and Kasprzyk, 1986). Such errors can also occur in population-based studies in which probability-based sample designs apply sampling weights to account for frame coverage, nonresponse, and sampling probabilities. Errors can occur in modifying data in these ways and can affect the results of the study.

Internet/online surveys. Internet surveys have numerous advantages over traditional survey methods. Data collection and coding can be completed rapidly over a large geographic area at a relatively low cost per survey. Because they are computer-based, moreover, Internet surveys allow for many capabilities not readily available with paper questionnaires, such as complex skip patterns, branching, and the inclusion of video and audio (e.g., Dillman et al., 2009). And the anonymity and accessibility of the Internet make it a particularly good medium for conducting sexuality research among otherwise underrepresented populations (Mustanski, 2001).

As a data collection mode, the Internet can be used with probability or nonprobability samples, depending on the existence of a sampling frame and the use of a probability-based method of sample selection (Couper, 2000). In organizational settings where Internet access is provided, such as academic and health care institutions, a sampling frame of research participants may be generated using personnel records, and members of the sample may be asked to complete a questionnaire online. Other methods, such as random-digit dialing, can also be used to obtain a probability sample for an Internet study if Web access is ensured for all. For example, Knowledge Networks has used random-digit dialing techniques to recruit members of an ongoing panel; Internet access and equipment are provided to panel members who lack them.

Most Internet studies, however, rely on nonprobability samples recruited through a variety of means. Samples recruited from the Internet are subject to bias because those without Internet access are excluded. In addition, the characteristics of individuals more likely to respond to Internet surveys could differ from those of the general population (Rosser et al., 2009). For instance, Internet survey participants may be more likely than respondents recruited in other venues to seek sexual partners online (Bolding et al., 2007). On the other hand, given that survey data gathered online reflect only the individuals who complete the survey, the data obtained may not reflect the complete population of individuals using the Internet to seek sexual partners. Studies of Web surveys conducted among men who have sex with men in the United States and the United Kingdom also have found that certain variables were associated with higher rates of questionnaire noncompletion in online sexuality research; these variables include nonwhite ethnicity, less openness about sexual orientation, self-identifying as heterosexual or bisexual, and in some cases younger age (Evans et al., 2008; Ross et al., 2004).

As with other nonprobability sampling methods, Internet-based research with samples of volunteers faces some special challenges related to the internal validity of the data. Verifying participants' identities can be difficult, raising concern about the honesty of responses and the possibility of multiple submissions from the same respondent. (It should be noted that similar problems arise in studies that distribute paper questionnaires throughout a community, such as in newspapers or magazines.) A number of solutions have been proposed for this problem, including directly asking participants not to respond more than once, collecting e-mails or Internet Protocol (IP) addresses, and placing tracking "cookies" (units of information stored by a user's Web browser) on the computers of individuals who have responded (Reips, 2000). While these strategies offer partial solutions, the collection of e-mail and IP addresses and the use of cookies also raise other methodological and ethical concerns (Mustanski, 2001; Riggle et al., 2005).

With the increasingly widespread use of Internet and mobile phone technology, it is worth noting that emerging technologies can play a role not only in recruitment of study participants but also in many other areas of research (e.g., surveillance, interventions, clinical trials). Technologies such as text messaging, e-mailing, web-based interventions, and geographic information systems are currently being used to identify and reach at-risk populations and offer promising opportunities for future studies (for example, see Bowen et al., 2008; Carpenter et al., 2010; Geanuracos et al., 2007).

Randomized controlled trials. Since the work of Fisher (1925) was published, it has been recognized that randomization lends credibility to estimates of causal relationships that cannot be matched by other research designs. RCTs measure an intervention's effect by randomly assigning individuals (or groups of individuals) to an intervention group or a control group. In health research, RCTs typically are used to assess the efficacy of a behavioral or clinical intervention, such as in a drug trial, or participation in a risk reduction program.

While RCTs, at their best, can have high internal validity, concerns invariably remain with regard to external validity. For example, a particular AIDS treatment that is found to be effective in an RCT conducted with middle-aged white men in the United States might be less effective for other subpopulations. An RCT of the efficacy of a behavioral intervention to prevent the acquisition of HIV among men who have sex with men in six U.S. cities over a period of 48 months, known colloquially as the EXPLORE study, used HIV infection as the primary efficacy outcome (HIV Prevention Trials Network, 2011). In a sample of 4,295 participants, 39.7 percent reported having a history of childhood sexual abuse (Mimiaga et al., 2009). In prior studies, rates of childhood sexual abuse reported by men who have sex with men ranged from 11 to 37 percent (Brennan et al., 2007), while the rate of such abuse among the general population of men had been estimated at 5 to 10 percent (Finkelhor, 1994). Analysis of data from EXPLORE showed that childhood sexual abuse was highly associated with HIV risk-taking behavior and infection among men who have sex with men who participated in the study.

Even when RCTs are impractical, their basic principles can be extended to other research. Suppose one wants to evaluate the effectiveness of a community-based training program designed to help LGBT high school dropouts transition to employment. Researchers clearly cannot establish credible estimates of a "treatment" (completion of the program) by comparing subsequent employment rates of program participants with those of nonparticipants. After all, youths with high motivation are more likely to stay with the program than youths with low motivation. Researchers might, however, credibly estimate the impact of the program by comparing employment rates of youths in neighborhoods where the program was made available (the "treatment" group) with those of youths in otherwise comparable neighborhoods that had no training program (the "control" group). Such credible program evaluations are important for understanding the treatment effects of social programs, and can be conducted even when the "treatment" choice (the neighborhood choice for the employment program) is not randomly assigned as in a proper RCT.

CDC's Diffusion of Effective Behavioral Interventions (DEBI) program is an example of how RCTs are being used to determine the most effective of two or more community-level or population-specific interventions. DEBI is a national-level strategy to provide high-quality training and ongoing technical assistance to state and community HIV/sexually transmitted infection (STI) program staff for selected evidence-based prevention interventions that focus on HIV, other STIs, and viral hepatitis. Initiated in 1999, the program includes evidence-based behavioral interventions identified in the *2009 Compendium of Evidence-Based HIV Prevention Interventions*, which were evaluated through a series of efficacy reviews, many of which involved RCTs (CDC, 2009). Development of a model for adapting evidence-based prevention interventions to groups not initially studied was initiated in 2004 (McKleroy et al., 2006). This effort supported increased funding for adapting and culturally tailoring evidence-based prevention interventions initially designed for gay men for use with other affected population groups.

Implementation of the DEBI program has been critically reviewed in the context of dissemination and technology transfer. Dworkin and colleagues (2008) emphasize the importance of adaptation and dissemination as a participatory process and conclude that additional strategies are needed to ensure that the experience and assistance of community stakeholders are effectively represented.

The view of RCTs as the gold standard for measuring an intervention's impact extends across many diverse fields of human inquiry, such as education, welfare and employment, medicine, and psychology. The impact of an intervention can be evaluated only for populations participating in these trials. A letter to the *New England Journal of Medicine* suggests that sexual minorities have, at times, been explicitly excluded from such trials (Egleston et al., 2010). There is a need for peer-reviewed research to explore this topic further. The inclusion of LGBT participants in efficacy trials of treatment interventions would help ensure that the needs of these populations are reflected in such research.

Longitudinal cohort studies. Longitudinal studies are often used in psychology to study developmental trends across the life span, in education to assess the outcomes of education or training, in sociology to study life events throughout lifetimes or generations, or in economics to study behavioral and attitudinal data on social and economic issues (Kasprzyk et al., 1989; Lynn, 2009). Unlike cross-sectional studies, longitudinal studies track the same analytic units, usually individuals, over time. Therefore, analyses of unit-level changes and analyses of the frequency, timing, or duration of specific events are of interest. The advantages of such studies are discussed by Lynn (2009). By providing repeated measures on the same characteristics and following the same individuals, these studies can observe changes more accurately than other approaches and develop an extensive set of analytic variables. One of the challenges with longitudinal studies is recruitment. LGBT participants are members of small populations and not always easy to identify. Another challenge is retention of participants. Since studies span a number of years, participants may move, lose interest, or otherwise become unreachable by researchers. In medicine, the design is used to uncover predictors of certain diseases. Results from longitudinal cohort studies have made a significant contribution to the understanding of LGB health concerns. Longitudinal designs may be employed with probability as well as nonprobability samples, the data may be qualitative or quantitative, and data collection can utilize any of the methods discussed in this chapter. Some examples of longitudinal cohort studies are presented in Box 3-5.

The Nurses' Health Study (NHS), initiated in 1976 by Dr. Frank Speizer, and the NHSII, initiated in 1989 by Dr. Walter Willett, are the most definitive long-term epidemiological studies conducted to date on older women's health. Married registered nurses who were aged 30–55 in 1976, who lived in the 11 most populous states, and whose nursing boards agreed to supply the researchers with their members' names and addresses were enrolled in the cohort if they responded to the baseline questionnaire. Approximately 122,000 nurses out of the 170,000 who received the questionnaire by mail responded. For the NHSII, the target population was women aged 25–42 in 1989. Over time, additional questions have been added, most notably a dietary assessment added to the original NHS in 1980. Sexual orientation

BOX 3-5
Examples of Longitudinal Cohort Studies

Nurses' Health Study, initiated in 1976, and Nurses' Health Study II, initiated in 1989

Cohort participation has been carefully maintained. Deaths, usually reported by kin or by postal authorities, have been followed up. Where possible and permitted, in cases suggestive of cardiovascular disease or coronary heart disease, the follow-up has gone beyond examining death certificates to include gathering available documentation from autopsy reports and other records. Mortality follow-up has been better than 98 percent.

The core NHS sample consisted of 121,700 female registered nurses. In 1995, when sexual orientation was measured, the sample size was 90,823.

Sexual Orientation Question

Whether or not you are currently sexually active, what is your sexual orientation or identity? (Please choose one answer). Heterosexual; Lesbian, gay or homosexual; Bisexual; None of these; Prefer not to answer.

Growing Up Today Study (GUTS)

GUTS is a longitudinal cohort study of adolescent girls and boys living throughout the United States. Study participants were recruited in 1996 from among NHSII participants who reported having at least one child aged 9–14. Sexual orientation was captured in 1999 with a sample size of 16,800.

Sexual Orientation Question

Which one of the following best describes your feelings? (1) Completely heterosexual (attracted to persons of the opposite sex); (2) mostly heterosexual; (3) bisexual (equally attracted to men and women); (4) mostly homosexual; (5) completely homosexual (gay/lesbian, attracted to persons of the same sex); and (6) not sure.

SOURCES: Channing Laboratory, 2011a,b.

was not assessed at study initiation but was added in 1995 in the NHSII (Case et al., 2004).

Corliss and colleagues (2008) analyzed data on 13,450 youth who had been followed for 7 or more years in the Growing Up Today Study (GUTS), a community-based prospective cohort study of adolescent girls and boys living throughout the United States. The researchers recruited 16,882 study participants in 1996 by identifying NHSII participants who reported having at least one child aged 9–14. A mail survey was used to collect data.

Use of patient-level data. Coupled with national health care reform initiatives, the growing awareness of health disparities among LGBT people and concerns about barriers to their care have generated increased attention to the importance of identifying sexual and gender minorities within patient populations. Although the rationale for collecting these data may be increasingly clear, the best ways to do so have not yet been clarified. Organizations that focus on services for LGBT people typically utilize information about sexual orientation entered within the patient's record by the physician; the physician may not be required to check a category that will become part of the patient's enduring record. Thus, disclosure is kept between patient and provider, and it is up to the patient to determine whether to share this information.

Gathering data about patients' sexual orientation and/or transgender identity has been a subject of considerable interest for at least a decade. In 2001–2002, an urban federally qualified health center with a specific focus on serving the LGBT community conducted a pilot study in which patients were asked at intake to complete a voluntary one-page survey that included sexual orientation and gender identity questions (Barrett et al., 2002). Respondent demographics closely matched those of the overall patient population. Information from this study was valuable for organizational management and development, leading to an ongoing discussion about the best way to gather this information on a routine basis without endangering the privacy of patients. With recent improvements in database design and the expectation that such data will be increasingly important for tracking services to this population, the health center has added sexual orientation measures to the standard patient-registration form. To identify transgender patients, the question "Do you identify as a transgender person?" was added 3 years ago, following the legal sex question with "male" or "female" options.

In 2010, the Joint Commission on Accreditation of Healthcare Organizations published the monograph *Advancing Effective Communication, Cultural Competence, and Patient- and Family-Centered Care: A Roadmap for Hospitals* to help hospitals integrate the concepts of effective communication and patient-centered care into their organizations. This monograph contains several recommendations specific to LGBT populations and identifies best practices and processes that can assist hospitals in meeting the needs of their LGBT patients (The Joint Commission, 2010). New accreditation requirements have been developed to assess hospital performance, including two that are specifically relevant to the care of LGBT people: the first addressing the patient's right to choose his or her support individuals; the second addressing prohibition of discrimination, encompassing that based on personal characteristics, including "sexual orientation and gender identity or expression." These new requirements will count toward a hospital's accreditation decision beginning July 1, 2011 (The Joint Commission, 2011).

As awareness of the health-related needs of LGBT people grows, it is reasonable to expect that opportunities for collecting patient-level data for these populations will continue to emerge. For example, the Agency for Healthcare Research and Quality's Practice Based Research Networks could be one way to collect, analyze, and disseminate data on LGBT health. It is also reasonable to expect that the inclusion of sexual- and gender-minority measures in databases will increase. Consistent with the overall thrust of this chapter, it will be important for standard measures to be developed and implemented according to procedures that have been tested and found effective for ensuring privacy and confidentiality at all levels of health care organizations, including education of patients and their support persons, as well as providers and administrators. The use of patient-level data holds great potential for yielding a better understanding of the health status and health-related needs of LGBT people and how these differ from those of other groups in the U.S. population.

Qualitative Methods

Qualitative research methods can bring unique strengths to efforts to understand LGBT health. Examples of qualitative research include one-on-one interviews, focus groups, and cognitive interviews. Qualitative studies cannot be used to assess the characteristics of an entire population, but they do allow for a more detailed account of individuals' experiences as members of LGBT populations (Binson et al., 2007). These accounts can help a researcher identify hypotheses that could be tested in another study and lay the groundwork for future research. This type of perspective is ordinarily unavailable from sample survey based research. In addition, qualitative research can assist in developing quantitative instruments for studying LGBT populations. Qualitative methods are particularly well suited to

- explore understudied areas of inquiry, social settings, behaviors, or groups;
- build knowledge of key issues to refine elements of research designs for subsequent quantitative study;
- understand thought processes, experiences, or meanings of phenomena;
- describe and explain complexity and situational context in lived experience; and
- generate novel understandings and formulate explanations of patterns of human experience.

In studies of LGBT health, qualitative research is particularly relevant in exploring and explaining meanings of sexual- and gender-minority status in specific, local, and historical contexts of lived experience. Qualitative methods, both on their own and in conjunction with quantitative methods, are essential tools for understanding LGBT health.

One-on-one interviews. One-on-one interviews can vary from structured interviews typically used by survey researchers to less structured interviews that tend to be used by researchers who collect qualitative data (Bates et al., 2008). In structured interviews, the interviewer follows scripted questions, with no deviations from a set order; in semistructured interviews, the interviewer initiates questions and probes in response to the participant's answers, and questions may be reordered; and unstructured interviews are like a free-flowing conversation, with no set order to any questions—the interviewer may answer questions and make clarifications and may add or delete questions between interviews. Qualitative interviews are a good choice when the research aims are to shed new light on puzzling questions, identify variables and frame hypotheses for future survey research, and unravel complex events and events that evolve over time. Jarama and colleagues (2007) used random-digit dialing to recruit a probability sample of black women to undergo personal interviews conducted by trained peers. The purpose of the interviews was to have participants describe in their own words their perceptions of HIV risks and how they were taught to think and behave about sexuality. Each of the interviews was guided by a common set of questions; while some interviews followed the questions in order, others took their own direction, circling back to cover questions that were not answered in order. Peer interviewers had been carefully trained to ensure that study data would be collected from each interview and in a manner that respected the flow of each participant's thought process and mode of expression.

Focus groups. Focus groups are often used as one component of a mixed-methods study in which the goal is to obtain quantitative data on a target population. During the first phase of the Virginia Transgender Health Initiative Study, for example, regional focus groups were conducted to inform the content of a phase two statewide survey of self-identified transgender residents. A team of facilitators including transgender researchers and community advocates was trained to conduct the interviews, which were developed in conjunction with a statewide task force created to guide and support the initiative. Results were disseminated to communities, and after feedback was received from community and professional audiences, the focus group findings were used in developing a conceptual framework and questions for the phase two statewide quantitative survey (Xavier and Bradford, 2005; Xavier et al., 2007). In another example, the Census Bureau recently used 18 focus groups distributed over seven locations to help develop a better understanding of how gay and lesbian couples think about and report their relationship and marital status (Bates et al., 2010).

Cognitive interviews. The cognitive interviewing approach to evaluating sources of response error in survey questionnaires was developed during the 1980s through an interdisciplinary effort involving survey methodologists and psychologists (NRC, 1984). This approach has the following general features (Willis, 2004):

- It focuses mainly on the questionnaire rather than on the entire survey administration process. That is, the focus is on survey questions, as opposed to administrative procedures such as computer-administered personal interviewing, mentioned earlier in this chapter.
- It focuses explicitly on the cognitive processes that respondents use to answer survey questions. Therefore, covert processes that are normally hidden, as well as overt, observable processes, are studied.
- For the conduct of the cognitive interview, volunteer subjects are recruited and are interviewed either in a laboratory environment or in some other private location. (In this application, the term "subject" refers to an individual who is tested through a cognitive interviewing procedure, and "respondent" defines someone who is interviewed in a fielded survey.)
- The recruitment of subjects targets persons with specific characteristics of interest (for example, the elderly, those who have used illicit drugs in the past 12 months, teenagers who have used chewing tobacco).

Clark and colleagues (2005) used cognitive interviews of a sample of 40 women to evaluate survey questions designed to measure sexual orientation and gender expression. Results of the interviews helped identify questions that may have been confusing to respondents and specific terms that needed additional clarification. Cognitive interviews are currently being used by the National Center for Health Statistics to develop and test measures for including LGBT questions on federal surveys.

DATA SOURCES

The relative lack of population-based data presents the greatest challenge to describing the health status and health-related needs of LGBT people. Although recommendations have been made for some time about collecting data on sexual and gender minorities (Westoff, 1973), only a limited number of publicly funded probability sample studies include measures of sexual orientation, and none measure gender identity. In 2000, Healthy People, the nation's health promotion and disease prevention program (HHS, 2000), included people defined by sexual orientation as a population group experiencing health disparities. At that time, only two federally funded data sets (the National Health and Nutrition Examination Survey and the National Household Survey on Drug Abuse) included measures of sexual orientation. Secondary analysis of these data sets was prominent in calling attention to significant differences in reported rates of mental health and substance abuse between LGB people and heterosexuals (Cochran and Mays, 2000; Cochran et al., 2000, 2004). In the past decade, sexual orientation measures have been included in additional federally funded surveys. Recurring federally funded surveys that include LGB measures are listed and their properties described in Table 3-2.

Not surprisingly, the limited number of studies that have used probability samples and rigorous methods and focused on sexual and gender minorities has contributed to the lack of an extensive published literature on LGBT health. A Medline database review of literature published during 1980–1999 found that only 0.1 percent of articles over this 20-year period had focused on LGBT people or same-sex behavior or attraction (Boehmer, 2002). This percentage is based on the contents of the entire Medline database; the study identified 3,777 articles that met its inclusion criteria. Most of these articles were focused on HIV/AIDS, substance abuse, and mental health to the exclusion of other topics (Gay and Lesbian Medical Association and LGBT Health Experts, 2010). Since 2008, the Center for Population Research in LGBT Health has maintained a publicly accessible bibliography of published literature on LGBT health, including journal articles, books, and reports published since 1990 and indexed in PubMed. As of this writing, the programmed search has yielded 12,928 journal articles. A chart of the number of publications meeting search criteria suggests an increase in annual scholarly output in LGBT health research, particularly in the last decade; when charted as a ratio of all PubMed[2] journal articles, however, growth in scholarly output in LGBT health appears to have been slower and more uneven (Figure 3-1).

BEST-PRACTICE PRINCIPLES ASSOCIATED WITH SAMPLE SURVEY AND RESEARCH STUDIES

Scientific and methodological challenges exist in the design and implementation of most sample surveys and research studies. This is

[2] These patterns may not reflect all published scientific research on sexual- and gender-minority populations insofar as PubMed and Medline do not index all social and behavioral science journals.

TABLE 3-2 Recurring Federally Funded Surveys That Include LGB Measures

Name/Study Website	Sexual Orientation/ Gender Identity Measures	Periodicity	Sample Size	Data Collection Mode	Topic Areas
American Community Survey census.gov/acs	Same-sex partner household	Annually	2009: 2,064,000 households	Mail (SAQ[a]), telephone (CATI[b]), and personal visits (CAPI[c])	Vary from year to year; for more information about subjects covered: census.gov/acs/www/data_documentation/pums_documentation/
Behavioral Risk Factor Surveillance System[d] cdc.gov/brfss/	Varies by state; states have included identity, behavior, transgender identity	Annually	Varies by state	Telephone (CATI)	Health risk behaviors, preventive health practices, and health care access related primarily to chronic disease and injury
Current Population Survey census.gov/cps/	Same-sex partner household	Monthly	2010: 97,263 households	Personal visits (CAPI), telephone (CATI)	Work status, earnings, hours of work, and other employment indicators; supplemental questions on diverse topics such as expectation of family size, tobacco use, computer use, and voting patterns are sometimes added
General Social Survey norc.uchicago.edu/GSS+Website/	Identity, behavior, same-sex partner household	Annually; sexual orientation only in 2008	2008: 2,000 individuals	Personal visits (CAPI)	Includes a standard "core" of demographic, behavioral, and attitudinal questions, plus topics of special interest
National Epidemiologic Survey of Alcohol and Related Conditions pubs.niaaa.nih.gov/publications/arh29-2/74-78.htm	Identity, behavior, attraction	Wave 1: 2001–2002; Wave 2: 2004–2005 (longitudinal)	43,100 individuals	Personal visits (CAPI)	Alcohol and drug use; alcohol and drug abuse and dependence; associated psychiatric and other medical comorbidities

National Health and Nutrition Examination Survey cdc.gov/nchs/nhanes.htm	Identity, behavior	Annually	2007–2008: 10,149 individuals	Personal visits (CAPI), health examination	Disease and chronic conditions, health risk factors, smoking, alcohol consumption, sexual practices, drug use, physical fitness and activity, weight, dietary intake, and reproductive health
National Health Interview Survey cdc.gov/nchs/nhis.htm	Same-sex partner household	Annually	2009: 33,856 households	Personal visits (CAPI)	Demographics, health status and limitations, injuries, health care access and utilization, health behaviors, health insurance, and income and assets
National Household Survey on Drug Abuse oas.samhsa.gov/nsduh.htm	Behavior	Annually; sexual orientation assessed only in 1996	1996: 18,300 individuals	Personal visits (SAQ until 1999, ACASI[e] thereafter)	Use of illicit drugs, alcohol, and tobacco; substance abuse treatment history; illegal activities; mental health; access to care; driving behavior; and demographics
National Survey of Family Growth cdc.gov/nchs/nsfg.htm	Identity, behavior, attraction	7 cycles collected since 1973; only the 2002 cycle included sexual orientation	2002: 12,600 individuals	Personal visits (including CAPI, ACASI, and interviewer observations)	Schooling, family background, marriage and divorce, fertility, family planning, sex education, sexual history, sexually transmitted diseases (STDs)/AIDS, and demographics
United States Census census.gov	Same-sex partner household	Decennially	2000: 115.9 million households	Mail (SAQ), personal visit follow-up	Age, sex, race, household relationships, tenure; the American Community Survey replaced the "long form" on the census

continued

TABLE 3-2 Continued

Name/Study Website	Sexual Orientation/ Gender Identity Measures	Periodicity	Sample Size	Data Collection Mode	Topic Areas
Youth Risk Behavior Surveillance System[f] cdc.gov/HealthyYouth/yrbs/	Varies; states have included identity, behavior, attraction, transgender identity	Biennially	Varies	SAQ	Adolescent health risk behaviors, including behaviors that contribute to unintentional injuries and violence, tobacco use, alcohol and other drug use, sexual behaviors that contribute to unintended pregnancy and STDs, unhealthy dietary behaviors, and physical inactivity

NOTES:
[a] SAQ = self-administered questionnaire.
[b] CATI = computer-assisted telephone interview.
[c] CAPI = computer-assisted personal interview.
[d] Locations that have historically measured sexual-minority status include Arkansas, California, Colorado, Connecticut, Georgia (Fulton County), Massachusetts, New York City, North Dakota, Ohio, Oregon, San Francisco, Vermont, Washington, and Wisconsin.
[e] ACASI = audio computer-assisted self-interview.
[f] Locations that have historically measured sexual-minority status include Boston, Chicago, Connecticut, Delaware, Hawaii, Illinois, Los Angeles, Maine, Massachusetts, Milwaukee, North Dakota, New Hampshire, New York City, Rhode Island, San Diego, San Francisco, Seattle, Vermont, Washington (DC), and Wisconsin. The Oregon Healthy Teens Survey and Minnesota Student Survey are similar surveys.

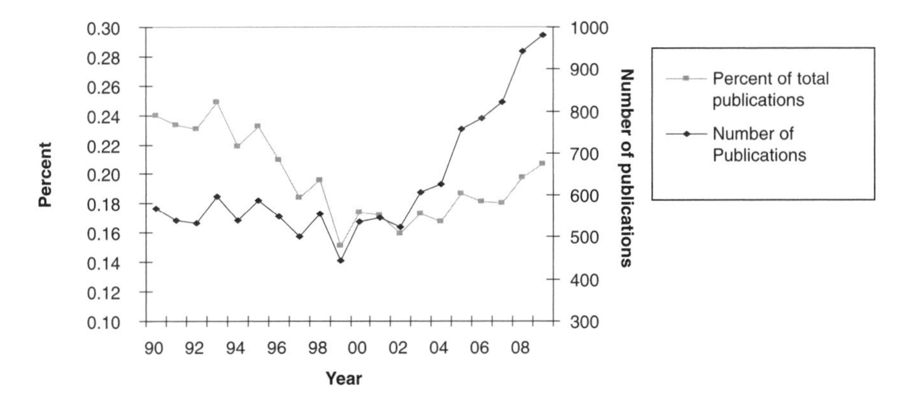

FIGURE 3-1 Publications in LGBT health indexed in PubMed.
SOURCE: Center for Population Research in LGBT Health (http://www.icpsr.umich.edu/icpsrweb/FENWAY/findings/index.jsp).

particularly true of studies of relatively small populations on topics construed by the respondent to be of a sensitive nature. Health research studies of LGBT populations are often viewed in this way. Methodological challenges, however, can be overcome when careful attention is paid to scientific rigor and respectful involvement of individuals who represent the target population. Scientific rigor includes incorporating and monitoring culturally competent study designs, such as the use of appropriate measures to identify participants and implementation processes adapted to unique characteristics of the study population. Respectful involvement of the study population, in this case LGBT people, refers to the involvement of individuals and community representatives in the research process, from decisions about the study purpose and methods, to ongoing consultation and data gathering, to dissemination of results (Minkler and Wallerstein, 2002).

The use of professionally accepted best practices that ensure scientific rigor in the design, conduct, and analysis of sample surveys and research studies is critical to the general acceptance of the results. As noted earlier in this report, the lack of demographic, economic, and health-related information on LGBT populations and their racial/ethnic subgroups makes it difficult to discuss health policy options intelligently. Identifying and adopting best practices for a sample survey or research study helps ensure that discussions about health policy do not become confounded with discussions about the nature of the data and the sample survey/study used to collect the data. Several textbooks concerned with methods for conducting sample surveys provide good examples of the issues a researcher must address to conduct such a survey with scientific rigor (Biemer and Lyberg,

2003; Czaja and Blair, 1996; Groves et al., 2004). These sources describe the key elements of sample surveys and design and implementation issues, sources of error, and ways of minimizing and controlling error. The American Association for Public Opinion Research (AAPOR), an association of survey methodologists, statisticians, and social science researchers, has identified best practices for its members to follow on its website (AAPOR, 2010). These practices, identified by a committee of survey methodologists, represent a valuable and thoughtful way to approach collecting information by means of a rigorous sample survey.

The principles relied upon to design and conduct scientifically rigorous sample surveys are critical as well to successful research studies, particularly community-based participatory research studies, in which scientific rigor and strong research community collaboration are critical. The contributions of such studies to research on LGBT and other minority and underserved populations have been acknowledged by numerous public agencies and private organizations (Buchting et al., 2008; SMART, 2009), including institutes within NIH that have allocated funding for this type of study with certain populations, including those defined by sexual orientation. For example, reviewing approaches to HIV surveillance, McFarland and Caceres (2001) emphasize the importance of ongoing formative research and alliances with key organizations and actors in communities of men who have sex with men to develop study measures and guide appropriate use of data.

Listed below are some general principles related to best practices for sample surveys and research studies. The intent is not to identify individual design decisions, such as the data collection mode, the reference period, or an appropriate sample or study design, as "best" since individual study goals, circumstances, and available resources will vary.

- Identify specific goals for the study—for example, to develop estimates with which to describe a population or certain relationships, or to study the effects of experimental treatments. If a community-based study, develop partnerships and collaborate actively on the study goals with representatives of the study population within the community.
- Identify and describe the study's target population.
- Identify or develop a sampling frame from which to select members of the target population for the study.
- Determine and implement an appropriate method for drawing a probability-based sample to represent the target population or a recruitment strategy for the study population in a nonprobability design.

- If the study will analyze the effects of a program or intervention, identify and implement an appropriate experimental design.
- Determine a data collection mode consistent with the nature of the study.
- Identify and develop the concepts to be measured, and, as appropriate, use cognitive interviews, focus groups, or expert panels to review draft questionnaires; for community-based research, developing a thorough knowledge of the local community, its culture, and its health-related needs is particularly important.
- If appropriate for the study, identify sponsors, respected community leaders, or interested parties who support the study, and develop materials for the respondents that enable them to understand the reasons for the study, its potential benefits, and the need for their participation.
- Pretest questionnaires on a sample of the study population.
- If interviewers are being used to conduct the study, ensure that they receive sufficient training.
- Develop procedures to maximize the data collection response rate, subject to availability of funds.
- Develop and implement data processing and editing specifications to ensure that data are consistent and outlier data are minimized.
- Develop and implement appropriate statistical methods to weight the data (if a probability sample) and to calculate variances for sample estimates.
- Use statistical methods appropriate to the analysis.
- Provide sufficient documentation on the survey, data collection, and statistical methods used (including response rates) to permit an independent reviewer to assess the quality of the data collection and analysis.
- Ensure the privacy and confidentiality of survey responses.
- Disseminate the results of the survey or research study widely, and in the case of community-based research, do so through meetings and presentations to the community and through partnership communication channels.

SUMMARY OF KEY FINDINGS AND RESEARCH OPPORTUNITIES

Findings

This chapter has addressed the challenges as well as the methodological issues associated with conducting research on LGBT populations and subpopulations. This discussion should provide a foundation for the review of the state of knowledge regarding LGBT health across the life course in the following chapters. Key findings presented in this chapter are listed below.

Research Challenges

A number of challenges are associated with conducting research on the health status of LGBT populations:

- The lack of standardized measures in federally funded surveys—Sexual orientation and gender nonconformity are multifaceted concepts, and a variety of methods have been used to identify them for research purposes.
- Small populations—Since LGBT populations represent a relatively small proportion of the U.S. population, creating a sufficiently large sample to provide reliable estimates of these populations requires considerable resources. A further challenge arises in obtaining a probability sample of LGBT participants that includes sufficient numbers of representatives of population subgroups, such as racial- and ethnic-minority individuals, to permit meaningful analyses.
- Barriers to identification as LGBT—Because of concerns about stigma and privacy, individuals may be reluctant to answer research questions about their same-sex sexual behavior or gender nonconformity.

Sampling

- Probability sampling allows findings based on the data to be generalized to the study's target population with a known margin of error. Some methods make it possible to improve the precision of estimates for small populations by combining two or more data sets. Although probability sampling is not used frequently in the study of LGBT health, some studies have obtained probability samples of LGBT participants, while others (such as federal health surveys and the U.S. census) have examined subsets of sexual and gender minorities using probability samples not designed specifically to study those individuals.
- The majority of studies addressing topics relevant to LGBT health have been conducted using nonprobability samples. Even though the extent to which their findings accurately characterize the entirety of LGBT populations is unknown, studies based on nonprobability samples have yielded valuable information. In addition to providing general descriptive data for LGBT populations and subgroups, they have served to demonstrate the existence of certain phenomena, to test experimentally the effectiveness of various be-

havioral and medical interventions, to assess relationships among variables, to identify differences among groups, and in general, to provide insights into the health-related challenges faced by LGBT people. In addition, in the absence of data from probability samples, researchers often develop approximations of population patterns when the findings from multiple methodologically rigorous studies with different nonprobability samples converge.

Methods

- Quantitative data can be collected through a variety of methods, including survey research, RCTs, longitudinal cohort studies, and patient-level data. Of these methods, survey research is particularly common in LGBT health studies, especially as a way to generate demographic data. There are four main sources of error associated with survey research: coverage, nonresponse, measurement, and processing errors (Table 3-1).
- RCTs measure an intervention's effects by randomly assigning individuals (or groups of individuals) to an intervention or control group. While these trials are considered the gold standard for measuring an intervention's impact, the results may not be generalizable to groups other than those who participated in the trials.
- Longitudinal cohort studies track individuals over time, allowing researchers to observe changes more accurately than is otherwise possible. The NHS and NHSII are examples of longitudinal cohort studies that have made significant contributions to understanding health.
- Research on LGBT populations using patient-level data is evolving, with discussion ongoing about how to collect sexual orientation and gender identity data in databases.
- Qualitative data can be collected through a variety of methods, including one-on-one interviews, focus groups, and cognitive interviews. These methods can be especially useful for generating hypotheses and laying the groundwork for future research.

Research Opportunities

A number of issues related to studying the health status of LGBT populations would benefit from additional research:

- Federally funded surveys do not measure sexual orientation or gender expression in a uniform and consistent way, limiting the ability to compare data across these surveys.

- The majority of LGBT literature relies exclusively on LGBT respondents, making it difficult to compare characteristics of LGBT populations with those of the entire U.S. population.
- Research into better methods for recruiting and retaining participants in longitudinal studies is needed.
- While valuable research has been conducted despite the limitations of available data sources, more national data must be collected if we are to fully understand the health needs of U.S. LGBT populations.
- Even if LGBT populations can be identified through national surveys, since these populations represent a relatively small proportion of the U.S. population, estimates will be relatively imprecise unless resources are available with which to collect large oversamples of LGBT individuals. Research is necessary on ways to improve the quality and understand the limitations of estimates obtained by combining independent data sets, or by combining direct sample-based estimates with model-based estimates derived from supplemental but related data.
- Guidelines need to be developed for maximizing the utility of available data through such mechanisms as aggregating data sets over time, adding supplemental samples or oversampling LGBT individuals for ongoing studies, and developing standards for recoding measures across multiple studies to achieve nationally representative data sets.

REFERENCES

AAPOR (American Association for Public Opinion Research). 2010. *Best practices*. https://www.aapor.org/Best_Practices.htm (accessed October 22, 2010).

Aaron, D. J., Y. F. Chang, N. Markovic, and R. E. LaPorte. 2003. Estimating the lesbian population: A capture-recapture approach. *Journal of Epidemiology & Community Health* 57(3):207–209.

Almeida, J., R. M. Johnson, H. L. Corliss, B. E. Molnar, and D. Azrael. 2009. Emotional distress among LGBT youth: The influence of perceived discrimination based on sexual orientation. *Journal of Youth & Adolescence* 38(7):1001–1014.

Austin, S. B., K. Conron, A. Patel, and N. Freedner. 2007. Making sense of sexual orientation measures: Findings from a cognitive processing study with adolescents on health survey questions. *Journal of LGBT Health Research* 3(1):55–65.

Balsam, K. F., T. P. Beauchaine, E. D. Rothblum, and S. E. Solomon. 2008. Three-year follow-up of same-sex couples who had civil unions in Vermont, same-sex couples not in civil unions, and heterosexual married couples. *Developmental Psychology* 44(1):102–116.

Barrett, K., J. Bradford, and J. Ellis. 2002. *Using mapping to facilitate development of a health care infrastructure*. Redlands, CA: ESRI Newsletter.

Bates, C., C. Droste, L. Cuba, and J. Swingle. 2008. *One-on-one interviews: A qualitative assessment approach*. Crawfordsville, IN: Center in Inquiry in the Liberal Arts at Wabash College.

Bates, N., T. J. Demaio, C. Robins, and W. Hicks. 2010. *Classifying relationship and marital status among same-sex couples*. Paper read at Proceedings of the Section on Survey Research Methods, July 31–August 10, 2010, Vancouver, British Columbia, Canada.

Bell, A. P., and T. S. Weinberg. 1978. *Homosexualities: A study of diversity among men and women*. New York: Simon and Schuster.

Biemer, P. P. 2010. Overview of design issues: Total survey error. In *Handbook on survey research* (2nd ed.), edited by P. V. Mardsen and J. D. Wright. Bingley, UK: Emerald Group Publishing Limited. Pp. 27–57.

Biemer, P. P., and L. Lyberg. 2003. *Introduction to survey quality*. Hoboken, NJ: Wiley & Sons, Inc.

Binson, D., J. Blair, D.M. Huebner, and W.J. Woods. 2007. Sampling in surveys of lesbian, gay, and bisexual people. In *The health of sexual minorities*, edited by I. H. Meyer and M. E. Northridge. New York: Springer. Pp. 375–418.

Black, D. A., G. Gates, S. G. Sanders, and L. J. Taylor. 2000. Demographics of the gay and lesbian population in the United States: Evidence from available systematic data sources. *Demography* 37(2):139–154.

Black, D. A., S. G. Sanders, and L. J. Taylor. 2007. The economics of lesbian and gay families. *The Journal of Economic Perspectives* 21:53–70.

Blair, J. 1999. A probability sample of gay urban males: The use of two-phase adaptive sampling. *Journal of Sex Research* 36(1):39–44.

Boehmer, U. 2002. Twenty years of public health research: Inclusion of lesbian, gay, bisexual, and transgender populations. *American Journal of Public Health* 92(7):1125–1130.

Boehmer, U., M. Clark, M. Glickman, A. Timm, M. Sullivan, J. Bradford, and D. J. Bowen. 2010. Using cancer registry data for recruitment of sexual minority women: Successes and limitations. *Journal of Women's Health* 19(7):1289–1297.

Bolding, G., M. Davis, G. Hart, L. Sherr, and J. Elford. 2007. Where young MSM meet their first sexual partner: The role of the Internet. *AIDS & Behavior* 11(4):522–526.

Bowen, A. M., M. L. Williams, C. M. Daniel, and S. Clayton. 2008. Internet based HIV prevention research targeting rural MSM: Feasibility, acceptability, and preliminary efficacy. *Journal of Behavioral Medicine* 31(6):463–477.

Bowen, D. J., J. B. Bradford, D. Powers, P. McMorrow, R. Linde, B. C. Murphy, J. Han, and J. Ellis. 2004. Comparing women of differing sexual orientations using population-based sampling. *Women & Health* 40(3):19–34.

Bradford, J., C. Ryan, and E. D. Rothblum. 1993. National Lesbian Health Care Survey: Implications for mental health care. *Journal of Consulting & Clinical Psychology* 62(2):228–242.

Brennan, D. J., W. L. Hellerstedt, M. W. Ross, and S. L. Welles. 2007. History of childhood sexual abuse and HIV risk behaviors in homosexual and bisexual men. *American Journal of Public Health* 97(6):1107–1112.

Brick, J. M., and G. Kalton. 1996. Handling missing data in survey research. *Statistical Methods in Medical Research* 5(3):215–238.

Buchting, F. O., Scout, P. Fagan, M. Pien, and A. Rose. 2008. *Lesbians, gays, bisexuals, and transgenders of color sampling methodology*. Scotts Valley, CA: ETR Associates.

Carpenter, C. 2003. Sexual orientation and body weight: Evidence from multiple surveys. *Gender Issues* 21(3):60–74.

Carpenter, C., and G. J. Gates. 2008. Gay and lesbian partnership: Evidence from California. *Demography* 45(3):573–590.

Carpenter, K., S. Stoner, A. Mikko, L. Dhanak, and J. Parsons. 2010. Efficacy of a web-based intervention to reduce sexual risk in men who have sex with men. *AIDS and Behavior* 14(3):549–557.

Case, P., S. B. Austin, D. J. Hunter, J. E. Manson, S. Malspeis, W. C. Willett, and D. Spiegelman. 2004. Sexual orientation, health risk factors, and physical functioning in the Nurses' Health Study II. *Journal of Women's Health* 13(9):1033–1047.

Catania, J. A., D. Binson, J. Canchola, L. M. Pollack, W. Hauck, and T. J. Coates. 1996. Effects of interviewer gender, interviewer choice, and item wording on responses to questions concerning sexual behavior. *Public Opinion Quarterly* 60(3):345–375.

Catania, J. A., D. Osmond, R. D. Stall, L. Pollack, J. P. Paul, S. Blower, D. Binson, J. A. Canchola, T. C. Mills, L. Fisher, K. H. Choi, T. Porco, C. Turner, J. Blair, J. Henne, L. L. Bye, and T. J. Coates. 2001. The continuing HIV epidemic among men who have sex with men. *American Journal of Public Health* 91(6):907–914.

CDC (Centers for Disease Control and Prevention). 2009. *2009 compendium of evidence-based HIV prevention interventions.* http://www.cdc.gov/hiv/topics/research/prs/evidence-based-interventions.htm (accessed October 27, 2010).

Channing Laboratory. 2011a. *Growing Up Today Study (GUTS).* http://nhs2survey.org/gutsweb/?page_id=2 (accessed March 7, 2011).

Channing Laboratory. 2011b. *The Nurses' Health Study.* http://www.channing.harvard.edu/nhs/ (accessed March 3, 2011).

Clark, M. A., G. Armstrong, and L. Bonacore. 2005. Measuring sexual orientation and gender expression among middle-aged and older women in a cancer screening study. *Journal of Cancer Education* 20(2):108–112.

Cochran, S. D., and V. M. Mays. 2000. Lifetime prevalence of suicide symptoms and affective disorders among men reporting same-sex sexual partners: Results from NHANES III. *American Journal of Public Health* 90(4):573–578.

Cochran, S. D., and V. M. Mays. 2007. Physical health complaints among lesbians, gay men, and bisexual and homosexually experienced heterosexual individuals: Results from the California Quality of Life Survey. *American Journal of Public Health* 97(11):2048–2055.

Cochran, S. D., and V. M. Mays. 2009. Burden of psychiatric morbidity among lesbian, gay, and bisexual individuals in the California Quality of Life Survey. *Journal of Abnormal Psychology* 118(3):647–658.

Cochran, S. D., C. Keenan, C. Schober, and V. M. Mays. 2000. Estimates of alcohol use and clinical treatment needs among homosexually active men and women in the U.S. population. *Journal of Consulting and Clinical Psychology* 68(6):1062–1071.

Cochran, S. D., J. G. Sullivan, and V. M. Mays. 2003. Prevalence of mental disorders, psychological distress, and mental health services use among lesbian, gay, and bisexual adults in the United States. *Journal of Consulting and Clinical Psychology* 71(1):53–61.

Cochran, S. D., D. Ackerman, V. M. Mays, and M. W. Ross. 2004. Prevalence of non-medical drug use and dependence among homosexually active men and women in the US population. *Addiction* 99(8):989–998.

Cochran, S. D., V. M. Mays, M. Alegria, A. N. Ortega, and D. Takeuchi. 2007. Mental health and substance use disorders among Latino and Asian American lesbian, gay, and bisexual adults. *Journal of Consulting and Clinical Psychology* 75(5):785–794.

Conron, K. J., Scout, and S. B. Austin. 2008. "Everyone has a right to, like, check their box:" Findings on a measure of gender identity from a cognitive testing study with adolescents. *Journal of LGBT Health Research* 4(1):1–9.

Conron, K. J., M. J. Mimiaga, and S. J. Landers. 2010. A population-based study of sexual orientation identity and gender differences in adult health. *American Journal of Public Health* 100(10):1953–1960.

Consolacion, T. B., S. T. Russell, and S. Sue. 2004. Sex, race/ethnicity, and romantic attractions: Multiple minority status adolescents and mental health. *Cultural Diversity & Ethnic Minority Psychology* 10(3):200–214.

Corliss, H. L., M. Rosario, D. Wypij, L. B. Fisher, and S. B. Austin. 2008. Sexual orientation disparities in longitudinal alcohol use patterns among adolescents: Findings from the Growing Up Today Study. *Archives of Pediatrics & Adolescent Medicine* 162(11):1071–1078.

Couper, M. P. 2000. Web surveys: A review of issues and approaches. *Public Opinion Quarterly* 64(4):464–494.

Czaja, R., and J. Blair, eds. 1996. *Designing surveys: A guide to decisions and procedures.* Thousand Oaks, CA: Pine Forge Press.

Deputy, N. P., and U. Boehmer. 2010. Determinants of body weight among men of different sexual orientation. *Preventive Medicine* 51(2):129–131.

Diamond, L. M. 1998. Development of sexual orientation among adolescent and young adult women. *Developmental Psychology* 34(5):1085.

Diamond, L. M. 2008. Female bisexuality from adolescence to adulthood: Results from a 10-year longitudinal study. *Developmental Psychology* 44(1):5–14.

Dillman, D. A., J. D. Smyth, and L. M. Christian. 2009. *Internet, mail, and mixed-mode surveys: The tailored design method* (3rd ed.). Hoboken, NJ: John Wiley & Sons, Inc.

Dworkin, S. L., R. M. Pinto, J. Hunter, B. Rapkin, and R. H. Remien. 2008. Keeping the spirit of community partnerships alive in the scale up of HIV/AIDS prevention: Critical reflections on the roll out of DEBI (Diffusion of Effective Behavioral Interventions). *American Journal of Community Psychology* 42(1–2):51–59.

Egleston, B. L., R. L. Dunbrack, Jr., and M. J. Hall. 2010. Clinical trials that explicitly exclude gay and lesbian patients. *New England Journal of Medicine* 362(11):1054–1055.

Elliott, M. N., D. F. McCaffrey, B. K. Finch, D. J. Klein, N. Orr, M. K. Beckett, and N. Lurie. 2009. Improving disparity estimates for rare racial/ethnic groups with trend estimation and Kalman filtering: An application to the National Health Interview Survey. *Health Services Research* 44(5 Pt. 1):1622–1639.

Evans, A. R., R. D. Wiggins, G. Bolding, and J. Elford. 2008. Characteristics of gay and bisexual men who drop out of a web survey of sexual behaviour in the UK. *AIDS & Behavior* 12(6):957–963.

Finkelhor, D. 1994. Current information on the scope and nature of child sexual abuse. *Future Child* 4(2):31–53.

Fisher, R. A. 1925. *Statistical methods for research workers.* London: Oliver and Boyd.

Galesic, M., R. Tourangeau, and M. Casper. 2006. Complementing random digit dial telephone surveys with other approaches to collecting data. *American Journal of Preventive Medicine* 31(5):437–443.

Gallagher, K. M., P. S. Sullivan, A. Lansky, and I. M. Onorato. 2007. Behavioral surveillance among people at risk for HIV infection in the U.S.: The National HIV Behavioral Surveillance System. *Public Health Reports* 122(Suppl. 1):32–38.

Garofalo, R., J. Deleon, E. Osmer, M. Doll, and G. W. Harper. 2006. Overlooked, misunderstood and at-risk: Exploring the lives and HIV risk of ethnic minority male-to-female transgender youth. *Journal of Adolescent Health* 38(3):230–236.

Gates, G. 2007. *Geographic trends among same-sex couples in the U.S. Census and the American Community Survey.* Los Angeles, CA: The Williams Institute.

Gates, G. 2009. *Same-sex spouses and unmarried partners in the American Community Survey, 2008.* Los Angeles, CA: The Williams Institute.

Gay and Lesbian Medical Association and LGBT Health Experts. 2010. *Healthy People 2010 companion document for lesbian, gay, bisexual, and transgender (LGBT) health.* San Francisco, CA: Gay and Lesbian Medical Association.

Geanuracos, C. G., S. D. Cunningham, G. Weiss, D. Forte, L. M. Reid, and J. M. Ellen. 2007. Use of geographic information systems for planning HIV prevention interventions for high-risk youths. *American Journal of Public Health* 97(11):1974–1981.

Grant, J. M., L. A. Mottet, J. Tanis, D. Min, J. L. Herman, J. Harrison, and M. Keisling. 2010. *National Transgender Discrimination Survey Report on Health and Health Care*. Washington, DC: National Center for Transgender Equality and the National Gay and Lesbian Task Force.

Gribble, J. N., H. G. Miller, S. M. Rogers, and C. F. Turner. 1999. Interview mode and measurement of sexual behaviors: Methodological issues. *Journal of Sex Research* 36(1):16–24.

Groves, R. M., F. J. Fowler, M. P. Couper, J. M. Lepkowski, E. Singer, and R. Tourangeau. 2004. *Survey methodology*. New York: John Wiley & Sons, Inc.

Hall, D., K. Meador, and H. Koenig. 2008. Measuring religiousness in health research: Review and critique. *Journal of Religion and Health* 47(2):134–163.

Hatzenbuehler, M. L., K. M. Keyes, and D. S. Hasin. 2009. State-level policies and psychiatric morbidity in lesbian, gay, and bisexual populations. *American Journal of Public Health* 99(12):2275–2281.

Hatzenbuehler, M. L., K. A. McLaughlin, K. M. Keyes, and D. S. Hasin. 2010. The impact of institutional discrimination on psychiatric disorders in lesbian, gay, and bisexual populations: A prospective study. *American Journal of Public Health* 100(3):452–459.

Herbenick, D., M. Reece, V. Schick, S. A. Sanders, B. Dodge, and J. D. Fortenberry. 2010. Sexual behavior in the United States: Results from a national probability sample of men and women ages 14–94. *The Journal of Sexual Medicine* 7:255–265.

Herek, G. M. 2009. Hate crimes and stigma-related experiences among sexual minority adults in the United States: Prevalence estimates from a national probability sample. *Journal of Interpersonal Violence* 24(1):54–74.

Herek, G. M. 2010. Sexual orientation differences as deficits: Science and stigma in the history of American psychology. *Perspectives on Psychological Science* 5.

Herek, G. M., J. R. Gillis, and J. C. Cogan. 1999. Psychological sequelae of hate-crime victimization among lesbian, gay, and bisexual adults. *Journal of Consulting and Clinical Psychology* 67(6):945–951.

Herek, G. M., A. Norton, T. Allen, and C. Sims. 2010. Demographic, psychological, and social characteristics of self-identified lesbian, gay, and bisexual adults in a US probability sample. *Sexuality Research and Social Policy* 7(3):176–200.

HHS (U.S. Department of Health and Human Services). 2000. *Healthy People 2010: Understanding and improving health*. Washington, DC: HHS.

HIV Prevention Trials Network. 2011. *Explore: A randomized clinical trial of the efficacy of a behavioral intervention to prevent acquisition of HIV among men who have sex with men (MSM)*. http://www.hptn.org/research_studies/hivnet015.asp (accessed March 7, 2011).

Holbrook, A. L., J. A. Krosnick, and A. Pfent. 2008. The causes and consequences of response rates in surveys by the news media and government contractor survey research firms. In *Advances in telephone survey methodology*, edited by C. T. J. Lepkowski, J. M. Brick, E. de Leeuw, L. Japec, P. J. Lavrakas, M. W. Link, and R. L. Sangster. New York: John Wiley & Sons, Inc. Pp. 499–528.

Jarama, S. L., F. Z. Belgrave, J. Bradford, M. Young, and J. A. Honnold. 2007. Family, cultural and gender role aspects in the context of HIV risk among African American women of unidentified HIV status: An exploratory qualitative study. *AIDS Care: Psychological and Socio-medical Aspects of AIDS/HIV* 19(3):307–317.

The Joint Commission. 2010. *Advancing effective communication, cultural competence, and patient- and family-centered care: A roadmap for hospitals*. Oakbrook Terrace, IL: The Joint Commission.

The Joint Commission. 2011. *Joint Commission Perspectives* 31 (3). Oakbrook Terrace, IL: The Joint Commission.

Kalman, R. E. 1960. A new approach to linear filtering and prediction problems. *Transactions of the ASME—Journal of Basic Engineering* 82 (Series D):35–45.

Kalton, G. 2009. Methods for oversampling rare subpopulations in social surveys. *Survey Methodology* 35(2):125–141.

Kalton, G., and D. Kasprzyk. 1986. The treatment of missing survey data. *Survey Methodology* 12(1):1–16.

Kasprzyk, D., G. Duncan, G. Kalton, and M. P. Singh, eds. 1989. *Panel surveys*. New York: John Wiley & Sons, Inc.

Keeter, S., C. Miller, A. Kohut, R. M. Groves, and S. Presser. 2000. Consequences of reducing nonresponse in a national telephone survey. *Public Opinion Quarterly* 64(2):125–148.

Kellstedt, L. A., and C. E. Smidt. 1996. Measuring fundamentalism: An analysis of different operational strategies. In *Religion and the culture wars: Dispatches from the front,* edited by J. C. Green, J. L. Guth, C. E. Smidt, and L. A. Kellstedt. Lanham, MD: Rowman & Littlefield. Pp. 193–218.

Kennamer, J. D., J. Honnold, J. Bradford, and M. Hendricks. 2000. Differences in disclosure of sexuality among African American and white gay/bisexual men: Implications for HIV/AIDS prevention. *AIDS Education & Prevention* 12(6):519–531.

Knight, K. 1999. Liberalism and conservatism. In *Measures of political attitudes*, Vol. 2, edited by J. P. Robinson, P. R. Shaver, and L. S. Wrightsman. San Diego, CA: Academic Press. Pp. 59–158.

Kurdek, L. A. 2004. Are gay and lesbian cohabiting couples really different from heterosexual married couples? *Journal of Marriage and the Family* 66(4):880–900.

Laumann, E. O., R. T. Michael, and J. H. Gagnon. 1994. A political history of the national sex survey of adults. *Family Planning Perspectives* 26(1):34–38.

Lee, R. M. 1993. *Doing research on sensitive topics*. Thousand Oaks, CA: SAGE Publications.

Lynn, P. 2009. *Methodology of longitudinal surveys*. New York: John Wiley & Sons, Inc.

Martin, J. L., and L. Dean. 1990. Developing a community sample of gay men for an epidemiologic study of AIDS. *American Behavioral Scientist* 33(5):546–561.

Massachusetts Department of Public Health. 2007. *Behavioral Risk Factor Survey 2007 Questionnaire*. Boston, MA: Massachusetts Department of Public Health.

Mays, V. M., and S. D. Cochran. 2001. Mental health correlates of perceived discrimination among lesbian, gay, and bisexual adults in the United States. *American Journal of Public Health* 91(11):1869–1876.

McFarland, W., and C. F. Caceres. 2001. HIV surveillance among men who have sex with men. *AIDS* 15(Suppl. 3):S23–S32.

McKleroy, V. S., J. S. Galbraith, B. Cummings, P. Jones, C. Harshbarger, C. Collins, D. Gelaude, and J. W. Carey. 2006. Adapting evidence-based behavioral interventions for new settings and target populations. *AIDS Education & Prevention* 18:59–73.

McLaughlin, K. A., M. L. Hatzenbuehler, and K. M. Keyes. 2010. Responses to discrimination and psychiatric disorders among black, Hispanic, female, and lesbian, gay, and bisexual individuals. *American Journal of Public Health* 100(8):1477–1484.

Meyer, I. H., and P. A. Wilson. 2009. Sampling lesbian, gay, and bisexual populations. *Journal of Counseling Psychology* 56(1):23–31.

Meyer, I. H., L. Rossano, J. M. Ellis, and J. Bradford. 2002. A brief telephone interview to identify lesbian and bisexual women in random digit dialing sampling. *Journal of Sex Research* 39(2):139–144.

Meyer, I. H., S. Schwartz, and D. M. Frost. 2008. Social patterning of stress and coping: Does disadvantaged social statuses confer more stress and fewer coping resources? *Social Science & Medicine* 67(3):368–379.

Mimiaga, M. J., E. Noonan, D. Donnell, S. A. Safren, K. C. Koenen, S. Gortmaker, C. O'Cleirigh, M. A. Chesney, T. J. Coates, B. A. Koblin, and K. H. Mayer. 2009. Childhood sexual abuse is highly associated with HIV risk-taking behavior and infection among MSM in the EXPLORE study. *Journal of Acquired Immune Deficiency Syndromes: JAIDS* 51(3):340–348.

Minkler, M., and N. Wallerstein, eds. 2002. *Community-based participatory research for health*. New York: Jossey-Bass.

Morris, J. F., and E. D. Rothblum. 1999. Who fills out a "lesbian" questionnaire? The interrelationship of sexual orientation, years "out," disclosure of sexual orientation, sexual experience with women, and participation in the lesbian community. *Psychology of Women Quarterly* 23(3):537–557.

Mosher, W. D., A. Chandra, and J. Jones. 2005. Sexual behavior and selected health measures: Men and women 15–44 years of age, United States, 2002. *Advanced Data* (362):1–55.

Muhib, F. B., L. S. Lin, A. Stueve, R. L. Miller, W. L. Ford, W. D. Johnson, and P. J. Smith. 2001. A venue-based method for sampling hard-to-reach populations. *Public Health Reports* 116(Suppl. 1):216–222.

Mustanski, B. S. 2001. Getting wired: Exploiting the Internet for the collection of valid sexuality data. *Journal of Sex Research* 38(4):292–301.

Nemoto, T., D. Operario, and J. Keatley. 2005. Health and social services for male-to-female transgender persons of color in San Francisco. In *Transgender health and HIV prevention: Needs assessment studies from transgender communities across the United States*, edited by W. Bockting and E. Avery. New York: The Haworth Medical Press. Pp. 5–19.

NIH (National Institutes of Health). 2011. *Certificates of confidentiality: Background information*. http://grants.nih.gov/grants/policy/coc/background.htm (accessed February 9, 2011).

NRC (National Research Council). 1984. *Cognitive aspects of survey methodology: Building a bridge between disciplines*. Washington, DC: National Academy Press.

NRC. 2004. *Understanding racial and ethnic differences in health in late life: A research agenda*. Washington, DC: The National Academies Press.

OMB (Office of Management and Budget). 2001. *Statistical policy working paper 31: Measuring and reporting sources of error in surveys*. Washington, DC: Federal Committee on Statistical Methodology.

Raghuhathan, T. E., D. Xie, N. Schenker, V. L. Parsons, W. W. Davis, K. W. Dodd, and E. J. Feuer. 2007. Combining information from two surveys to estimate county-level prevalence rates of cancer risk factors and screening. *Journal of the American Statistical Association* 102(478):474–486.

Rao, J. N. K. 2003. *Small area estimation*. New York: John Wiley & Sons, Inc.

Reips, U. 2000. The web experiment method: Advantages, disadvantages, and solutions. In *Psychological experiments on the Internet*, edited by M. H. Birnbaum. San Diego, CA: Academic Press. Pp. 89–117.

Reisner, S. L., M. J. Mimiaga, C. V. Johnson, S. Bland, P. Case, S. A. Safren, and K. H. Mayer. 2010. What makes a respondent-driven sampling "seed" productive? Example of finding at-risk Massachusetts men who have sex with men. *Journal of Urban Health* 87(3):467–479.

Riggle, E. D., S. S. Rostosky, and C. Reedy. 2005. Online surveys for BGLT research: Issues and techniques. *Journal of Homosexuality* 49(2):1–21.

Rosenfeld, M. J. 2010. Nontraditional families and childhood progress through school. *Demography* 47(3):755–775.

Ross, M. W., B. R. S. Rosser, and J. Stanton. 2004. Beliefs about cybersex and Internet-mediated sex of Latino men who have Internet sex with men: Relationships with sexual practices in cybersex and in real life. *AIDS Care* 16(8):1002–1011.

Rosser, B. R. S., M. H. Miner, W. O. Bockting, M. W. Ross, J. Konstan, L. Gurak, J. Stanton, W. Edwards, S. Jacoby, A. Carballo-Dieguez, R. Mazin, and E. Coleman. 2009. HIV risk and the Internet: Results of the Men's Internet Sex (MINTS) Study. *AIDS & Behavior* 13(4):746–756.

Rothblum, E. D., and R. Factor. 2001. Lesbians and their sisters as a control group: Demographic and mental health factors. *Psychological Science* 12(1):63–69.

Rothblum, E. D., K. F. Balsam, and R. M. Mickey. 2004. Brothers and sisters of lesbians, gay men, and bisexuals as a demographic comparison group: An innovative research methodology to examine social change. *Journal of Applied Behavioral Science* 40(3):283–301.

Schenker, N., and T. E. Raghunathan. 2007. Combining information from multiple surveys to enhance estimation of measures of health. *Statistics in Medicine* 26(8):1802–1811.

Schenker, N., J. F. Gentleman, D. Rose, E. Hing, and I. M. Shimizu. 2002. Combining estimates from complementary surveys: A case study using prevalence estimates from national health surveys of households and nursing homes. *Public Health Reports* 117(4):393–407.

Sirken, M. G. 2004. Network sample surveys of rare and elusive populations: A historical review paper read at Symposium 2004: Innovative Methods for Surveying Difficult-to-Reach Populations.

SMART (Self-Monitoring, Analysis, and Reporting Technology). 2009. *Best practices for asking questions about sexual orientation on surveys.* Los Angeles, CA: The Williams Institute.

Smith, T. W. 1995. Some aspects of measuring education. *Social Science Research* 24(3):215–242.

Solarz, A. 1999. Lesbian health care issues. Exploring options for expanding research and delivering care. *AWHONN Lifelines* 3(5):13–14.

Stephan, C. W., and W. G. Stephan. 2000. The measurement of racial and ethnic identity. *International Journal of Intercultural Relations* 24(5):541–552.

Tang, H., G. L. Greenwood, D. W. Cowling, J. C. Lloyd, A. G. Roeseler, and D. G. Bal. 2004. Cigarette smoking among lesbians, gays, and bisexuals: How serious a problem? (United States). *Cancer Causes & Control* 15(8):797–803.

Tourangeau, R., and T. Yan. 2007. Sensitive questions in surveys. *Psychological Bulletin* 133(5):859–883.

Tourangeau, R., L. J. Rips, and K. A. Rasinski. 2000. *The psychology of survey response.* Cambridge, England: Cambridge University Press.

Villarroel, M. A., C. F. Turner, E. Eggleston, A. Al-Tayyib, S. M. Rogers, A. M. Roman, P. C. Cooley, and H. Gordek. 2006. Same-gender sex in the United States: Impact of T-ACASI on prevalence estimates. *Public Opinion Quarterly* 70(2):166–196.

Volz, E., and D. Heckathorn. 2008. Probability based estimation theory for respondent driven sampling. *Journal of Official Statistics* 24(1):79–97.

Westoff, C. F. 1973. The commission on population growth and the American future: Its origins, operations, and aftermath. *Population Index* 39(4):491–507.

Wienke, C., and G. J. Hill. 2009. Does the "marriage benefit" extend to partners in gay and lesbian relationships? Evidence from a random sample of sexually active adults. *Journal of Family Issues* 30(2):259–289.

Willis, G. B. 2004. *Cognitive interviewing revisited: A useful technique, in theory? Methods for testing and evaluating survey questionnaires.* Hoboken, NJ: John Wiley & Sons, Inc.

Xavier, J. M., and J. Bradford. 2005. *Transgender health access in Virginia: Focus group report.* Richmond, VA: Virginia Department of Health.

Xavier, J. M., M. Bobbin, B. Singer, and E. Budd. 2005. A needs assessment of transgendered people of color living in Washington, DC. *International Journal of Transgenderism* 8(2/3):31–47.

Xavier, J. M., J. Bradford, and J. Honnold. 2007. *The health, health-related needs, and life-course experiences of transgender Virginians.* Richmond, VA: Virginia Department of Health.

4

Childhood/Adolescence

To understand the context of a person's life course, it is critical to understand the age cohort to which that individual belongs. Youth growing up today will see changes that earlier generations of lesbians and gay men would never have expected in their lifetimes, including politicians, business leaders, and educators who are openly gay; marriage between same-sex couples; and an evolving popular and artistic culture that provides many positive portrayals of lesbian and gay characters in movies and plays, on television, and in literature. Today's youth are able to use the Internet to retrieve online information about LGBT issues, providing social networking opportunities and access to knowledge in a way that was not available to older cohorts. At the same time, young LGBT people searching the Internet and interacting with their peers will be aware of the pervasive negative views of sexual and gender minorities.

Likewise, many transgender elders did not even know as children that other transgender people existed, and certainly received little acknowledgment of their transgender feelings. By contrast, many transgender children and adolescents today have role models (either in the media or in real life), and their gender-variant expression is often sufficient for parents to obtain more information and access existing networks of families with gender-variant children. Moreover, transgender youth today have access to early medical intervention to alleviate any gender dysphoria (defined as discomfort with one's sex assigned at birth) they might experience.

In this report, childhood and adolescence encompasses the life course through the emergence of adulthood, generally understood by the committee to occur in the early 20s. During this phase of life, a person, regardless of his or her sexual orientation or gender identity, develops from a child who must be cared for to a self-reliant individual. The developmental changes that occur are complex, particularly with the onset of puberty. LGBT youth face the same challenges as their heterosexual peers, but also stigma that may contribute to the identified disparities in health status between sexual- and gender-minority youth and heterosexual youth.

The ability to address these disparities is hampered by our lack of knowledge about LGBT youth. One of the challenges of discussing the development of children and adolescents who are LGBT is that beliefs and biases have often precluded substantive research. Not long ago, for example, a prevailing notion was that one's sexual identity and orientation did not emerge until late adolescence and that an attraction to people of the same sex was likely a passing phase (Money, 1990). Moreover, efforts to survey young people about their sexual orientation have been fraught with difficulties at both the institutional review board and community levels. These barriers have impeded important developmental research.

While the current state of knowledge regarding the health of LGBT youth is derived from limited research, it is worth noting that much of this research has focused on mental health; little research has been conducted on the physical health of LGBT youth because, like most other youth, they generally do not struggle with chronic diseases that impact their physical health. As mentioned in previous chapters, the disparities in both mental and physical health that are seen between LGBT and heterosexual and non-gender-variant youth are influenced largely by their experiences of stigma and discrimination during the development of their sexual orientation and gender identity and throughout the life course.

This chapter begins with a discussion of the development of sexual orientation and gender identity in LGBT youth. The chapter then reviews the research on mental health and then physical health in these youth. Risk and protective factors and health services are then addressed in turn. The chapter next examines contextual influences, such as demographic characteristics and the role of the family. The chapter concludes with a summary of key findings and research opportunities. Of note, the chapter emphasizes adolescence rather than childhood because of the limited research available on younger children's and pre-adolescents' awareness of, feelings about, and experiences with being LGBT.

DEVELOPMENT OF SEXUAL ORIENTATION AND GENDER IDENTITY

Adolescents are engaged in an ongoing process of sexual development (Rosario et al., 2008); many adolescents may be unsure of their sexual orientation, while others have been clear about it since childhood. This ongoing process suggests that for some adolescents, self-identification of sexual orientation and the sex of sexual partners may change over time and may not necessarily be congruent (Saewyc et al., 2004).

The development of sexual identity in lesbian, gay, and bisexual individuals is a unique process that has been widely reported in the scientific literature and popular culture but has received surprisingly little empirical attention. Early models of sexual identity development were generated on the basis of retrospective descriptions by adults. Models of homosexual identity development proposed by Cass (1979) and Troiden (1989) describe a staged process that (1) recognizes the impact of stigma that affects both the formation and expression of homosexual identity, (2) unfolds over a period of time, (3) involves increasing acceptance of a homosexual identity, and (4) includes disclosure to other persons. However, these models were developed at a time in which access to information about sexual orientation was limited; negative attitudes about homosexuality were more prevalent; and few resources existed for the study of LGB populations, particularly adolescents. Furthermore, the development of these theoretical models was based on the retrospective experiences of white adults.

The first study to explore the development of adolescent lesbian and gay identity in depth included 202 LGB adolescents, more than half of whom were racial minority youth (Herdt and Boxer, 1993). The mean age of self-identification as lesbian or gay was 16.7 years for males and 16 years for females. Gay males were, on average, aware of same-sex attraction at about age 9; the average age for lesbians was 10. Based on the results of their study, the researchers concluded that sexual identity development should be viewed as an ongoing process rather than as a series of stages or phases.

Investigators who conducted early work on the development of sexual orientation identity argued that coming out or self-identifying as lesbian or gay during adolescence may be a developmental process seen only in contemporary LGB youth—one that may have unique consequences for later life-course development compared with lesbian and gay adults who did not come out during adolescence (Boxer and Cohler, 1989). Herdt and Boxer (1993) document the process of transition from a heterosexual to a gay identity in the context of LGB cultural supports (social institutions, a gay youth program, lesbian and gay adult role models). Boxer and Cohler (1989) observe that one of the major developmental tasks for lesbian and gay youth is the deconstruction of previously internalized heterosexual expectations and the construction of a new set of future expectations of the gay and lesbian life course.

A range of investigators have focused on "milestones" as indicators of sexual identity development among LGB adolescents. These include age of awareness of sexual attraction; age of self-labeling as lesbian, gay, or bisexual; age of disclosure of same-sex orientation; and age of first sexual experience. Research subsequent to Herdt and Boxer's early work found comparable ages of first awareness of sexual attraction (i.e., approximately age 10) (e.g., D'Augelli, 2006; D'Augelli and Hershberger, 1993; Rosario et al., 1996).

"Coming out" or self-identifying and subsequently sharing that identity with others is a process that occurs in a social and historical context. Earlier literature indicates that this experience may be especially challenging for young people who come out during adolescence, given the need to integrate an LGB identity with other aspects of identity development in the context of social stigma and discrimination. However, little current research is available to show how this process might differ for contemporary adolescents as a result of increased awareness, greater access to information, and changes in media representation of LGB people. More research is needed to understand the process of coming out for diverse populations of LGB youth.

Similarly, little research has focused on sexual identity development among ethnically diverse LGB adolescents. Development experiences may differ as adolescents negotiate both ethnic and sexual orientation identity. One community-based study of 145 white, black, and Latino LGB youth aged 14–21 found no differences in sexual identity, current sexual orientation, or comfort with and acceptance of sexual identity among the three racial groups (Rosario et al., 2004). However, black youth were involved in fewer gay-related social activities, were less comfortable with others knowing about their sexual identity, and disclosed their sexual orientation to fewer persons than their white peers. While Latino youth disclosed their LGB identity to fewer people than white or black youth, they were more comfortable with others knowing about their LGB identity than members of the other racial groups.

More recent research examined ethnic and sexual identity development during adolescence among 22 black and Latino gay youth aged 16–22 (Jamil et al., 2009). The researchers found that ethnic and sexual identity developed concurrently during adolescence, but the processes were different and not related. Ethnic identity development was shaped by growing awareness of the youth's ethnic and cultural heritage and was supported by peers; family members; and cultural markers such as food, music, and holidays. Sexual identity development was supported by community-based organizations, peers, and information from the Internet. Sexual identity development was described as a private process, while ethnic identity development was viewed as a more public process.

The ongoing process of sexual development among adolescents presents challenges to the collection of data on the size of the population of LGB youth, although some studies using large samples of adolescents have examined the prevalence of same-sex attraction, same-sex sexual behavior, and LGB identities. In the 1999 wave of the Growing Up Today Study (n = 10,685), a national survey of adolescents aged 12–17, approximately 1 percent of adolescents identified as homosexual or bisexual (n = 103), with 5 percent identifying as mostly heterosexual (n = 511) and 2 percent identifying as unsure (n = 226) (Austin et al., 2004a). In the first wave of the National Longitudinal Study of Adolescent Health, conducted among 7th- through 12th-grade adolescents (n = 11,940), 5 percent of females and about 7.3 percent of males reported same-sex romantic or sexual attractions (Russell and Joyner, 2001). DuRant and colleagues (1998), reporting on the prevalence of reported same-sex sexual behavior using the 1995 wave of the Vermont Youth Risk Behavior Survey (n = 3,886 sexually active 8th- through 12th-grade males), found that 8.7 percent of high school males reported having had at least one same-sex partner (DuRant et al., 1998).

Similar to sexual orientation identity, gender expression is not necessarily constant throughout childhood development. Gender variance, as it relates to expressing and exploring gender identity and gender roles, is a part of normal development. A relatively small percentage of gender-variant children develop an adult transgender identity (Green, 1987; Wallien and Cohen-Kettenis, 2008; Zucker and Bradley, 1995). However, research shows that the majority of adolescents with a gender-variant identity develop an adult transgender identity (Wallien and Cohen-Kettenis, 2008). Data on the prevalence of childhood gender-variant or transgender identities are severely limited, largely because there is no national database available to collect such data. A relatively small number of studies using nonprobability samples have attempted to assess the incidence of childhood gender-variant identities. One such study, discussed in Chapter 2, found that 1 percent of parents of boys aged 4–11 reported that their son wished to be of the other sex; for girls, the percentage was 3.5 percent (Zucker et al., 1997).

Other studies using small nonprobability samples have documented trends in referrals to gender identity clinics by gender and persistence of gender identity concerns into adolescence and adulthood. One study examining children aged 3–12 with gender identity issues in a Toronto clinic (n = 358) and a Utrecht clinic (n = 130) showed that boys were referred more often and at an earlier age than girls for such concerns (Cohen-Kettenis et al., 2003). In another small study (n = 77) examining psychosexual outcomes of gender-dysphoric children at age of referral and then at follow-up approximately 10 years later, 27 percent of those with childhood gender identity concerns were still gender dysphoric (Wallien and Cohen-Kettenis, 2008). (It should be noted that at follow-up, 30 percent of the sample failed to respond to recruitment letters or were not traceable.) Research with small clinical samples of gender-variant children has shown that, compared with controls, gender-variant children have more difficulties with peer relationships (Zucker et al., 1997); this is the case particularly for boys compared with girls (Cohen-Kettenis et al., 2003). Poor peer relations was found to be the strongest predictor of behavior problems in both gender-variant boys and girls (Cohen-Kettenis et al., 2003). One small study showed that children with gender identity disorder (n = 25) may have a more anxious nature than gender-conforming children (n = 25) (Wallien et al., 2007).

Grossman and D'Augelli (2006) conducted focus groups with young self-identified transgender males and females aged 15–21 and explored factors related to physical and mental health. In this qualitative study, most of the youth reported experiences of family and peers reacting negatively toward their gender-atypical behaviors. Therapy or counseling that aims to change an individual's sexual orientation, often based on the presumption that LGBT orientation/identity is abnormal or unhealthy, is known as conversion or reparative therapy (Just the Facts Coalition, 2008). The nation's most prominent medical and mental health professional organizations, including the American Medical Association, the American Psychiatric Association, and the American Psychological Association, oppose the use of conversion therapy with both youth and adults (AMA, 2010; American Psychiatric Association, 2000a). The American Psychological Association formed a task force to review peer-reviewed studies on efforts to change sexual orientation. The task force concluded that evidence is lacking for the effectiveness of efforts to change sexual orientation and that conversion therapy may cause harm to LGBT individuals by increasing internalized stigma, distress, and depression (American Psychological Association, 2009). Instead, the task force expressed support for the use of affirmative, culturally competent therapy that helps those facing distress related to their sexual orientation cope with social and internalized stigma and strengthen their social support networks (American Psychological Association, 2009).

MENTAL HEALTH STATUS

As noted, most of the research conducted among LGBT youth has examined their mental health status. Although a small amount of the literature explores the process of sexual orientation and gender identity development among LGBT youth (see the preceding section), a greater portion of the literature focuses on sexual-minority youth's risk for suicidality and depression; few studies examine the prevalence of mood, anxiety, or eating disorders in these populations. As discussed below, the lack of data in many areas of mental health demonstrates the need for further research on the mental health status of LGBT youth.

It is important to note that LGBT youth are typically well adjusted and mentally healthy. Research based on probability samples with LGB youth consistently indicates that the majority do not report mental health problems (Mustanski et al., 2010b; Russell and Joyner, 2001). Regarding transgender youth, although no data from national probability samples are available, studies with sizable convenience samples indicate that many, if not most, of these youth do not report mental health problems (Clements-Nolle et al., 2001; Nuttbrock et al., 2010).

Mood and Anxiety Disorders

Most of the research that has been conducted on mental health disorders among LGBT youth has relied on symptom or distress scales rather than formal clinical diagnoses (Mustanski et al., 2010b). To the committee's knowledge, only two published studies have assessed LGBT adolescents diagnostically. Fergusson and colleagues (1999) conducted a study in New Zealand on the risk of psychiatric disorder and suicidal behavior using data from a birth cohort. They found that, relative to youth who identified as heterosexual, youth who identified as lesbian, gay, or bisexual were between 1.8 and 2.9 times more likely to experience generalized anxiety disorder, major depression, and conduct disorder. It should be noted, however, that of the 1,007 youth surveyed, only 28 self-identified as LGB or described past relationships with same-sex partners (Fergusson et al., 1999).

More recently, Mustanski and colleagues (2010b) administered a structured diagnostic interview to a community sample of 246 LGBT youth. They found that, although the youth in the sample showed a higher prevalence of *Diagnostic and Statistical Manual of Mental Disorders*, 4th edition (DSM-IV) diagnoses compared with national data, the prevalence was similar to that among another sample of urban, ethnically diverse youth from the same geographic area.

Depression and Suicidality

Over the past decade, an increasing number of studies based on large probability samples have consistently found that LGB youth and youth who report same-sex romantic attraction are at increased risk for suicidal ideation and attempts, as well as depressive symptoms, in comparison with their heterosexual counterparts. These include both school-based, state-based, and national studies (Almeida et al., 2009; Birkett et al., 2009; Bontempo and D'Augelli, 2002; Garofalo et al., 1999; Jiang et al., 2010; Russell and Joyner, 2001; Saewyc et al., 2007). The results of these studies suggest increased rates of suicidal ideation and attempts among LGB youth in comparison with heterosexual youth even after controlling for potentially confounding factors such as substance use and depression. These population-based studies followed more than two decades of community-based studies of LGB youth that showed elevated reported rates of suicidal ideation and attempts and identified predictors of suicidality in these populations, although it should be noted that, much as with the larger population of young people, it is a small group of LGB youth who report suicidal behavior.

With few exceptions, the increased rate of suicidality among LGB youth in comparison with heterosexual youth is consistent across age groups (i.e., middle school, high school, and young adult populations), gender (i.e., male, female, transgender), race/ethnicity (e.g., white, black, Latino, Asian/Pacific Islander, American Indian/Alaska Native), and differing definitions of sexual orientation (i.e., same-sex attraction, self-identification, and behavior) (Almeida et al., 2009; Birkett et al., 2009; Bontempo and D'Augelli, 2002; Faulkner and Cranston, 1998; Garofalo et al., 1998, 1999; Jiang et al., 2010; Saewyc et al., 2007). However, evidence from longitudinal studies on suicidality over time among LGB youth is lacking.

Some older evidence disputes the idea of increased rates of completed suicide among LGB youth. Two studies using postsuicide data found no association between suicide and sexual orientation (Rich et al., 1986; Shaffer et al., 1995). However, capturing information about sexual orientation is especially difficult postsuicide since adolescents who are highly conflicted about their sexual orientation may not share these concerns with others. Moreover, these studies examined completed suicides from more than 20 years ago, when it was more difficult to be openly gay during adolescence. In addition, results of two community-based studies suggest that some of the suicide attempts reported by LGB youth may not be life-threatening, but rather low-risk suicidal ideation or plans (Savin-Williams, 2001). These studies have been challenged for potentially drawing on relatively low-risk populations, however (Russell, 2003).

Many risk factors, both general and LGB-specific, have been implicated in the increased rates of suicidal behavior among LGB youth (see the detailed discussion of risk factors for the health of LGBT youth later in this chapter). General risk factors have been implicated in suicidal behavior in the larger population of youth and tend to be high among LGB youth. They include depression, substance use, early sexual initiation, not feeling safe at school, cigarette smoking, and inadequate social support. These factors may partially mediate the increased risk of suicidality for LGB youth, although results of studies on this association are mixed (Fergusson et al., 1999; Garofalo et al., 1999; Russell and Joyner, 2001). Specific factors related to sexual-minority status, including homophobic victimization and stress (Huebner et al., 2004; Safren and Heimberg, 1999; Savin-Williams and Ream, 2003), are associated with suicidal behavior. In a study of 528 self-identified LGB youth aged 15–19, D'Augelli and colleagues (2005) found that recognizing same-sex attraction, initiating same-sex sexual activity, or appearing gender nonconforming at earlier ages was associated with reported suicide attempts in LGB youth; this association may be exacerbated by experiences of victimization and maltreatment (Corliss et al., 2009; Friedman et al., 2006).

Family rejection due to sexual orientation may also be associated with increased risk of suicidality. In the previously mentioned study of 528 LGB youth, greater childhood parental psychological abuse and parental efforts to discourage gender-atypical behavior were associated with increased risk of suicide attempts (D'Augelli et al., 2005). Similarly, a study of 224 self-identified LGB youth aged 21–25 found that higher rates of family rejection were associated with increased rates of reports of attempted suicide, high levels of depression, and risk behaviors (Ryan et al., 2009). Conversely, findings from a study of 245 Latino and non-Latino white self-identified LGBT youth (aged 21–25) suggest that family acceptance of and supportive reactions to an adolescent's LGBT identity may be protective against depression and suicidal ideation and attempts (Ryan et al., 2010). Using data from the 2004 Minnesota Student Survey of 9th and 12th graders (n = 21,927), Eisenberg and Resnick (2006) found that family connectedness, adult caring, and school safety may also be protective against suicidal ideation and attempts.

Evidence from several large samples of middle and high school students suggests that the above LGB-specific factors, including victimization and perceived discrimination, largely mediate the association between sexual-minority status and both depressive symptoms and suicidal behavior (Almeida et al., 2009; Birkett et al., 2009; Bontempo and D'Augelli, 2002).

Because large data sets have not measured whether people are transgender, information on suicidal behavior and depressive symptoms among transgender youth is limited to relatively small convenience samples. In a nonprobability sample of 515 transgender people (n = 392 male-to-female and n = 123 female-to-male), Clements-Nolle and colleagues (2006) found that 47 percent of participants younger than 25 (n = 66) had a history of attempted suicide. Another study, of 55 transgender youth aged 15–21, found that 45 percent seriously thought about taking their lives, and 26 percent reported a history of life-threatening behavior (Grossman and D'Augelli, 2007). These studies suggest there is an elevated risk for depression and attempted suicide among transgender youth.

Limited cross-sectional research has explored mental health–related disparities among urban samples of transgender youth. Nuttbrock and colleagues (2010) examined the life course of 571 transgender females aged 19–59 (separated into two age groups: 19–39 and 40–59). The authors found that gender-related interpersonal abuse was a significant health problem in the sample. Among the younger group of transgender women, 15.6 percent reported an attempted suicide during adolescence. Among the older group, 23.5 percent experienced major depression during adolescence. In addition, interpersonal abuse associated with gender atypicality, not infrequently at the hands of parents or other family members, was associated with both major depression and suicidality as defined by DSM-IV. These associations, particularly with depression, were extremely strong during adolescence, and tended to decline over time but remain significant over the life course.

Interventional approaches to prevent suicidality among LGBT youth have not been widely tested. The published literature includes suggestions to encourage greater awareness and appropriate treatment by health care providers (Kitts, 2005), psychotherapists (Hart, 2001), and school personnel (Bontempo and D'Augelli, 2002); to educate and counsel parents and families to decrease rejecting and increase supportive behaviors (Ryan et al., 2010); or to use specific media to reach isolated youth, such as Web-based social networks (Silenzio et al., 2009). To the committee's knowledge, however, no specific interventions have been tested. In addition, little research has examined suicidality by race/ethnicity.

Eating Disorders/Body Image

A large cohort study provides some evidence that eating disorders follow gender-specific patterns among LGB youth. In data from the previously mentioned 1999 Growing Up Today Study (n = 10,583 youth), lesbian and bisexual girls, who were combined in the study (n = 59), were found to be more content with their bodies and less likely to report trying to look like images of women in the media than were heterosexual girls. On the other hand, the study found that gay and bisexual boys, also combined in the study (n = 38), were more likely than heterosexual boys to report trying to look like images of men in the media (Austin et al., 2004b). In another study, using the 1998–2005 waves of the Growing Up Today Study (n = 13,795), youth who described themselves as lesbian/gay, bisexual, and "mostly" heterosexual had higher rates of binge eating than their heterosexual peers, and all subgroups with the exception of lesbians had higher rates of purging (vomiting and/or using laxatives to control weight) throughout adolescence (Austin et al., 2009a). While these are provocative findings, they come from only two studies; more research is required to either confirm or refute them. Additionally, if these findings are accurate, more research is needed to understand the mechanisms that put these youth at increased risk for eating disorders.

Results of one study using data from the 1995 and 1997 waves of the Vermont (n = 14,623) and Massachusetts (n = 8,141) Youth Risk Behavior Surveys suggest that youth who reported having sex with both males and females were at greatest risk for a variety of problem behaviors, including disordered eating. In Vermont, 25.6 percent of youth with sexual partners of both sexes reported using unhealthy weight control practices, compared with 12.3 percent of those with exclusively same-sex sexual partners and 7.1 percent of those with exclusively opposite-sex sexual partners. In Massachusetts these practices were reported by 37.4 percent of students with sexual partners of both sexes, compared with 15.3 percent of those with exclusively same-sex sexual partners and 7.0 percent of those with exclusively opposite-sex sexual partners. This study was based on sexual behavior, not identity (Robin et al., 2002).

The literature on eating disorders among LGBT youth is based on large data sets, unlike most of the literature on these populations, which often relies on small convenience samples. However, the research on eating disorders in these populations is still sparse.

Transgender-Specific Mental Health Status

DSM-IV includes diagnoses of gender identity disorder for children as well as for adolescents (and adults) (American Psychiatric Association, 2000b). The criteria for diagnosis of childhood gender identity disorder are listed in Box 4-1. This diagnosis has been controversial, particularly when applied to children. One objection raised is that including this phenomenon as a psychiatric diagnosis identifies gender-variant identity and expression as pathological, even though many gender-variant children do not report emotional distress; rather, distress may be related to the reaction of the social environment to the child's gender variance. Also, as noted earlier in this chapter, most children with gender-variant expression do not develop an adolescent or adult transgender identity (Wallien and Cohen-Kettenis, 2008), and many adults with a transgender identity do not report symptoms of childhood gender identity disorder (Lawrence, 2010). More specifically, this diagnosis has been criticized for conflating gender-variant expression with gender-variant identity. At least four of the five criteria are required to qualify for the diagnosis, and only one of these explicitly refers to cross-gender identification, allowing children with gender-variant expression but without a variant gender identity to qualify for the diagnosis (see also Bockting and Ehrbar, 2006).

The approach to treatment of gender identity disorder among children includes early therapeutic interventions with the child, and perhaps with the family, school, and/or community, to broaden the child's gender role interests and behavior and/or provide a safe environment to allow gender identity to develop while preventing rejection, ridicule, and abuse from peers (Benestad, 2009; Brill and Pepper, 2008; Menvielle and Tuerk, 2002; Meyer-Bahlburg, 2002; Rosenberg, 2002; Zucker, 2008). The approach to treatment of gender identity disorder among adolescents includes

BOX 4-1
Criteria for Diagnosis of Childhood Gender Identity Disorder

A. A strong and persistent crossgender identification, manifested in 4 or more of the following:

1. Repeatedly stated desire to be, or insistence that he or she is, the other sex;
2. In boys, preference for cross-dressing or simulating female attire; in girls, insistence on wearing only stereotypical masculine clothing;
3. Strong and persistent preferences for cross-sex roles in make-believe play or persistent fantasies of being the other sex;
4. Intense desire to participate in the stereotypical games and pastimes of the other sex;
5. Strong preference for playmates of the other sex.

In adolescents, it is manifested by symptoms such as a stated desire to be the other sex, frequent passing as the other sex, desire to live or be treated as the other sex, or the conviction that he or she has the typical feelings and reactions of the other sex.

B. Persistent discomfort with his or her sex or sense of inappropriateness in the gender role of that sex, manifested by any of the following:

1. In boys, assertion that his penis or testes are disgusting or will disappear or assertion that it would be better not to have a penis, or aversion toward rough-and-tumble play and rejection of male stereotypical toys, games, and activities;
2. In girls, rejection of urinating in a sitting position, assertion that she has or will grow a penis, or assertion that she does not want to grow breasts or menstruate, or marked aversion toward normative feminine clothing.

In adolescents, the disturbance is manifested by symptoms such as preoccupation with getting rid of primary and secondary sex characteristics (e.g., request for hormones, surgery, or other procedures to physically alter sexual characteristics to simulate the other sex) or belief that he or she was born the wrong sex.

C. The disturbance is not concurrent with a physical intersex condition.

D. The disturbance causes clinically significant distress or impairment in social, occupational, or other important areas of functioning.

SOURCE: DSM IV (American Psychiatric Association, 2000b).

therapeutic interventions to assist the adolescent and his or her family to explore and understand gender variance and cope with the related stress and social adjustment, which may include a gender role transition (Di Ceglie, 2009; Meyer et al., 2001). In addition, early medical intervention is available for carefully selected youth who have persistent gender dysphoria that has increased with the initial stages of puberty and who have support from their parents for such intervention (Cohen-Kettenis et al., 2008; Hembree et al., 2009; Meyer et al., 2001). The intervention consists of administering puberty-delaying hormones (such as gonadotropin-releasing hormone [GnRH] analogs) as early as Tanner Stage II of puberty (a development stage marked by certain physical milestones as opposed to age) and cross-sex hormones as early as age 16. The puberty-delaying hormones allow for more time to monitor the development of the youth's gender identity while reducing the dysphoria associated with the pubertal development of incongruent sex characteristics, an approach that has been shown to be beneficial (Cohen-Kettenis and van Goozen, 1997; de Vries et al., 2010; Delemarre-van de Waal and Cohen-Kettenis, 2006; Smith et al., 2001, 2005).

PHYSICAL HEALTH STATUS

As noted earlier, for most people, including LGBT youth, childhood and adolescence are times of good physical health. It is not surprising, then, that few studies have examined the physical health of children and adolescents who are LGBT.

Teen Pregnancy/Reproductive Health

Very little research has been conducted on the relationship between teen pregnancy and sexual orientation, although there is some indication that lesbian and bisexual adolescents may have at least the same and possibly an increased likelihood of pregnancy compared with heterosexual adolescents. Saewyc and colleagues (1999) conducted a secondary analysis of a subsample of 12- to 19-year-old young women from the 1987 Minnesota Adolescent Health Survey (n = 3,816) and found that self-identified lesbians and bisexual females (samples combined for analysis, n = 182) were just as likely as their heterosexual counterparts (n = 1,881) to have heterosexual intercourse but much more likely to have gotten pregnant.

In 2008, Saewyc and colleagues (2008) performed secondary analyses on three different waves of the British Columbia Adolescent Health Survey (1992, 1998, and 2003 waves). Sexual orientation in 7th- to 12th-grade youth was measured by means of self-assessment in a paper-and-pencil survey. Gay and bisexual male students were more likely than heterosexual male students to have ever had sexual intercourse. They were also more likely to have been responsible for a pregnancy, to report having had two or more sexual partners, and to report first intercourse before age 14. Lesbian and bisexual female students were more likely than heterosexual female students to have ever had heterosexual intercourse, had higher odds of having been pregnant, were more likely to have had heterosexual intercourse before age 14, and were more likely to have had two or more sexual partners.

A more recent study using a community-based convenience sample of young women who have sex with women (n = 137, ages 16–24) found that 20 percent had been pregnant (Herrick et al., 2010). Although this is only one study, it is worth noting that this pregnancy rate is comparable to that among all girls. Providers may assume that young women who have sex with women are less likely to get pregnant, but findings from several studies suggest that this may not be the case even for those who self-identify as lesbians.

Aside from the studies conducted by Saewyc and colleagues (1998, 2008), most studies in this area have not included males. Although LGBT youth have indicated an interest in parenting (D'Augelli et al., 2006/2007), a discussion of parenting options and parenting/reproductive issues is largely absent in the literature on LGBT youth.

Obesity

Childhood obesity rates have risen dramatically in the United States in the past few decades (Ogden et al., 2010). As discussed in the following chapter, some research suggests a higher prevalence of obesity among lesbians than among heterosexual women. However, almost no research has examined weight-related patterns among LGBT youth. One study, drawing on data from the 1998–2005 waves of the Growing Up Today Study (n = 13,785, ages 12–23), found that self-identified sexual-minority adolescent females had elevated body mass indexes (BMIs) compared with their heterosexual peers (Austin et al., 2009b). The same study also found a relationship between sexual orientation and age among males, with heterosexual adolescents showing steeper increases in BMI from early to late adolescence than nonheterosexual adolescents. More research is needed to document whether these disparities are generalizable, to understand the interaction between sexual orientation/identity and body weight among adolescents, and to develop appropriate interventions.

HIV/AIDS and Other Sexually Transmitted Infections

In the United States, the burden of HIV infection among young people falls disproportionately on young men under age 25 who have sex with men, particularly those who belong to racial/ethnic minority groups. Young men who have sex with men account for almost 60 percent of HIV diagnoses among all young people and represent twice as many diagnoses as young women across all risk categories (CDC, 2009). The Young Men's Survey, administered by the Centers for Disease Control and Prevention (CDC) in seven urban areas (n = 3,492, ages 15–22), found that 7.2 percent of the young men who have sex with men who were surveyed were HIV-positive; among these youth, prevalence increased with age (from 5.6 percent among those aged 15–19 to 8.6 percent among those aged 20–22) (Valleroy et al., 2000). Waldo and colleagues (2000), using a subsample of the Young Men's Survey from three counties in San Francisco (n = 719), found that while those aged 15–17 reported fewer overall sex partners in the past 6 months than those aged 18–22, they reported similar levels of other sexual risk behaviors. National surveillance data from CDC for 2001–2006 showed that young men who have sex with men were the only risk group with an increasing number of HIV/AIDS diagnoses; the increase was an alarming 93 percent among young black men (CDC, 2008). Compared with their white peers in the United States in 2006, more than twice as many black young men who have sex with men were diagnosed with HIV; black and Latino young men who have sex with men were more likely to become infected at younger ages (CDC, 2008).

Agronick and colleagues (2004) examined HIV risk behavior among 441 Latino young men and found differences in partnership characteristics between those who self-identified as bisexual and those who self-identified as gay. The bisexual young men were more likely to report more than 1 male sex partner in the past 3 months and were less likely to report being in an exclusive sexual relationship with a primary male partner. The authors also found differences in sexual risk behaviors. The bisexual young men were more likely to report having unprotected insertive anal intercourse during their last sexual encounter with a nonprimary male partner, as well as using drugs or alcohol during their last sexual encounter with either a primary or nonprimary male partner.

Few studies have examined the correlates that might explain the racial/ethnic differences in HIV seroprevalence or HIV risk (Garofalo et al., 2010; Harawa et al., 2004). According to Peterson and Jones (2009), the racial/ethnic disparities in HIV seroprevalence are likely due to the intersection of race, sexual orientation, and other social determinants. Millett and colleagues (2007) conducted a meta-analysis comparing black and white men who have sex with men and concluded that behavioral risks, such as unprotected anal intercourse, commercial sex work, sex with a known HIV-positive partner, or HIV testing history may not fully explain racial disparities. While results were generalized across all ages, studies of youth were included in the analysis. For Asian/Pacific Islander youth, very limited data are available (Choi et al., 2005; Do et al., 2005).

Almost no data on HIV risk for young women exist except for a few isolated studies from convenience samples of urban women who have sex with women regarding increased risks for HIV and other sexually transmitted infections (STIs). One statewide survey using the 1995–2001 waves of the Massachusetts Youth Risk Behavior Survey examined the associations among self-identified sexual orientation (heterosexual, lesbian/gay, bisexual, or not sure), sex of partners, and HIV-related risk behavior among sexually experienced 9th- to 12th-grade females (n = 3,973). Goodenow and colleagues (2008) found that respondents' self-identification of their sexual orientation was frequently inconsistent with their reports of the sex of their sexual partners. They also found that self-identifying as lesbian, bisexual, or "not sure" or having any same-sex sexual experiences was associated with a greater probability of HIV-related risk behavior. There have been a few studies, using convenience samples, of HIV and STI prevalence and risk among transgender youth. Although these studies are quite limited (Garofalo et al., 2006; Wilson et al., 2009), they suggest that male-to-female transgender youth may face a risk for HIV similar to or even higher than that of young men who have sex with men.

Some studies of urban samples of young men who have sex with men have begun to look at the potential correlates or underlying mechanisms of HIV risk (Garofalo et al., 2007a, 2008; Koblin et al., 2006; Mustanski, 2007). There is an evolving literature on sexual contexts (for example, older partners and the Internet) as promoters of HIV risk (Mustanski, 2007; Mustanski et al., 2010a). One study involving a convenience sample (n = 120) found that among transgender women, the likelihood of HIV risk behaviors varied according to the nature of the relationship with their sexual partner (either main, casual, or commercial) (Wilson et al., 2010). It should be noted that, while much of the research has focused on sexual risk behaviors, there has been much less research on the actual acquisition of STIs other than HIV among young people. Exceptions are some research on hepatitis B (Diamond et al., 2003; MacKellar et al., 2001) and the work of Valleroy and colleagues (2000) based on the Young Men's Survey.

Although a fair amount of research has been conducted on the association between sexual orientation and HIV and other STIs, particularly using epidemiological data, the data still have limitations. For example, few studies have examined epidemiological data on multisite or representative national samples (Guenther-Grey et al., 2005; Valleroy et al., 2000). Much of the representative, population-based data still comes from the 1995–1999 Massachusetts Youth Risk Behavior Surveillance System. The first study using these data to examine the association between sexual orientation and health risk behaviors was published in *Pediatrics* in 1998 (Garofalo et al., 1998).

Few longitudinal or natural history studies of high-risk groups such as young men who have sex with men or young transgender women have been conducted. Filling these gaps in the literature may elucidate underlying mechanisms of risk and ultimately help in designing much-needed interventions, an area in which perhaps the greatest gap in the literature exists.

Despite alarming epidemiological data on the HIV risk faced by young men who have sex with men, there has been no commensurate response in terms of designing and implementing interventions to reduce this risk. The vast majority of youth-specific HIV prevention programs in the published literature are focused on heterosexual young people (Johnson et al., 2003; Mullen et al., 2002; Pedlow and Carey, 2004; Robin et al., 2004). A recent meta-analysis of HIV behavioral interventions targeting men who have sex with men reported not a single randomized controlled trial in which the mean age was less than 23 (Herbst et al., 2005). Similarly, in a community-based HIV prevention program targeting young men who have sex with men (n = 300 men who have sex with men), the mean age was 23 (Herbst et al., 2005; Kegeles et al., 1996).

Transgender-Specific Physical Health Status

Although some literature addresses the process of gender identity development among transgender youth, little of this literature is supported by empirical evidence or longitudinal data. The lack of available cohort data on the relationship between developmental issues and general health status represents a distinct gap in the literature. In addition, although some small, largely European studies in children and adolescents have examined the effects and consequences of hormone administration and/or blocking of puberty with GnRH analogs, empirical data on how these medical interventions affect overall physical health and well-being remain extremely limited. While some preliminary animal studies have suggested that GnRH analog therapy can affect sex-specific brain development, no comparable research has been done in humans.

RISK AND PROTECTIVE FACTORS

The literature addresses a number of risk factors that affect the health of LGBT youth. Conversely, little research has been conducted on protective factors for these populations.

Risk Factors

Risk factors affecting the health of LGBT youth examined in the literature include harassment, victimization, and violence; substance use; homelessness; and childhood abuse.

Harassment, Victimization, and Violence

Compared with heterosexual youth, LGBT youth report experiencing higher levels of harassment, victimization, and violence, including verbal, physical, and sexual abuse. These experiences are related to increased substance use (see below), mental health problems, and sexual risk-taking behavior (Birkett et al., 2009).

School-based harassment, bullying, and peer victimization are the most common topics in the literature on LGB youth. This emphasis may be due to the role of schools in child and adolescent socialization and development and the increasing focus over the past 20 years on schools as a primary site of conflict, victimization, and activism for young people who are known or perceived to be LGBT.

School victimization based on known or perceived sexual orientation and gender identity has been documented consistently in studies of LGB and, more recently, transgender adolescents. A community-based study of LGB youth aged 21 or younger (n = 350) (D'Augelli et al., 2002) found that school-based victimization was widespread for LGB youth and that an association existed between this victimization and mental health and posttraumatic stress symptoms. The study results showed that earlier recognition of same-sex feelings, self-identification as LGB, and disclosure of sexual orientation were correlated with increased high school victimization. Similarly, youth who were open about their sexual orientation or exhibited gender-atypical behavior were targets for victimization. Likewise, a series of community school climate surveys conducted since 1999 has documented extensive verbal and physical harassment and discrimination among LGBT students in schools (Kosciw et al., 2007, 2008).

Population-based surveys of high school students have shown that those with same-sex sexual experience (DuRant et al., 1998; Faulkner and Cranston, 1998; Robin et al., 2002) and those who identify as LGB (Garofalo et al., 1998) are more likely than their heterosexual peers to be threatened or injured with a weapon at school and to skip school because they feel unsafe. (Few population-based studies have assessed risk factors affecting the health of LGBT youth beyond violence. Those that have [Garofalo et al., 1998; O'Shaughnessy et al., 2004] have found significantly higher rates of health problems among LGB youth compared with their heterosexual peers.)

Concerns about their safety have consequences for the academic achievement of LGBT youth. O'Shaughnessy and colleagues (2004) examined data from the 2002 California Healthy Kids Survey (n = 237,544) and the 2003 Preventing School Harassment Survey (n = 634) and found that, compared with other students, LGBT students and students perceived to be sexual minorities were more likely to report low grades, to miss school because they felt unsafe, and to report less support from teachers and other adults. Similarly, using data from the 1995 wave of the National Longitudinal Study of Adolescent Health, Russell and colleagues (2001) found that, compared with heterosexual girls, sexual-minority girls as identified by same-sex attraction may hold less positive attitudes about school and may be more likely to have school problems. Both bisexual-attracted boys and girls appear to be significantly more likely to have school troubles and lower grade point averages. The study did not find significant differences in school outcomes or attitudes between heterosexual boys and boys reporting exclusively same-sex attraction.

Using data from waves 1 and 3 of the National Longitudinal Study of Adolescent Health, Himmelstein and Bruckner (2010) examined both school and criminal punishments received by LGB youth. They found that sexual-minority adolescents were 1.25 to 3 times more likely than their heterosexual peers to receive punishment from schools, police, or courts. The authors note that this greater likelihood of punishment is not explained by greater engagement in troublesome behaviors and suggest that LGB youth may be targeted for punishment or that mitigating factors such as self-defense may be overlooked.

Although less research has focused on nonschool settings, LGBT youth experience victimization and violence in their homes, communities, and other institutions. In a 1998 study of 105 LGB youth aged 14–21, family-based victimization, including verbal and physical abuse, was related to disclosure of and openness about sexual orientation (D'Augelli et al., 1998). In addition, results from a convenience sample of 521 LGB youth aged 13–22 suggest that LGB youth experience dating and intimate partner violence at rates that may be similar to those for heterosexual youth (Freedner et al., 2002).

Other than studies in small LGBT-specific journals, very little literature includes or focuses on transgender or gender-variant youth's experience of victimization or violence (Garofalo et al., 2006; McGuire et al., 2010). This lack of attention may be due to limited access to data sets that include transgender youth. Nonetheless, gender-based harassment and victimization clearly are a reality for transgender and gender-variant youth and are directly related to physical and emotional health outcomes. For example, a recent study of school victimization of gender-variant LGBT youth showed that the association between adolescent gender nonconformity and psychosocial adjustment in young adults is impacted by victimization as a result of perceived or actual LGBT status (Toomey et al., 2010).

Substance Use

Disparities in rates of substance use exist between LGB and heterosexual youth, with sexual minority youth reporting increased substance use and initiation of use at younger ages (Corliss et al., 2010; Marshal et al., 2009). The trajectory of substance use also appears to increase more rapidly for LGB youth compared with those who self-identify as heterosexual.

A study using data from the 1994–1996 wave of the National Longitudinal Study of Adolescent Health (n = 12,603) found that sexual-minority adolescent males and females had a higher prevalence of smoking than heterosexual youth (Easton et al., 2008). In a large cohort study using data from the 1999 Growing Up Today Study (n = 10,685), lesbian and bisexual girls (n = 62) were 9.7 times more likely than heterosexual girls (n = 5,475) to have smoked at least weekly in the past year. While there was no significant difference in the likelihood of smoking between gay and bisexual boys (n = 41) and heterosexual boys (n = 3,821), gay and bisexual boys were less likely to have tobacco dependence. In this study, lesbian and bisexual girls were combined for analysis, as were gay and bisexual boys (Austin et al., 2004a).

Another study examining substance use among college students (n = 9,161) found that both self-identified and behaviorally bisexual women had significantly higher odds of cigarette smoking (McCabe et al., 2005). Eisenberg and Wechsler (2003a) examined substance use and sexual behavior in a national sample of sexually active college students (n = 10,301) and found that women with both-sex partners were significantly more likely to smoke than women with exclusively other-sex partners. A significantly increased risk for smoking was not found among women and men with same-sex partners only or men with both-sex partners.

In addition to smoking, LGB youth may be at greater risk than their heterosexual peers for alcohol consumption. Almost a quarter of a community-based sample of young men who have sex with men aged 18–24 (n = 526) reported binge drinking (Wong et al., 2008). Three national studies using data from the National Longitudinal Study of Adolescent Health, the Growing Up Today Study, and the 1999 College Alcohol Study showed that adolescent males and females who indicated they had "both-sex" attractions were more likely to drink alcohol than their heterosexual counterparts (Russell et al., 2002; Ziyadeh et al., 2007). In the previously mentioned study by McCabe and colleagues (2005), no difference in heavy episodic drinking was found between self-identified bisexual and heterosexual females, but there were significantly higher rates of heavy episodic drinking among behaviorally bisexual than behaviorally heterosexual females. In contrast, self-identified and behaviorally bisexual males were significantly less likely than heterosexual males to engage in heavy episodic drinking (McCabe et al., 2005).

Differences in drug use and abuse based on sex may exist among LGB youth. In the previously mentioned study by Ford and Jasinski (2006), bisexual females were more likely than either heterosexual or homosexual students to have used marijuana and other illicit drugs. Other studies support this finding, with self-identified and behaviorally bisexual students, especially females, being more likely than any other group (e.g., lesbian, gay, heterosexual) to report drug use (Eisenberg and Wechsler, 2003a; Russell et al., 2002). On the other hand, McCabe and colleagues (2005) did not find a significant difference in rates of illicit drug use among homosexual, bisexual, and heterosexual college males.

In a community-based sample of 310 young men who have sex with men aged 16–24, methamphetamine use was identified as correlated with high-risk sexual behavior as well as with specific sexualized social contexts (for example, the Internet, bathhouses) (Garofalo et al., 2007b).

The literature highlights a number of potential mediators of substance use in LGB youth. In a study of 156 LGB youth aged 14–21, receiving a rejecting reaction to disclosure of sexual orientation was associated with use and abuse of alcohol, cigarettes, and marijuana (Rosario et al., 2009). Tucker and colleagues (2008) examined other psychosocial factors that may predict substance use among young women. Results of a longitudinal survey of approximately 1,600 young women based on self-reported sexual orientation as either bisexual or heterosexual (participants identifying as lesbian were not included in the analysis) suggest that as adolescents, bisexual women were more likely to have been substance users. Self-identified bisexual participants were also more likely than self-identified heterosexual participants to report holding beliefs in support of drugs, greater perceived parental approval of substance use, increased exposure to peers who used substances, and poorer mental health. By age 23, bisexual women in the study had higher rates of current substance use, greater quantity and frequency of use, and more problematic use (Tucker et al., 2008).

Almost no research has examined substance use among transgender youth. In one study, using a convenience sample of male-to-female transgender youth (n = 51) aged 16–24 from racial and ethnic minority communities, 65 percent reported alcohol use in the last year (Garofalo et al., 2006).

Although self-identified LGB youth engage in greater substance use and earlier initiation of use than heterosexual youth, sufficient evidence does not exist in the literature to determine whether this trend levels out with age. The committee was unable to locate longitudinal or natural history studies examining issues of substance use in these populations. Such studies would be helpful in discerning how patterns of use change over time and whether greater use relative to heterosexual youth levels off as these young people age into adulthood. There also has been little research on interventions specifically targeting substance use in LGBT youth.

Homelessness

Lesbian, gay, and bisexual youth are disproportionately represented among the homeless youth population. Studies of homelessness using a variety of samples have reported that 22–35 percent of their samples comprise sexual-minority youth (Cochran et al., 2002; Rew et al., 2002; Van Leeuwen et al., 2006). Studies specific to sexual minorities suggest that LGB youth are at increased risk of homelessness (Cochran et al., 2002; Gwadz et al., 2004; Milburn et al., 2006; Rew et al., 2002; Whitbeck et al., 2004). Furthermore, Gwadz and colleagues (2004) report that, in their sample of 569 young men who have sex with men, the probability of becoming homeless increased with age. Additionally, compared with young men who have sex with men who self-identified as homosexual or gay, the likelihood of homelessness was four times greater for those young men who have sex with men who identified as heterosexual, three times greater for those who identified as bisexual, and twice as likely for those who identified as transgender. The literature tends to define sexual orientation by behavior rather than by identity or attractions, thereby failing to account for the unique challenges faced by youth who engage in same-sex survival sex (sex for money, food, etc.) or the complex impact sexual identity may have on risk factors. Therefore, these findings are especially useful in helping to identify how sexual identity (as opposed to sexual behavior) may impact risk.

A review by Coker and colleagues (2010) highlights that the general risks associated with homelessness are exacerbated for LGB youth. In studies examining both sexual-minority and heterosexual homeless youth, the sexual-minority youth were shown to be at significantly greater risk for mental health issues (Cochran et al., 2002; Gangamma et al., 2008; Noell and Ochs, 2001; Whitbeck et al., 2004), including suicidal ideation and/or suicide attempts (Leslie et al., 2002; Noell and Ochs, 2001; Van Leeuwen et al., 2006).

In a study examining homeless adolescents (n = 227), LGB youth (n = 37) were significantly more likely than heterosexual youth to report discrimination due to being homeless (Milburn et al., 2006) and to have been sexually and/or physically victimized while homeless (Cochran et al., 2002; Whitbeck et al., 2004). Likewise, although homeless or street-involved LGB youth appear to be more likely than homeless heterosexual youth to be tested for HIV and other STIs (Rew et al., 2005; Solorio et al., 2006; Van Leeuwen et al., 2006), they also appear to engage in more sexual risk behaviors (Kipke et al., 2007), making them more likely to contract such infections (Gangamma et al., 2008; Marshall et al., 2010). And various studies have found that young men who have sex with men are significantly more likely than young heterosexual men to engage in survival sex after becoming homeless (Gangamma et al., 2008; Marshall et al., 2010; Russell et al., 2001; Van Leeuwen et al., 2006; Whitbeck et al., 2004). The literature also suggests that homeless young men who have sex with men are more likely than nonhomeless young men who have sex with men to use controlled substances (Clatts et al., 2005) and to have a lifetime history of substance use (Clatts et al., 2005). Therefore, it is apparent from the literature not only that LGB youth are at greater risk for homelessness than their heterosexual peers, but also that once homeless, LGB youth are more likely to experience multiple risk factors and significantly more negative outcomes.

Research on LGB homelessness has utilized both cross-sectional and longitudinal designs, and most studies have occurred in large, urban settings. The majority of samples have been recruited through venue-based convenience sampling and with the assistance of social service agencies. To the best of the committee's knowledge, there has been no published research on interventions directed at decreasing homelessness or alleviating negative outcomes among homeless LGB youth.

More problematic is that there has been very little research focused directly on the specific needs of homeless youth who are LGBT. Given the magnitude of the risks to which sexual- and gender-minority homeless youth are exposed, the scholarship on this particular issue lacks the depth needed to fully assess the problem or to inform the development of interventions. For example, the majority of studies provide comparisons of homeless LGB and heterosexual youth, outlining the basic risks without examining the mechanisms of those risks in depth. Understanding the mechanisms of risks is critically important, as highlighted by the case study of HIV in Chapter 2. In the case of HIV, the failure to examine mechanisms of risk among LGBT youth, specifically young men who have sex with men and young transgender women, has hindered the development of interventions for these high-risk groups.

There is almost no literature examining the risks of homelessness faced by transgender youth. The limited research that has been done on transgender females using small convenience samples suggests that they are at significant risk for homelessness (Garofalo et al., 2006; Wilson et al., 2009). There are hardly any data on homelessness among transgender males.

Childhood Abuse

Most of the literature on childhood abuse is based on adults reporting retrospectively about their childhood and/or adolescence. Chapters 5 and 6 present some of that literature. However, in secondary analyses of data from seven population-based high school health surveys in the United States and Canada, Saewyc and colleagues (2006) found that the prevalence of sexual and physical abuse was significantly higher for sexual minorities than for their heterosexual peers in nearly all of the surveys. In a survey of 391 young women aged 18–24, Austin and colleagues (2008) found that, compared with heterosexual females, "mostly heterosexual females" reported higher rates of childhood sexual abuse. More research is needed to determine what impact childhood emotional, physical, and sexual abuse has on LGBT youth, including how disclosure or nondisclosure of sexual identity relates to this abuse; when the abuse is taking place; and what interventions might be appropriate.

Protective Factors

While some may view the absence of risk factors as protective, there is, as noted earlier, a paucity of data on specific protective factors that affect the health of LGBT youth. When examining protective factors, it is important to focus on multiple levels: the individual level, interactional levels (e.g., family, school, or peers), and the broader systems level. The few studies that have examined protective factors for LGBT youth have considered individual and interactional factors, such as self-esteem (Savin-Williams, 1989a,b), school support, and family relatedness (Eisenberg and Resnick, 2006). Saewyc and colleagues (2009), using data from six large-scale school-based surveys, compared family connectedness, school connectedness, and religious involvement among bisexual adolescents with the same protective factors among heterosexual, mostly heterosexual, and homosexual adolescents. The results showed that in almost all of the cohorts, bisexual adolescent boys and girls tended to report lower levels of family and school connectedness compared with heterosexual adolescents. Similarly, Sheets and Mohr (2009) examined the relationship between social support and psychosocial functioning in 210 self-identified bisexual college students aged 18–25 and found that the level of support of both family and friends predicted depression, life satisfaction, and internalized negative feelings about bisexuality. Using data from the previously mentioned 2004 Minnesota Student Survey (n = 21,927), Eisenberg and Resnick (2006) studied four protective factors (family connectedness, teacher caring, other adult caring, and school safety) and their association with suicidal ideation and attempts among high school students with same-sex sexual experience. Based on their sex partners, the students were classified as LGB or non-LGB, and data on the LGB students were analyzed as a whole. The researchers found that family connectedness, adult caring, and school safety were significantly protective against suicidal ideation and attempts.

The systemic exposure to stigma that LGBT children and adolescents experience from early ages calls for studying protective factors that are unique to LGBT youth in addition to those that can be found among heterosexual youth (Russell, 2005). While little research has focused on protective factors unique to LGB youth, several studies may provide insight. For example, an association was found between high self-esteem among young gay men (n = 214) and their being open about their gay identity with their mothers (Savin-Williams, 1989a), as well as holding positive attitudes about homosexuality (Savin-Williams, 1989b). These findings may warrant further research. Another potential protective factor may be disclosure of sexual identity. In one study of 156 LGB youth participating in an HIV prevention program, youth who disclosed their sexual identity to more people in their support networks were less likely to have high levels of distress related to their sexual identity, which has been associated with mental health problems in LGB youth (Wright and Perry, 2006). However, disclosure of identity is a multifaceted issue, and as noted in the above discussion of risk factors, may also lead to harassment and victimization (D'Augelli, 2002). Ryan and colleagues (2010) found protective effects related to specific accepting family reactions to adolescents' LGBT identity—such as advocating for the youth when they were discriminated against or welcoming their LGBT friends and partners to family events and activities. In their community sample of LGBT young adults (n = 245), those who experienced high levels of family acceptance reported significantly lower rates of depression, substance abuse, and suicidal ideation and attempts compared with those who reported no or low levels of family acceptance. Unique protective factors for LGBT youth warrant further study, particularly to inform services and approaches to caring for LGBT adolescents.

A small body of research has begun to evaluate the impact of school policies and procedures on the experiences of LGB students (Szalacha, 2003). Blake and colleagues (2001), using data (n = 4,159) from the 1995 Massachusetts Youth Risk Behavior Survey, found an association between LGB students who attended schools with gay-sensitive HIV instruction and less sexual risk taking than their LGB peers in other schools. Goodenow and colleagues (2006) analyzed data from the 1999 Massachusetts Youth Risk Behavior Survey and a 1998 state survey of high school principals to examine the relationship among school supports, victimization, and suicidality among LGB youth. They found that LGB students (n = 202) who attended schools with supportive staff, antibullying policies, and gay–straight alliance clubs were less likely to report being victimized, skipping school because of fear of victimization, or attempting suicide compared with those in other schools. They also found that sexual-minority youth in larger schools with more low-income and ethnically diverse students experienced lower rates of victimization and suicidality. In the previously mentioned study by O'Shaughnessy and colleagues (2004), results showed that students at schools with antiharassment policies reported feeling safer and less likely to be harassed. Similarly, students were less likely to report being harassed or feeling unsafe at schools with gay–straight alliance clubs and teachers who intervened to stop harassment. Another study comparing sexual minorities at colleges with and without LGB resources found that sexual-minority women were less likely to smoke at colleges with LGB resources, but sexual-minority men were more likely to binge drink at these same colleges (Eisenberg and Wechsler, 2003b). These conflicting findings indicate the need for further study to understand protective factors.

HEALTH SERVICES

In addition to addressing specific needs related to sexual orientation and gender identity, primary care for LGBT adolescents, as for all adolescents, should be sensitive, comprehensive, and high-quality. Preventive health and health maintenance visits should include periodic, private, and confidential discussions of a range of health and health-related issues, including sexuality and sex (Frankowski and American Academy of Pediatrics Committee on Adolescence, 2004). These discussions should address identity-related feelings and concerns, as well as behaviors and experiences that can affect health and development.

Access and Utilization

With the recent implementation of health care reform, access to health services has increased for many youth since they can now be covered under their parents' insurance until age 26. However, this increased access may be less relevant for those LGBT youth who are not cared for by their families.

In some U.S. cities, specialized health care centers are available to provide comprehensive care to LGB youth. In addition to primary care services, these centers provide other services, such as case management, counseling, and support groups. Organizations such as the Gay and Lesbian Medical Association have websites that offer listings of health care professionals who are able to provide appropriate care to LGB patients. However, not all LGB youth have access to such centers or health care professionals; most receive health care from providers in their own community who also provide care to non-LGB youth. Nationally, family physicians are the primary care providers for the majority of youth aged 15–24, and overall they are insufficiently trained to provide care to LGBT youth (IOM, 2009).

In a study of the experiences of transgender youth with physical and mental health services (n = 26), the youth reported a lack of access to health care for the prevention and treatment of STIs, transition-related health services, and mental health services; they attributed this lack of access to discrimination by providers (Grossman and D'Augelli, 2006). As with LGB youth, while centers exist that specialize in providing care to transgender patients, not all transgender youth have access to these centers.

Quality of Care

Studies utilizing convenience samples of LGBT youth show that they value the same health provider characteristics as other youth. Specifically, they wish to receive private and confidential services, to be treated with respect and honesty, and to be seen by providers who are well trained and have good listening and communication skills (Ginsburg et al., 2002; Hoffman et al., 2009).

Whether LGB or straight, adolescents often are uncomfortable with initiating discussions about sex (including sexual orientation) with their providers; thus, it is incumbent on those who provide health services to youth to initiate such discussions. Studies of LGB youth (using small convenience samples) show that substantial percentages have not disclosed their sexual orientation to their physician; these include youth who describe themselves as being out to almost everyone in their lives (Allen et al., 1998; Meckler et al., 2006). In a sample of 60 pediatricians and adolescent medicine specialists responding to a mailed survey, more than half reported that they do not usually include sexual orientation in their sexual histories, and a large majority had some reservations about broaching the issue with patients (East and El Rayess, 1998). In a more recent self-administered survey, most physicians reported that they did not discuss sexual orientation, sexual attraction, or gender identity with their adolescent patients. A majority of respondents indicated they would not address sexual orientation even if their patient were depressed, had suicidal thoughts, or had attempted suicide. Physicians reported that they did not feel they could adequately address sexual orientation issues with their patients (Kitts, 2010). In a similar study, 70 percent of physicians reported that they did not discuss sexual orientation with their adolescent patients. Many of those physicians reported a fear of offending patients and a lack of knowledge about the treatment needs of sexual-minority patients (Lena et al., 2002). Furthermore, data from a variety of samples suggest that many clinicians may have negative attitudes toward LGBT individuals. These attitudes may affect clinicians' ability to provide appropriate care to these populations (Kaiser Family Foundation, 2002; Klamen et al., 1999; Sanchez et al., 2006; Smith and Mathews, 2007).

CONTEXTUAL INFLUENCES

The health of LGBT children and adolescents is shaped by contextual influences such as sociodemographic and familial factors. Limited research exploring these factors has been conducted.

Sociodemographic Factors

Few recent population-based studies have published substantive sociodemographic findings on LGBT youth. However, studies with smaller samples suggest that sociodemographic factors play a role in the lives of LGBT youth. For example, in a community-based sample of 145 sexual-minority youth aged 14–21, Rosario and colleagues (2004) found racial and ethnic differences in the timing of the coming out process. Similarly, a recent retrospective study of a community-based sample of 245 LGBT young adults on family acceptance during their adolescence found an association between family acceptance and parental job status, with highly accepting families having higher parental job status (Ryan et al., 2010). The same study also explored religion as a factor in family acceptance and found that participants who reported a religious affiliation in childhood also reported lower family acceptance compared with participants with no childhood religious affiliation (Ryan et al., 2010).

Drawing on population-based data obtained from students in 7th through 12th grades in British Columbia, Poon and Saewyc (2009) compared adolescents from rural and urban areas. They found differences between the groups on some health outcomes (for example, rural sexual-minority youth were more likely than their urban peers to binge drink) and further noted that the interaction between gender and location produced different outcomes. Rural boys were more likely to have considered or attempted suicide in the past year than rural girls or urban boys, and rural girls were more likely than urban girls or rural boys to have been physically assaulted at school.

More community-based and population-based research on the lives of LGBT adolescents is needed to document the role of sociodemographic factors and their impact on health. Community-based research can help inform the questions in this area for population-based surveys.

Familial Factors

Although connections to family have been shown to be protective against major health risk behaviors, the literature on LGB youth and families has been very limited in scope and quantity, and has focused mainly on negative aspects of the relationships between LGB youth and their parents. Little research has examined the family experiences of transgender youth. Exceptions include research conducted by Grossman and colleagues (Grossman and D'Augelli, 2006; Grossman et al., 2005) as part of a larger study of LGBT youth using a convenience sample and Ryan and colleagues' (2010) research on LGBT adolescents, young adults, and families.

Family-related research has been based on reports of LGBT youth themselves and rarely on reports of parents or other family members, especially among ethnically diverse groups. Research has continued to document fear of coming out to parents (D'Augelli et al., 1998), which remains a persistent concern for LGB youth (D'Augelli et al., 2010) despite considerable social changes over the past two decades.

Other research has measured parental rejection and support among LGBT adolescents and young adults in several ways. Rosario and colleagues (2009) examined substance use among LGB youth (n = 156) and asked the youth whether they perceived reactions to their LGB identity from a range of people (including family members, coaches, teachers, and friends) to be accepting, neutral, or rejecting. The number of perceived rejecting reactions was found to predict substance use. Although accepting reactions did not directly reduce substance use, such reactions buffered the link between rejecting reactions and alcohol use.

Needham and Austin (2010) assessed the relationship between LGB young adults' perceived family support (e.g., general closeness, warmth, and enjoying time together) and depression, substance use, and suicidality using data on young adults from wave 3 of the National Longitudinal Study of Adolescent Health (n = 11,153). They found that parental support either partially or fully mediated associations related to suicidal thoughts, recent drug use, and depressive symptomatology.

Ryan and colleagues (2009) measured specific parental rejecting behaviors in a sample of 224 LGB young adults, recruited from community organizations, who were open about their LGB identity to at least one parent or caregiver during adolescence. They found associations between parental rejection and use of illegal drugs, depression, attempted suicide, and sexual health risk. A subsequent study of specific parental and caregiver supportive behaviors during adolescence found that family acceptance during adolescence predicted increased self-esteem, social support, and general health status, and also protected against depression, substance abuse, and suicidal ideation and behaviors among LGB young adults (Ryan et al., 2010).

Results of the above studies provide evidence to inform family interventions aimed at reducing risk and promoting well-being among LGBT children and adolescents, thereby reducing health disparities and affecting outcomes across the life course.

Little research has focused on LGBT youth in custodial care—foster care or juvenile justice—although reports from providers have noted a high proportion of LGBT youth in these systems over many years. Researchers and providers have documented the experiences of LGBT individuals involved in these systems in a series of listening forums across the United States (Child Welfare League of America, 2006). In addition, experts have developed model standards for care of LGBT youth in foster care and juvenile justice settings that are informed by research (Wilbur et al., 2006).

SUMMARY OF KEY FINDINGS AND RESEARCH OPPORTUNITIES

Findings

Although the data on LGBT youth are scarce, the available research offers a number of important findings about the health status of these populations. Key findings are presented below.

Development of Sexual Orientation and Gender Identity

- As a result of the ongoing process of sexual development and awareness among adolescents, self-identification of sexual orientation and the sex of sexual partners may change over time and may not necessarily be congruent.
- Some research examining sexual identity development among ethnically diverse sexual-minority adolescents suggests that the process may differ as adolescents negotiate both ethnic and sexual orientation identity.
- A relatively small percentage of gender-variant children may develop an adult transgender identity.
- Gender-variant children may have more difficulties with peer relationships and behavioral problems than non-gender-variant children.

Mental Health Status

- LGB youth are at increased risk for suicidal ideation, attempted suicide, and depression. This increased risk appears to be consistent across age group, gender, race, and self-identified orientation. A few studies with small nonprobability samples suggest the same is true for transgender youth.
- Potential risk factors for increased rates of suicidal ideation and suicide attempts specific to LGB youth include sexual-minority status, homophobic victimization and stress, and family rejection.
- A few studies show that LGB youth may demonstrate higher rates of disordered eating than heterosexual youth.

Physical Health Status

- Pregnancy rates may be the same or possibly even higher for lesbian and bisexual girls than for heterosexual girls.

- Self-identified sexual-minority females may have elevated BMIs relative to their heterosexual peers.
- While GnRH analogs may be used to alleviate gender dysphoria among adolescents, a paucity of empirical data exists concerning how these medical interventions affect overall physical health and well-being.
- The burden of HIV infection falls disproportionately on young men who have sex with men, particularly young black men who have sex with men. These racial disparities are likely due to the intersection of race, sexual orientation, and other social determinants. Additionally, interventions are lacking for this group of LGBT youth.
- Limited studies suggest that male-to-female transgender youth may face a risk for HIV similar to or even higher than that faced by young men who have sex with men.

Risk and Protective Factors

- LGBT youth report experiencing elevated levels of harassment, victimization, and violence. School-based victimization due to known or perceived identity has been documented, although very little literature exists on violence experienced by young lesbians, bisexual women, or transgender people.
- Compared with other students, sexual-minority youth may be more likely to report feeling unsafe at school, being offered weaker support by school staff, and receiving lower grades.
- Rates of substance use, including smoking and alcohol consumption, may be higher among LGB than heterosexual youth. Almost no research has examined substance use among transgender youth. Few interventions have been developed to address these disparities.
- The homeless youth population comprises a disproportionate number of LGB youth. Some research suggests that young transgender women are also at significant risk for homelessness. There are almost no data on homelessness among young transgender men. Interventions designed to decrease homelessness are lacking, and limited research on the specific health needs of homeless LGBT youth has been conducted.
- The prevalence of childhood abuse may be higher among sexual-minority youth compared with their heterosexual peers.
- The few studies that have examined protective factors for LGBT youth suggest that family connectedness and school safety are two possible areas for intervention research.

- Limited studies evaluating the impact of school polices on the experiences of LGB students indicate that students attending schools with antiharassment policies report that they feel safer and are less likely to be harassed.
- Family acceptance among LGBT youth may be a protective factor against depression, substance use, and suicidal ideation and attempts.

Health Services

- LGBT youth may lack access to health care professionals who are able to provide appropriate care to LGBT patients.
- Small studies suggest that many LGB youth have not disclosed their sexual orientation to their physician. Similarly, there appears to be some unease among physicians about addressing sexual orientation with their adolescent patients.

Contextual Influences

- Population-level data on sociodemographic factors that affect LGBT youth are lacking. Studies with small samples suggest that sociodemographic factors, including race, ethnicity, geography, religion, and socioeconomic status, play a role in the lives of LGBT youth.
- While research on families suggests that family support may be protective, most research has focused on negative interactions with families. Results of this research suggest that family rejection may be associated with negative mental health outcomes.

Research Opportunities

Research on all adolescents, regardless of their sexual orientation or gender identity, is limited. However, research on the health status of LGBT youth is particularly challenging. Other than small studies based on convenience samples, the committee found no studies addressing health and health care for subgroups of LGBT youth, such as racial and ethnic minorities, or health and health care for transgender youth. While a few studies on LGBT health have included bisexual youth, research examining health and health care for this group specifically is quite limited. Both cross-sectional and longitudinal research is especially needed to explore the demographic realities of LGBT youth in an intersectional and social ecology framework, and to illuminate the mechanisms of both risk and resilience so that appropriate interventions for LGBT youth can be developed. These parameters could be brought to bear in research in the following areas:

- **Demographic and descriptive information**, including the percentage of adolescents who are LGBT and how that percentage varies by demographic characteristics such as race, ethnicity, socioeconomic status, geography, and religion; also, the general experiences and health status of LGBT adolescents and how these vary by demographic characteristics.
- **Family and interpersonal relations**, including the family life of LGBT youth from diverse backgrounds (e.g., race/ethnicity, socioeconomic status) and school and social life concomitants of LGBT identity and attraction, with special attention to protective factors at the individual, interactional (family, school, peers), and systems levels; also patterns and experiences of homelessness among LGBT youth, as well as intrafamily and domestic violence (e.g., sexual abuse, abuse by parents, intimate partner violence) and anti-LGBT victimization.
- **Health services**, including barriers to access (particularly related to identity disclosure and interactions with providers), utilization rates, and quality of care received.
- **Mental health**, including the diagnosis of disorders among LGBT youth, their rates of suicidal behavior and suicidality, identity-related issues and experiences of stigma and discrimination, and eating disorders.
- **Physical health**, including obesity and substance use (including smoking and alcohol use).
- **Sexual and reproductive health**, including sexual development, sexual health, reproductive health, risk behaviors, pregnancy, STIs, and HIV rates and interventions (with a focus on natural history studies of high-risk groups).
- **Transgender-specific health care**, including the effects, benefits, and risks of puberty-delaying hormone therapy.

REFERENCES

Agronick, G., L. O'Donnell, A. Stueve, A. S. Doval, R. Duran, and S. Vargo. 2004. Sexual behaviors and risks among bisexually- and gay-identified young Latino men. *AIDS & Behavior* 8(2):185–197.

Allen, L. B., A. D. Glicken, R. K. Beach, and K. E. Naylor. 1998. Adolescent health care experience of gay, lesbian, and bisexual young adults. *Journal of Adolescent Health* 23(4):212–220.

Almeida, J., R. M. Johnson, H. L. Corliss, B. E. Molnar, and D. Azrael. 2009. Emotional distress among LGBT youth: The influence of perceived discrimination based on sexual orientation. *Journal of Youth & Adolescence* 38(7):1001–1014.

AMA (American Medical Association). 2010. *Health care needs of the homosexual population. AMA policy regarding sexual orientation.* http://www.ama-assn.org/ama/pub/about-ama/our-people/member-groups-sections/glbt-advisory-committee/ama-policy-regarding-sexual-orientation.shtml (accessed September 2, 2010).

American Psychiatric Association. 2000a. *Therapies focused on attempts to change sexual orientation (reparative or conversion therapies): Position statement.* http://www.psych.org/Departments/EDU/Library/APAOfficialDocumentsandRelated/PositionStatements/200001.aspx (accessed September 2, 2010).

American Psychiatric Association. 2000b. *Diagnostic and Statistical Manual of Mental Disorders (Fourth Edition) (DSM-IV-TR).* Washington, DC: American Psychiatric Association.

American Psychological Association. 2009. *Report of the task force on appropriate therapeutic responses to sexual orientation.* Washington, DC: American Psychological Association.

Austin, S. B., N. Ziyadeh, L. B. Fisher, J. A. Kahn, G. A. Colditz, and A. L. Frazier. 2004a. Sexual orientation and tobacco use in a cohort study of US adolescent girls and boys. *Archives of Pediatrics & Adolescent Medicine* 158(4):317–322.

Austin, S. B., N. Ziyadeh, J. A. Kahn, C. A. Camargo, Jr., G. A. Colditz, and A. E. Field. 2004b. Sexual orientation, weight concerns, and eating-disordered behaviors in adolescent girls and boys. *Journal of the American Academy of Child & Adolescent Psychiatry* 43(9):1115–1123.

Austin, S. B., A. L. Roberts, H. L. Corliss, and B. E. Molnar. 2008. Sexual violence victimization history and sexual risk indicators in a community-based urban cohort of "mostly heterosexual" and heterosexual young women. *American Journal of Public Health* 98(6):1015–1020.

Austin, S., N. J. Ziyadeh, H. L. Corliss, M. Rosario, D. Wypij, J. Haines, C. A. Camargo, Jr., and A. E. Field. 2009a. Sexual orientation disparities in purging and binge eating from early to late adolescence. *Journal of Adolescent Health* 45(3):238–245.

Austin, S. B., N. J. Ziyadeh, H. L. Corliss, J. Haines, H. R. Rockett, D. Wypij, and A. E. Field. 2009b. Sexual orientation disparities in weight status in adolescence: Findings from a prospective study. *Obesity* 17(9):1776–1782.

Benestad, E. E. P. 2009. Addressing the disturbed, like ripples in water: Intervention with the social networks of children who transe. *Sexual and Relationship Therapy* 24(2):207–216.

Birkett, M., D. L. Espelage, and B. Koenig. 2009. LGB and questioning students in schools: The moderating effects of homophobic bullying and school climate on negative outcomes. *Journal of Youth & Adolescence* 38(7):989–1000.

Blake, S. M., R. Ledsky, T. Lehman, C. Goodenow, R. Sawyer, and T. Hack. 2001. Preventing sexual risk behaviors among gay, lesbian, and bisexual adolescents: The benefits of gay-sensitive HIV instruction in schools. *American Journal of Public Health* 91(6):940–946.

Bockting, W. O., and R. Ehrbar. 2006. Commentary: Gender variance, dissonance, or identity disorder. *Journal of Psychology and Human Sexuality* 17(3/4):125–134.

Bontempo, D. E., and A. R. D'Augelli. 2002. Effects of at-school victimization and sexual orientation on lesbian, gay, or bisexual youths' health risk behavior. *Journal of Adolescent Health* 30(5):364–374.

Boxer, A. M., and B. J. Cohler. 1989. The life course of gay and lesbian youth: An immodest proposal for the study of lives. *Journal of Homosexuality* 17(3-4):315–355.

Brill, S. A., and A. Pepper. 2008. *The transgender child: A handbook for families and professionals.* Berkeley, CA: Cleis Press.

Cass, V. C. 1979. Homosexual identity formation: A theoretical model. *Journal of Homosexuality* 4(3):219–235.

CDC (Centers for Disease Control and Prevention). 2008. Trends in HIV/AIDS diagnoses among men who have sex with men—33 states, 2001–2006. *Morbidity and Mortality Weekly Report* 57(25):681–686.

CDC. 2009. Sexual and reproductive health of persons aged 10–24 years—United States, 2002–2007. http://www.cdc.gov/mmwr/preview/mmwrhtml/ss5806a1.htm (accessed July 17, 2009).

Child Welfare League of America. 2006. *Out of the margins: A report on regional listening forums highlighting the experiences of lesbian, gay, bisexual and transgender youth in care*. Washington, DC: Child Welfare League of America.

Choi, K.-H., D. Operario, S. E. Gregorich, W. McFarland, D. MacKellar, and L. Valleroy. 2005. Substance use, substance choice, and unprotected anal intercourse among young Asian American and Pacific Islander men who have sex with men. *AIDS Education & Prevention* 17(5):418–429.

Clatts, M. C., L. Goldsamt, H. Yi, and M. V. Gwadz. 2005. Homelessness and drug abuse among young men who have sex with men in New York City: A preliminary epidemiological trajectory. *Journal of Adolescence* 28(2):201–214.

Clements-Nolle, K., R. Marx, R. Guzman, and M. Katz. 2001. HIV prevalence, risk behaviors, health care use, and mental health status of transgender persons: Implications for public health intervention. *American Journal of Public Health* 91(6):915–921.

Clements-Nolle, K., R. Marx, and M. Katz. 2006. Attempted suicide among transgender persons: The influence of gender-based discrimination and victimization. *Journal of Homosexuality* 51(3):53–69.

Cochran, B. N., A. J. Stewart, J. A. Ginzler, and A. M. Cauce. 2002. Challenges faced by homeless sexual minorities: Comparison of gay, lesbian, bisexual, and transgender homeless adolescents with their heterosexual counterparts. *American Journal of Public Health* 92(5):773–777.

Cohen-Kettenis, P. T., and S. H. M. van Goozen. 1997. Sex reassignment of adolescent transsexuals: A follow-up study. *Journal of the American Academy of Child & Adolescent Psychiatry* 36(2):263.

Cohen-Kettenis, P. T., A. Owen, V. G. Kaijser, S. J. Bradley, and K. J. Zucker. 2003. Demographic characteristics, social competence, and behavior problems in children with gender identity disorder: A cross-national, cross-clinic comparative analysis. *Journal of Abnormal Child Psychology* 31(1):41.

Cohen-Kettenis, P. T., H. A. Delemarre-van de Waal, and L. J. G. Gooren. 2008. The treatment of adolescent transsexuals: Changing insights. *The Journal of Sexual Medicine* 5(8):1892–1897.

Coker, T. R., S. B. Austin, and M. A. Schuster. 2010. The health and health care of lesbian, gay, and bisexual adolescents. *Annual Review of Public Health* 31:457–477.

Corliss, H. L., S. D. Cochran, V. M. Mays, S. Greenland, and T. E. Seeman. 2009. Age of minority sexual orientation development and risk of childhood maltreatment and suicide attempts in women. *American Journal of Orthopsychiatry* 79(4):511–521.

Corliss, H. L., M. Rosario, D. Wypij, S. A. Wylie, A. L. Frazier, and S. B. Austin. 2010. Sexual orientation and drug use in a longitudinal cohort study of U.S. adolescents. *Addictive Behaviors* 35(5):517–521.

D'Augelli, A. R. 2002. Mental health problems among lesbian, gay, and bisexual youths ages 14 to 21. *Clinical Child Psychology and Psychiatry* 7(3):433–456.

D'Augelli, A. R. 2006. Developmental and contextual factors and mental health among lesbian, gay, and bisexual youths. In *Sexual orientation and mental health: Examining identity and development in lesbian, gay, and bisexual people*, edited by A. M. Omoto and H. S. Kurtzman. Washington, DC: American Psychological Association. Pp. 37–53.

D'Augelli, A. R., and S. L. Hershberger. 1993. Lesbian, gay, and bisexual youth in community settings: Personal challenges and mental health problems. *American Journal of Community Psychology* 21(4):421–448.

D'Augelli, A. R., S. L. Hershberger, and N. W. Pilkington. 1998. Lesbian, gay, and bisexual youth and their families: Disclosure of sexual orientation and its consequences. *American Journal of Orthopsychiatry* 68(3):361–371.

D'Augelli, A. R., N. W. Pilkington, and S. L. Hershberger. 2002. Incidence and mental health impact of sexual orientation victimization of lesbian, gay, and bisexual youths in high school. *School Psychology Quarterly* 17(2):148–167.

D'Augelli, A. R., A. H. Grossman, N. P. Salter, J. J. Vasey, M. T. Starks, and K. O. Sinclair. 2005. Predicting the suicide attempts of lesbian, gay, and bisexual youth. *Suicide & Life-Threatening Behavior* 35(6):646–660.

D'Augelli, A. R., J. H. Rendina, K. O. Sinclair, and A. H. Grossman. 2006/2007. Lesbian and gay youth's aspirations for marriage and raising children. *Journal of LGBT Issues in Counseling* 1(4):77–98.

D'Augelli, A. R., A. H. Grossman, M. T. Starks, and K. O. Sinclair. 2010. Factors associated with parents' knowledge of gay, lesbian, and bisexual youths' sexual orientation. *Journal of LGBT Family Studies* 6(2):178–198.

de Vries, A. L., T. D. Steensma, T. A. Doreleijers, and P. T. Cohen-Kettenis. 2010. Puberty suppression in adolescents with gender identity disorder: A prospective follow-up study. *Journal of Sexual Medicine*. http://onlinelibrary.wiley.com/doi/10.11.11/j.1743-6109.2010.09143.x/full (accessed May 25, 2011).

Delemarre-van de Waal, H. A., and P. T. Cohen-Kettenis. 2006. Clinical management of gender identity disorder in adolescents: A protocol on psychological and paediatric endocrinology aspects. *European Journal of Endocrinology* 155(Suppl. 1):S131–137.

Di Ceglie, D. 2009. Engaging young people with atypical gender identity development in therapeutic work: A developmental approach. *Journal of Child Psychotherapy* 35(1):3–12.

Diamond, C., H. Thiede, T. Perdue, G. M. Secura, L. Valleroy, D. Mackellar, L. Corey, and T. Seattle Young Men's Survey. 2003. Viral hepatitis among young men who have sex with men: Prevalence of infection, risk behaviors, and vaccination. *Sexually Transmitted Diseases* 30(5):425–432.

Do, T. D., S. Chen, W. McFarland, G. M. Secura, S. K. Behel, D. A. MacKellar, L. A. Valleroy, and K. H. Cho. 2005. HIV testing patterns and unrecognized HIV infection among young Asian and Pacific Islander men who have sex with men in San Francisco. *AIDS Education & Prevention* 17(6):540–554.

DuRant, R. H., D. P. Krowchuk, and S. H. Sinal. 1998. Victimization, use of violence, and drug use at school among male adolescents who engage in same-sex sexual behavior. *Journal of Pediatrics* 133(1):113–118.

East, J. A., and F. El Rayess. 1998. Pediatricians' approach to the health care of lesbian, gay, and bisexual youth. *Journal of Adolescent Health* 23(4):191–193.

Easton, A., K. Jackson, P. Mowery, D. Comeau, and R. Sell. 2008. Adolescent same-sex and both-sex romantic attractions and relationships: Implications for smoking. *American Journal of Public Health* 98(3):462–467.

Eisenberg, M. E., and M. D. Resnick. 2006. Suicidality among gay, lesbian and bisexual youth: The role of protective factors. *Journal of Adolescent Health* 39(5):662–668.

Eisenberg, M. E., and H. Wechsler. 2003a. Substance use behaviors among college students with same-sex and opposite-sex experience: Results from a national study. *Addictive Behaviors* 28(5):899–913.

Eisenberg, M. E., and H. Wechsler. 2003b. Social influences on substance-use behaviors of gay, lesbian, and bisexual college students: Findings from a national study. *Social Science & Medicine* 57(10):1913–1923.

Faulkner, A. H., and K. Cranston. 1998. Correlates of same-sex sexual behavior in a random sample of Massachusetts high school students. *American Journal of Public Health* 88(2):262–266.

Fergusson, D. M., L. J. Horwood, and A. L. Beautrais. 1999. Is sexual orientation related to mental health problems and suicidality in young people? *Archives of General Psychiatry* 56(10):876–880.

Ford, J. A., and J. L. Jasinski. 2006. Sexual orientation and substance use among college students. *Addictive Behaviors* 31(3):404–413.

Frankowski, B. L., and American Academy of Pediatrics Committee on Adolescence. 2004. Sexual orientation and adolescents. *Pediatrics* 113(6):1827–1832.

Freedner, N., L. H. Freed, Y. W. Yang, and S. B. Austin. 2002. Dating violence among gay, lesbian, and bisexual adolescents: Results from a community survey. *Journal of Adolescent Health* 31(6):469–474.

Friedman, M. S., G. F. Koeske, A. J. Silvestre, W. S. Korr, and E. W. Sites. 2006. The impact of gender-role nonconforming behavior, bullying, and social support on suicidality among gay male youth. *Journal of Adolescent Health* 38(5):621–623.

Gangamma, R., N. Slesnick, P. Toviessi, and J. Serovich. 2008. Comparison of HIV risks among gay, lesbian, bisexual and heterosexual homeless youth. *Journal of Youth & Adolescence* 37(4):456–464.

Garofalo, R., R. C. Wolf, S. Kessel, S. J. Palfrey, and R. H. DuRant. 1998. The association between health risk behaviors and sexual orientation among a school-based sample of adolescents. *Pediatrics* 101(5):895–902.

Garofalo, R., R. C. Wolf, L. S. Wissow, E. R. Woods, and E. Goodman. 1999. Sexual orientation and risk of suicide attempts among a representative sample of youth. *Archives of Pediatrics & Adolescent Medicine* 153(5):487–493.

Garofalo, R., J. Deleon, E. Osmer, M. Doll, and G. W. Harper. 2006. Overlooked, misunderstood and at-risk: Exploring the lives and HIV risk of ethnic minority male-to-female transgender youth. *Journal of Adolescent Health* 38(3):230–236.

Garofalo, R., A. Herrick, B. S. Mustanski, and G. R. Donenberg. 2007a. Tip of the iceberg: Young men who have sex with men, the internet, and HIV risk. *American Journal of Public Health* 97(6):1113–1117.

Garofalo, R., B. S. Mustanski, D. J. McKirnan, A. Herrick, and G. R. Donenberg. 2007b. Methamphetamine and young men who have sex with men: Understanding patterns and correlates of use and the association with HIV-related sexual risk. *Archives of Pediatrics & Adolescent Medicine* 161(6):591–596.

Garofalo, R., B. Mustanski, and G. Donenberg. 2008. Parents know and parents matter: Is it time to develop family-based HIV prevention programs for young men who have sex with men? *Journal of Adolescent Health* 43(2):201–204.

Garofalo, R., B. Mustanski, A. Johnson, and E. Emerson. 2010. Exploring factors that underlie racial/ethnic disparities in HIV risk among young men who have sex with men. *Journal of Urban Health* 87(2):318–323.

Ginsburg, K. R., R. J. Winn, B. J. Rudy, J. Crawford, H. Zhao, and D. F. Schwarz. 2002. How to reach sexual minority youth in the health care setting: The teens offer guidance. *Journal of Adolescent Health* 31(5):407–416.

Goodenow, C., L. Szalacha, and K. Westheimer. 2006. School support groups, other school factors, and the safety of sexual minority adolescents. *Psychology in the Schools* 43(5): 573–589.

Goodenow, C., L. A. Szalacha, L. E. Robin, and K. Westheimer. 2008. Dimensions of sexual orientation and HIV-related risk among adolescent females: Evidence from a statewide survey. *American Journal of Public Health* 98(6):1051–1058.

Green, R. 1987. *The "sissy boy syndrome" and the development of homosexuality*. New Haven, CT: Yale University Press.

Grossman, A. H., and A. R. D'Augelli. 2006. Transgender youth: Invisible and vulnerable. *Journal of Homosexuality* 51(1):111–128.

Grossman, A. H., and A. R. D'Augelli. 2007. Transgender youth and life-threatening behaviors. *Suicide & Life-Threatening Behavior* 37(5):527–537.

Grossman, A. H., A. R. D'Augelli, T. J. Howell, and S. Hubbard. 2005. Parents' reactions to transgender youths' gender nonconforming expression and identity. *Journal of Gay and Lesbian Social Services* 18(1):3–16.

Guenther-Grey, C. A., S. Varnell, J. I. Weiser, R. M. Mathy, L. O'Donnell, A. Stueve, G. Remafedi, and Community Intervention Trial for Youth Study. 2005. Trends in sexual risk-taking among urban young men who have sex with men, 1999–2002. *Journal of the National Medical Association* 97(Suppl. 7):S38–S43.

Gwadz, M. V., M. C. Clatts, N. R. Leonard, and L. Goldsamt. 2004. Attachment style, childhood adversity, and behavioral risk among young men who have sex with men. *Journal of Adolescent Health* 34(5):402–413.

Harawa, N. T., S. Greenland, T. A. Bingham, D. F. Johnson, S. D. Cochran, W. E. Cunningham, D. D. Celentano, B. A. Koblin, M. LaLota, D. A. MacKellar, W. McFarland, D. Shehan, S. Stoyanoff, H. Thiede, L. Torian, and L. A. Valleroy. 2004. Associations of race/ethnicity with HIV prevalence and HIV-related behaviors among young men who have sex with men in 7 urban centers in the United States. *Journal of Acquired Immune Deficiency Syndromes: JAIDS* 35(5):526–536.

Hart, T. 2001. Lack of training in behavior therapy and research regarding lesbian, gay, bisexual, and transgendered individuals. *The Behavior Therapist* 24(10):217–218.

Hembree, W. C., P. Cohen-Kettenis, H. A. Delemarre-van de Waal, L. J. Gooren, W. J. Meyer, III, N. P. Spack, V. Tangpricha, and V. M. Montori. 2009. Endocrine treatment of transsexual persons: An endocrine society clinical practice guideline. *Journal of Clinical Endocrinology & Metabolism* 94(9):3132–3154.

Herbst, J. H., R. T. Sherba, N. Crepaz, J. B. DeLuca, L. Zohrabyan, R. D. Stall, C. M. Lyles, and HIV/AIDS Prevention Research Synthesis Team. 2005. A meta-analytic review of HIV behavioral interventions for reducing sexual risk behavior of men who have sex with men. *Journal of Acquired Immune Deficiency Syndromes: JAIDS* 39(2):228–241.

Herdt, G., and A. Boxer. 1993. *Children of horizons: How gay and lesbian teens are leading a new way out of the closet.* Boston, MA: Beacon Press.

Herrick, A. L., A. K. Matthews, and R. Garofalo. 2010. Health risk behaviors in an urban sample of young women who have sex with women. *Journal of Lesbian Studies* 14(1):80–92.

Himmelstein, K. E. W., and H. Bruckner. 2010. Criminal-justice and school sanctions against nonheterosexual youth: A national longitudinal study. *Pediatrics* 2009–2306.

Hoffman, N. D., K. Freeman, and S. Swann. 2009. Healthcare preferences of lesbian, gay, bisexual, transgender and questioning youth. *Journal of Adolescent Health* 45(3):222–229.

Huebner, D. M., G. M. Rebchook, and S. M. Kegeles. 2004. Experiences of harassment, discrimination, and physical violence among young gay and bisexual men. *American Journal of Public Health* 94(7):1200–1203.

IOM (Institute of Medicine). 2009. *Adolescent health services: Missing opportunities.* Washington, DC: The National Academies Press.

Jamil, O. B., G. W. Harper, and M. I. Fernandez. 2009. Sexual and ethnic identity development among gay-bisexual-questioning (GBQ) male ethnic minority adolescents. *Cultural Diversity and Ethnic Minority Psychology* 15(3):203–214.

Jiang, Y., D. K. Perry, and J. E. Hesser. 2010. Adolescent suicide and health risk behaviors: Rhode Island's 2007 Youth Risk Behavior Survey. *American Journal of Preventive Medicine* 38(5):551–555.

Johnson, B. T., M. P. Carey, K. L. Marsh, K. D. Levin, and L. A. J. Scott-Sheldon. 2003. Interventions to reduce sexual risk for the human immunodeficiency virus in adolescents, 1985–2000: A research synthesis. *Archives of Pediatrics & Adolescent Medicine* 157(4):381–388.

Just the Facts Coalition. 2008. *Just the facts about sexual orientation and youth: A primer for principals, educators, and school personnel.* Washington, DC: American Psychological Association.

Kaiser Family Foundation. 2002. *National Survey of Physicians Part I: Doctors on disparities in medical care*. Washington, DC: The Kaiser Family Foundation.

Kegeles, S. M., R. B. Hays, and T. J. Coates. 1996. The mpowerment project: A community-level HIV prevention intervention for young gay men. *American Journal of Public Health* 86(8):1129–1136.

Kipke, M. D., K. Kubicek, G. Weiss, C. Wong, D. Lopez, E. Iverson, and W. Ford. 2007. The health and health behaviors of young men who have sex with men. *Journal of Adolescent Health* 40(4):342–350.

Kitts, R. L. 2005. Gay adolescents and suicide: Understanding the association. *Adolescence* 40(159):621–628.

Kitts, R. L. 2010. Barriers to optimal care between physicians and lesbian, gay, bisexual, transgender, and questioning adolescent patients. *Journal of Homosexuality* 57(6):730–747.

Klamen, D. L., L. S. Grossman, and D. R. Kopacz. 1999. Medical student homophobia. *Journal of Homosexuality* 37(1):53–63.

Koblin, B. A., M. J. Husnik, G. Colfax, Y. Huang, M. Madison, K. Mayer, P. J. Barresi, T. J. Coates, M. A. Chesney, and S. Buchbinder. 2006. Risk factors for HIV infection among men who have sex with men. *AIDS* 20(5):731–739.

Kosciw, J. G., E. S. Byard, S. N. Fischer, and C. Joslin. 2007. Gender equity and lesbian, gay, bisexual, and transgender issues in education. In *Handbook for achieving gender equity through education* (2nd ed.), edited by S. S. Klein, B. Richardson, D. A. Grayson, L. H. Fox, C. Kramarae, D. S. Pollard, and C. A. Dwyer. Mahwah, NJ: Lawrence Erlbaum Associates Publishers. Pp. 553–571.

Kosciw, J. G., A. Diaz, and E. A. Greytak. 2008. *2007 National School Climate Survey: The experiences of lesbian, gay, bisexual and transgender youth in our nation's schools*. New York: The Gay, Lesbian and Straight Education Network.

Lawrence, A. A. 2010. Sexual orientation versus age of onset as bases for typologies (subtypes) for gender identity disorder in adolescents and adults. *Archives of Sexual Behavior* 39(2):514–545.

Lena, S. M., T. Wiebe, S. Ingram, and M. Jabbour. 2002. Pediatricians' knowledge, perceptions, and attitudes towards providing health care for lesbian, gay, and bisexual adolescents. *Annals of the Royal College of Physicians & Surgeons of Canada* 35(7):406–410.

Leslie, M. B., J. A. Stein, and M. J. Rotheram-Borus. 2002. Sex-specific predictors of suicidality among runaway youth. *Journal of Clinical Child & Adolescent Psychology* 31(1):27–40.

MacKellar, D. A., L. A. Valleroy, G. M. Secura, W. McFarland, D. Shehan, W. Ford, M. LaLota, D. D. Celentano, B. A. Koblin, L. V. Torian, H. Thiede, and R. S. Janssen. 2001. Two decades after vaccine license: Hepatitis B immunization and infection among young men who have sex with men. *American Journal of Public Health* 91(6):965–971.

Marshal, M. P., M. S. Friedman, R. Stall, and A. L. Thompson. 2009. Individual trajectories of substance use in lesbian, gay and bisexual youth and heterosexual youth. *Addiction* 104(6):974–981.

Marshall, B. D. L., K. Shannon, T. Kerr, R. Zhang, and E. Wood. 2010. Survival sex work and increased HIV risk among sexual minority street-involved youth. *Journal of Acquired Immune Deficiency Syndromes: JAIDS* 53(5):661–664.

McCabe, S. E., T. L. Hughes, W. Bostwick, and C. J. Boyd. 2005. Assessment of difference in dimensions of sexual orientation: Implications for substance use research in a college-age population. *Journal of Studies on Alcohol & Drugs* 66(5):620–629.

McGuire, J. K., C. R. Anderson, R. B. Toomey, and S. T. Russell. 2010. School climate for transgender youth: A mixed method investigation of student experiences and school responses. *Journal of Youth & Adolescence* 39:1175–1188.

Meckler, G. D., M. N. Elliott, D. E. Kanouse, K. P. Beals, and M. A. Schuster. 2006. Nondisclosure of sexual orientation to a physician among a sample of gay, lesbian, and bisexual youth. *Archives of Pediatrics & Adolescent Medicine* 160(12):1248–1254.

Menvielle, E. J., and C. Tuerk. 2002. A support group for parents of gender-nonconforming boys. *Journal of the American Academy of Child & Adolescent Psychiatry* 41(8): 1010–1013.

Meyer, W. J. I., W. Bockting, P. Cohen-Kettenis, C. Coleman, D. DiCeglie, H. Devor, L. Gooren, J. J. Hage, S. Kirk, B. Kuiper, D. Laub, A. A. Lawrence, Y. Menard, S. Monstrey, J. Patton, L. Schaefer, A. Webb, and C. C. Wheeler. 2001. *Standards of care for gender identity disorders, sixth version.* http://www.wpath.org/Documents2/socv6.pdf (accessed March 25, 2011).

Meyer-Bahlburg, H. F. L. 2002. Gender identity disorder in young boys: A parent- and peer-based treatment protocol. *Clinical Child Psychology and Psychiatry* 7(3):360–376.

Milburn, N. G., G. Ayala, E. Rice, P. Batterham, and M. J. Rotheram-Borus. 2006. Discrimination and exiting homelessness among homeless adolescents. *Cultural Diversity and Ethnic Minority Psychology* 12(4):658–672.

Millett, G. A., S. A. Flores, J. L. Peterson, and R. Bakeman. 2007. Explaining disparities in HIV infection among black and white men who have sex with men: A meta-analysis of HIV risk behaviors. *AIDS* 21(15):2083–2091.

Money, J. 1990. *Gay, straight, and in-between: The sexology of erotic orientation.* New York: Oxford University Press.

Mullen, P. D., G. Ramirez, D. Strouse, L. V. Hedges, and E. Sogolow. 2002. Meta-analysis of the effects of behavioral HIV prevention interventions on the sexual risk behavior of sexually experienced adolescents in controlled studies in the United States. *Journal of Acquired Immune Deficiency Syndromes: JAIDS* 30(Suppl. 1):S94–S105.

Mustanski, B. S. 2007. Are sexual partners met online associated with HIV/STI risk behaviours? Retrospective and daily diary data in conflict. *AIDS Care* 19(6):822–827.

Mustanski, B. S., T. Lyons, and S. C. Garcia. 2010a. Internet use and sexual health of young men who have sex with men: A mixed-methods study. *Archives of Sexual Behavior* [Epub ahead of print].

Mustanski, B. S., R. Garofalo, and E. M. Emerson. 2010b. Mental health disorders, psychological distress, and suicidality in a diverse sample of lesbian, gay, bisexual, and transgender youths. *American Journal of Public Health* 100(12):2426–2432.

Needham, B. L., and E. L. Austin. 2010. Sexual orientation, parental support, and health during the transition to young adulthood. *Journal of Youth & Adolescence* 39(10):1189–1198.

Noell, J. W., and L. M. Ochs. 2001. Relationship of sexual orientation to substance use, suicidal ideation, suicide attempts, and other factors in a population of homeless adolescents. *Journal of Adolescent Health* 29(1):31–36.

Nuttbrock, L., S. Hwahng, W. Bockting, A. Rosenblum, M. Mason, M. Macri, and J. Becker. 2010. Psychiatric impact of gender-related abuse across the life course of male-to-female transgender persons. *Journal of Sex Research* 47(1):12–23.

Ogden, C. L., M. D. Carroll, L. R. Curtin, M. M. Lamb, and K. M. Flegal. 2010. Prevalence of high body mass index in us children and adolescents, 2007–2008. *Journal of the American Medical Association* 303(3):242–249.

O'Shaughnessy, M., S. Russell, K. Heck, C. Calhoun, and C. Laub. 2004. *Safe place to learn: Consequences of harassment based on actual or perceived sexual orientation and gender non-conformity and steps for making schools safer.* San Francisco, CA: California Safe Schools Coalition.

Pedlow, C., and M. Carey. 2004. Developmentally appropriate sexual risk reduction interventions for adolescents: Rationale, review of interventions, and recommendations for research and practice. *Annals of Behavioral Medicine* 27(3):172–184.

Peterson, J. L., and K. T. Jones. 2009. HIV prevention for black men who have sex with men in the United States. *American Journal of Public Health* 99(6):976–980.

Poon, C. S., and E. M. Saewyc. 2009. Out yonder: Sexual-minority adolescents in rural communities in British Columbia. *American Journal of Public Health* 99(1):118–124.

Rew, L., R. T. Fouladi, and R. D. Yockey. 2002. Sexual health practices of homeless youth. *Journal of Nursing Scholarship* 34(2):139–145.

Rew, L., T. A. Whittaker, M. A. Taylor-Seehafer, and L. R. Smith. 2005. Sexual health risks and protective resources in gay, lesbian, bisexual, and heterosexual homeless youth. *Journal for Specialists in Pediatric Nursing* 10(1):11–19.

Rich, C. L., R. C. Fowler, D. Young, and M. Blenkush. 1986. San Diego suicide study: Comparison of gay to straight males. *Suicide & Life-Threatening Behavior* 16(4):448–457.

Robin, L., N. D. Brener, S. F. Donahue, T. Hack, K. Hale, and C. Goodenow. 2002. Associations between health risk behaviors and opposite-, same-, and both-sex sexual partners in representative samples of Vermont and Massachusetts high school students. *Archives of Pediatrics & Adolescent Medicine* 156(4):349–355.

Robin, L., P. Dittus, D. Whitaker, R. Crosby, K. Ethier, J. Mezoff, K. Miller, and K. Pappas-Deluca. 2004. Behavioral interventions to reduce incidence of HIV, STD, and pregnancy among adolescents: A decade in review. *Journal of Adolescent Health* 34(1):3–26.

Rosario, M., H. F. L. Meyer-Bahlburg, J. Hunter, T. M. Exner, M. Gwadz, and A. M. Keller. 1996. The psychosexual development of urban lesbian, gay, and bisexual youths. *Journal of Sex Research* 33(2):113–126.

Rosario, M., E. W. Schrimshaw, and J. Hunter. 2004. Ethnic/racial differences in the coming-out process of lesbian, gay, and bisexual youths: A comparison of sexual identity development over time. *Cultural Diversity and Ethnic Minority Psychology* 10(3):215–228.

Rosario, M., E. W. Schrimshaw, and J. Hunter. 2008. Predicting different patterns of sexual identity development over time among lesbian, gay, and bisexual youths: A cluster analytic approach. *American Journal of Community Psychology* 42(3-4):266–282.

Rosario, M., E. W. Schrimshaw, and J. Hunter. 2009. Disclosure of sexual orientation and subsequent substance use and abuse among lesbian, gay, and bisexual youths: Critical role of disclosure reactions. *Psychology of Addictive Behaviors* 23(1):175–184.

Rosenberg, M. 2002. Children with gender identity issues and their parents in individual and group treatment. *Journal of the American Academy of Child & Adolescent Psychiatry* 41(5):619–621.

Russell, S. T. 2003. Sexual minority youth and suicide risk. *American Behavioral Scientist* 46(9):1241–1257.

Russell, S. T. 2005. Beyond risk: Resilience in the lives of sexual minority youth. *Journal of Gay & Lesbian Issues in Education* 2(3):5–18.

Russell, S. T., and K. Joyner. 2001. Adolescent sexual orientation and suicide risk: Evidence from a national study. *American Journal of Public Health* 91(8):1276–1281.

Russell, S. T., H. Seif, and N. L. Truong. 2001. School outcomes of sexual minority youth in the United States: Evidence from a national study. *Journal of Adolescence* 24(1):111–127.

Russell, S. T., A. K. Driscoll, and N. Truong. 2002. Adolescent same-sex romantic attractions and relationships: Implications for substance use and abuse. *American Journal of Public Health* 92(2):198–202.

Ryan, C., D. Huebner, R. M. Diaz, and J. Sanchez. 2009. Family rejection as a predictor of negative health outcomes in white and Latino lesbian, gay, and bisexual young adults. *Pediatrics* 123(1):346–352.

Ryan, C., S. T. Russell, D. M. Huebner, R. Diaz, and J. Sanchez. 2010. Family acceptance in adolescence and the health of LGBT young adults. *Journal of Child and Adolescent Psychiatric Nursing* 23(4):205–213.

Saewyc, E. M., C. L. Skay, L. H. Bearinger, R. W. Blum, and M. D. Resnick. 1998. Sexual orientation, sexual behaviors, and pregnancy among American Indian adolescents. *Journal of Adolescent Health* 23(4):238–247.

Saewyc, E. M., L. H. Bearinger, R. W. Blum, and M. D. Resnick. 1999. Sexual intercourse, abuse and pregnancy among adolescent women: Does sexual orientation make a difference? *Family Planning Perspectives* 31(3):127–131.

Saewyc, E. M., G. R. Bauer, C. L. Skay, L. H. Bearinger, M. D. Resnick, E. Reis, and A. Murphy. 2004. Measuring sexual orientation in adolescent health surveys: Evaluation of eight school-based surveys. *Journal of Adolescent Health* 35(4):345 e1–e15.

Saewyc, E. M., C. L. Skay, S. L. Pettingell, E. A. Reis, L. Bearinger, M. Resnick, A. Murphy, and L. Combs. 2006. Hazards of stigma: The sexual and physical abuse of gay, lesbian, and bisexual adolescents in the United States and Canada. *Child Welfare* 85(2):195–213.

Saewyc, E. M., C. L. Skay, P. Hynds, S. Pettingell, L. H. Bearinger, M. D. Resnick, and E. Reis. 2007. Suicidal ideation and attempts in North American school-based surveys: Are bisexual youth at increasing risk? *Journal of LGBT Health Research* 3(2):25–36.

Saewyc, E. M., C. S. Poon, Y. Homma, and C. L. Skay. 2008. Stigma management? The links between enacted stigma and teen pregnancy trends among gay, lesbian, and bisexual students in british columbia. *Canadian Journal of Human Sexuality* 17(3):123–139.

Saewyc, E. M., Y. Homma, C. L. Skay, L. H. Bearinger, M. D. Resnick, and E. Reis. 2009. Protective factors in the lives of bisexual adolescents in North America. *American Journal of Public Health* 99(1):110–117.

Safren, S. A., and R. G. Heimberg. 1999. Depression, hopelessness, suicidality, and related factors in sexual minority and heterosexual adolescents. *Journal of Consulting & Clinical Psychology* 67(6):859–866.

Sanchez, N. F., J. Rabatin, J. P. Sanchez, S. Hubbard, and A. Kalet. 2006. Medical students' ability to care for lesbian, gay, bisexual, and transgendered patients. *Family Medicine* 38(1):21–27.

Savin-Williams, R. C. 1989a. Coming out to parents and self-esteem among gay and lesbian youths. *Journal of Homosexuality* 18(1):1–35.

Savin-Williams, R. C. 1989b. Parental influences on the self-esteem of gay and lesbian youths: A reflected appraisals model. *Journal of Homosexuality* 17(1/2):93–109.

Savin-Williams, R. C. 2001. Suicide attempts among sexual-minority youths: Population and measurement issues. *Journal of Consulting & Clinical Psychology* 69(6):983–991.

Savin-Williams, R. C., and G. L. Ream. 2003. Suicide attempts among sexual-minority male youth. *Journal of Clinical Child & Adolescent Psychology* 32(4):509–522.

Shaffer, D., P. Fisher, R. H. Hicks, M. Parides, and M. Gould. 1995. Sexual orientation in adolescents who commit suicide. *Suicide & Life-Threatening Behavior* 25(Suppl.):64–71.

Sheets, R. L., Jr., and J. J. Mohr. 2009. Perceived social support from friends and family and psychosocial functioning in bisexual young adult college students. *Journal of Counseling Psychology* 56(1):152–163.

Silenzio, V. M., P. R. Duberstein, W. Tang, N. Lu, X. Tu, and C. M. Homan. 2009. Connecting the invisible dots: Reaching lesbian, gay, and bisexual adolescents and young adults at risk for suicide through online social networks. *Social Science & Medicine* 69(3):469–474.

Smith, D. M., and W. C. Mathews. 2007. Physicians' attitudes toward homosexuality and HIV: Survey of a California medical society-revisited (PATHH-II). *Journal of Homosexuality* 52(3–4):1–9.

Smith, Y. L., S. H. van Goozen, and P. T. Cohen-Kettenis. 2001. Adolescents with gender identity disorder who were accepted or rejected for sex reassignment surgery: A prospective follow-up study. *Journal of the American Academy of Child & Adolescent Psychiatry* 40(4):472–481.

Smith, Y. L. S., S. H. M. Van Goozen, A. J. Kuiper, and P. T. Cohen-Kettenis. 2005. Sex reassignment: Outcomes and predictors of treatment for adolescent and adult transsexuals. *Psychological Medicine* 35(1):89–99.

Solorio, M. R., N. G. Milburn, R. E. Weiss, and P. J. Batterham. 2006. Newly homeless youth STD testing patterns over time. *Journal of Adolescent Health* 39(3):443 e449–443 e416.

Szalacha, L. A. 2003. Safer sexual diversity climates: Lessons learned from an evaluation of Massachusetts safe schools program for gay and lesbian students. *American Journal of Education* 110(1):58–88.

Toomey, R., C. Ryan, R. Diaz, N. A. Card, and S. T. Russell. 2010. Gender nonconforming lesbian, gay, bisexual, and transgender youth: School victimization and young adult psychosocial adjustment. *Developmental Psychology* 46(6):1580–1589.

Troiden, R. R. 1989. The formation of homosexual identities. *Journal of Homosexuality* 17(1–2):43–73.

Tucker, J. S., P. L. Ellickson, and D. J. Klein. 2008. Understanding differences in substance use among bisexual and heterosexual young women. *Womens Health Issues* 18(5):387–398.

Valleroy, L. A., D. A. MacKellar, J. M. Karon, D. H. Rosen, W. McFarland, D. A. Shehan, S. R. Stoyanoff, M. LaLota, D. D. Celentano, B. A. Koblin, H. Thiede, M. H. Katz, L. V. Torian, and R. S. Janssen. 2000. HIV prevalence and associated risks in young men who have sex with men. Young Men's Survey Study Group. *Journal of the American Medical Association* 284(2):198–204.

Van Leeuwen, J. M., S. Boyle, S. Salomonsen-Sautel, D. Baker, J. Garcia, A. Hoffman, and C. J. Hopfer. 2006. Lesbian, gay, and bisexual homeless youth: An eight-city public health perspective. *Child Welfare Journal* 85(2):151–170.

Waldo, C. R., W. McFarland, M. H. Katz, D. MacKellar, and L. A. Valleroy. 2000. Very young gay and bisexual men are at risk for HIV infection: The San Francisco Bay Area Young Men's Survey II. *Journal of Acquired Immune Deficiency Syndromes: JAIDS* 24(2):168–174.

Wallien, M. S. C., and P. T. Cohen-Kettenis. 2008. Psychosexual outcome of gender-dysphoric children. *Journal of the American Academy of Child & Adolescent Psychiatry* 47(12):1413–1423.

Wallien, M. S. C., S. H. M. Van Goozen, and P. T. Cohen-Kettenis. 2007. Physiological correlates of anxiety in children with gender identity disorder. *European Child & Adolescent Psychiatry* 16(5):309–315.

Whitbeck, L. B., X. Chen, D. R. Hoyt, K. A. Tyler, and K. D. Johnson. 2004. Mental disorder, subsistence strategies, and victimization among gay, lesbian, and bisexual homeless and runaway adolescents. *Journal of Sex Research* 41(4):329–342.

Wilbur, S., C. Ryan, and J. Marksamer. 2006. *Serving LGBT youth in out-of-home care: Best practices guide*. Washington, DC: Child Welfare League of America.

Wilson, E. C., R. Garofalo, R. D. Harris, A. Herrick, M. Martinez, J. Martinez, and M. Belzer. 2009. Transgender female youth and sex work: HIV risk and a comparison of life factors related to engagement in sex work. *AIDS & Behavior* 13(5):902–913.

Wilson, E. C., R. Garofalo, D. R. Harris, and M. Belzer. 2010. Sexual risk taking among transgender male-to-female youths with different partner types. *American Journal of Public Health* 100(8):1500–1505.

Wong, C. F., M. D. Kipke, and G. Weiss. 2008. Risk factors for alcohol use, frequent use, and binge drinking among young men who have sex with men. *Addictive Behaviors* 33(8):1012–1020.

Wright, E. R., and B. L. Perry. 2006. Sexual identity distress, social support, and the health of gay, lesbian, and bisexual youth. *Journal of Homosexuality* 51(1):81–110.

Ziyadeh, N. J., L. A. Prokop, L. B. Fisher, M. Rosario, A. E. Field, C. A. Camargo, Jr., and S. B. Austin. 2007. Sexual orientation, gender, and alcohol use in a cohort study of U.S. adolescent girls and boys. *Drug & Alcohol Dependence* 87(2–3):119–130.

Zucker, K. J. 2008. Children with gender identity disorder: Is there a best practice? *Neuropsychiatrie de l'Enfance et de l'Adolescence* 56(6):358–364.

Zucker, K. J., and S. J. Bradley. 1995. *Gender identity disorder and psychosexual problems in children and adolescents*. New York: Guilford Press.

Zucker, K. J., S. J. Bradley, and M. Sanikhani. 1997. Sex differences in referral rates of children with gender identity disorder: Some hypotheses. *Journal of Abnormal Child Psychology* 25(3):217.

5

Early/Middle Adulthood

Those belonging to the current cohort of adults would have witnessed the genesis of the gay rights movement during their childhood. They would have experienced the explosion of the HIV/AIDS epidemic as they transitioned into adulthood, and as adults they would have seen the U.S. Supreme Court strike down all sodomy laws in *Lawrence v. Texas* in 2003 and, in 2004, Massachusetts become the first state to legalize marriage between same-sex couples.

Early/middle adulthood, defined roughly in this report as the period of life from the 20s to the 60s, is ushered in by a transition from adolescence generally thought to involve a number of physiological, work, family, and social life milestones. These include the physical changes associated with puberty and growth in adulthood, as well as the completion of formal education, issues of career choice and efforts to establish financial independence, the selection of a mate (often with the introduction of children into the relationship), the launching of friendships and other interpersonal relationships, and community involvement. During the adult years, these physiological, work, family, and social life domains continue to evolve. The journey through adulthood is often characterized by the physical manifestations of midlife, career achievements and transitions, relationship and family development and changes, and changes in interpersonal ties and community participation. These same domains and issues characterize the experiences of LGBT adults, albeit often in different forms. People who are LGBT engage in educational and career pursuits in ways that are similar to those of their heterosexual peers (even if levels and outcomes may differ). Other domains, however, particularly marriage and parenthood, may be affected by larger cultural and legal forces. Personal relationships, social support, and community involvement may also assume different forms, similarly affected by cultural influences.

The last two decades have seen a growing recognition of the unique health needs of LGBT individuals. Research, however, is still sparse on the developmental life stage of adulthood with regard to the specific health issues confronted by the LGBT community broken down by race/ethnicity and socioeconomic status, with the largest body of work focusing on HIV/AIDS.

The following sections describe research on LGBT adults in the areas of the development of sexual orientation and gender identity; mental health status; physical health status; risk and protective factors; health services; and contextual influences, including demographic characteristics and the role of the family. The final section presents a summary of key findings and research opportunities. It is important to note that some of the literature presented in this chapter may also appear in the following chapter on later adulthood because studies do not always delineate their findings according to the age ranges used in this report, and certain studies may present findings that are relevant to both early/middle and later adulthood.

DEVELOPMENT OF SEXUAL ORIENTATION AND GENDER IDENTITY

The process of sexual orientation development and of "coming out" is different for each LGBT individual. As individuals come out, they reach various milestones in the process: they experience their first awareness of same-sex attraction, they have their first same-sex sexual experience, they self-identify as LGB, and they choose to disclose their sexual orientation identity to others. Depending on contextual factors in their lives, LGB individuals may choose to come out at many different times throughout the life course, and the stage at which they come out will influence their experiences. Moreover, the association between sexual orientation identity, or coming out, and mental health is not invariant across LGBT populations in the United States. Multiple social, cultural, and psychological influences affect the extent to which members of homosexually active populations experience favorable consequences from self-identity as lesbian or gay. Thus, the assumption of a universal positive link between coming out and mental health appears unwarranted.

Gates (2010) examined the relationship between demographic factors and coming out among different age cohorts using data from the 2008 General Social Survey, a nationally representative sample of 2,023 adults aged 18 and older. Of the 1,773 respondents providing information about sexual orientation and behavior, 58 self-identified as LGB, and 104 reported same-sex partners. The authors found that relative to individuals younger than 30, adults aged 30–54 were 16 times more likely to be closeted.

In their analysis of a nonprobability sample of 2,001 women (mean age = 40) who self-identified as lesbian or bisexual or reported sexual activity with or attraction to other women, Corliss and colleagues (2009) found that on average, the women reported first awareness of same-sex sexual attractions at age 16, first coming out to another person at age 23, and first sexual encounter with another woman at age 21. They also found that women who were aware of their same-sex attractions before age 12 were more likely to be Latina or black, more likely to come from families with less parental education, and more likely to self-identify as a lesbian than as a bisexual woman. Those who reported coming out and having a sexual experience with another female before age 18 were more likely to be younger and less educated than other women in the sample.

Factors such as race, ethnicity, and education may affect the coming-out process differently for nonwhite and white members of sexual minorities in the United States. In a review of the effects of social context on black homosexual males, Peterson and Jones (2009) note that studies reveal that, relative to men of other racial groups, black men experience higher levels of internalized homophobia, are less likely to disclose their homosexual orientation, and are more likely to perceive that their friends and neighbors disapprove of homosexuality. While the effects of race, ethnicity, and education may be widespread, they are likely even more salient among low-income than middle-class nonwhite LGB individuals. Moreover, the resources and social support typically received by nonwhite LGBT individuals from their racial/ethnic communities before they come out may often be jeopardized if they come out, and this may create significant barriers to the coming out process for these individuals. In addition, black LGBT individuals may experience racism in mainstream gay and lesbian communities. In a survey of 2,645 LGBT individuals at "black gay pride" festivals across the United States, nearly half of the participants believed that racism was a problem within primarily white LGBT communities. Such experiences pose further obstacles to coming out for these individuals (Battle et al., 2002).

For LGB individuals who come out during adulthood, factors such as marital status and parenthood may also influence the coming out process. For example, Morris and colleagues (2002) compared developmental milestones among 2,431 self-identified lesbians and bisexual women who had children before coming out (n = 313, mean age = 44.8) or after coming out (n = 187, mean age = 39.7) or did not have children (n = 1,919, mean age = 34.6). They found that mothers who had children before coming out reached developmental milestones at older ages than both other groups. Mothers who had children before coming out reached each milestone in the coming out process approximately 7 to 12 years later than mothers who had children after coming out and approximately 6 to 8 years later than nonmothers.

As society continues to change, the timing of coming out and achieving developmental milestones also changes. In 1994 Drasin and colleagues (2008) published a survey in *The Advocate* and examined data from 2,402 self-identified gay men aged 18–83 (mean age = 38.3) to determine whether trends in developmental, psychological, and sexual developmental milestones differed by age cohort and whether those trends had changed over time. Recognizing that this sample may have omitted younger men who identify as gay later in life and that readers of *The Advocate* may be more likely to identify as gay, the authors performed conservative sensitivity tests on the data and made conservative corrections accordingly. They found that of those who were aged 50 or older at the time of the survey (16 percent of the sample), 57 percent had realized they were gay by age 18, 22 percent had done so by age 22, and 9 percent had not done so by age 30. In examining the social, sexual, and psychological milestones for their sample, the authors found that the milestones occurred at an earlier age in younger cohorts, but the changes in age at occurrence by cohort are occurring at different rates. For instance, while sexual behavior milestones (age at first sexual contact with another male) are changing slowly, individual psychological milestones (age at first awareness of same-sex attraction, self-identification as gay) are changing more rapidly, and social milestones (age at first coming out, frequenting a gay bar) are changing even more rapidly. Even with the corrections performed by the authors, results showed that coming out to a family member has changed from occurring at age 40 among those who reached age 18 before 1953, to the mid-30s for those who reached age 18 between 1953 and 1962, to the mid- to late 20s in the 1963 to 1982 cohort, to around age 21 for those who reached 18 after 1982.

The existing literature examines some of the factors that influence the timing of the coming out process among LGB adults. Further research is needed to elucidate the ways in which the timing of the coming out process influences the health status of LGB people and their specific health needs.

Transgender individuals are coming out to affirm their gender identity at younger and younger ages (Makadon et al., 2007). Transgender men tend to come out at earlier ages than transgender women (Zucker and Lawrence, 2009). Transgender women can generally be divided into two groups: those who have been gender nonconforming since childhood in both role and identity and those who have been gender conforming in role, but may or may not have been aware of feelings of cross-gender identity in childhood or adolescence (Bockting and Coleman, 2007; Lawrence, 2010). The latter individuals typically report cross-dressing in private, which initially is often accompanied by sexual arousal; their feelings of cross-gender identity may be expressed in sexual fantasy (Bockting and Coleman, 2007), particularly among older-generation white transgender women (Nuttbrock et al., 2009a). Transgender women who did not conform to gender roles in childhood tend to come out at an early age, either before or during early adulthood, and if so desired, change gender roles and feminize their body through hormone therapy and/or surgery (Bockting and Coleman, 2007; Lawrence, 2010). By contrast, transgender women who were gender role conforming in childhood tend to come out during mid- or later life (Bockting and Coleman, 2007; Lawrence, 2010), and their developmental challenges may vary as a result. Whereas gender role–nonconforming individuals must develop resilience in the face of enacted stigma early in life (Nuttbrock et al., 2010), gender role–conforming individuals may protect themselves against enacted stigma by keeping their transgender feelings private, yet are likely to experience felt stigma and, in isolation, may not benefit from the support a community of similar others can provide (Meyer, 2007).

Several authors have attempted to describe the process of transgender identity development or to adapt stage models of gay and lesbian coming out (Minton and McDonald, 1983) to the coming out process of transgender individuals. Bockting and Coleman (2007) describe five stages (precoming out, coming out, exploration, intimacy, and identity integration) based on Erikson's (1950) model of social development and their extensive clinical experience in working with transgender individuals. Devor (2004) defines 14 possible stages of transgender identity development based on sociological field research and in-depth interviews with transgender men. Gagne and colleagues (1997) define four stages (early transgender experiences, coming out to one's self, coming out to others, and resolution of identity) based on a qualitative study of transgender women. Lewins (1995) describes six stages of becoming a (transgender) woman (abiding anxiety, discovery, purging and delay, acceptance, surgical reassignment, and invisibility) based on interviews with transsexual women. Finally, based on her clinical experience and a review of the scientific literature, Lev (2004) describes six stages of transgender emergence: awareness; seeking information/reaching out; disclosure to significant others; exploration, identity, and self-labeling; exploration, transition issues, and possible body modification; and integration, acceptance, and posttransition issues. Although informed by formative research, these stage models have not been tested empirically and systematically.

MENTAL HEALTH STATUS

LGBT adults are typically well adjusted and mentally healthy. Studies based on probability samples of LGB populations indicate that the majority of LGB adults do not report mental health problems (Cochran and Mays,

2006; Herek and Garnets, 2007). While national probability samples of transgender adults are not available, data from convenience samples similarly show that many, if not most, transgender adults do not report mental health problems (Clements-Nolle et al., 2001; Nuttbrock et al., 2010).

Nonetheless, disparities in mental health do exist among some sexual-minority groups. In a meta-analysis of research on mental health among LGB people published between 1966 and 2005, King and colleagues (2008) examined the prevalence of a number of mental health outcomes. They found that LGB individuals had a 1.5 times higher risk for depression and anxiety disorders over a period of 12 months or a lifetime than heterosexual individuals. Other findings revealed that the risk for suicide attempts over a lifetime among lesbian, gay, and bisexual individuals was more than twice as great as that among heterosexual individuals.

The evidence is not conclusive, however. A study comparing lesbians and their heterosexual sisters as a control group found no difference in the prevalence of mental health problems between the lesbian–heterosexual sister pairs (n = 184 pairs), but found that the lesbians had significantly higher self-esteem than their heterosexual sisters (Rothblum and Factor, 2001). Horowitz and colleagues (2003) examined specific quality-of-life indicators by behaviorally defined sexual orientation categories (heterosexual, homosexual, bisexual since age 18 and within the last 12 months) (n = 11,536). They found that there were no significant differences among heterosexual, homosexual, and bisexual men and women with respect to general happiness, perceived health, or job satisfaction since age 18 or within the last 12 months.

For transgender people, the available studies generally suggest high rates of negative mental health outcomes. Most of these studies, however, are limited by the use of nonprobability samples, and few compare the mental health of transgender people and nontransgender controls. A clinical sample of 31 male-to-females reported significantly more symptoms on the General Severity Index (GSI) of the Brief Symptom Inventory relative to nontransgender men (n = 57). Further analyses of the data indicated clinically significant levels of anxiety and depression, along with increased feelings of self-consciousness and distrust of other people (Derogatis et al., 1978). A clinical sample of 20 female-to-males showed no clinically significant differences on the GSI in comparison with nontransgender females (n = 143); however, scores on subscales of anxiety and interpersonal sensitivity were elevated (Derogatis et al., 1981). There also appear to be mental health differences among lesbian, gay, bisexual, and transgender populations. For instance, in a chart review of 223 lesbians and bisexual women presenting to a mental health clinic, Rogers and colleagues (2003) found that the lesbians were more likely than the bisexual women to present at intake with suicidal ideation, while the bisexual women were more likely to present with stressors related to social environment and health care access. Similarly, Page (2004) explored the experiences with mental health services of self-identified bisexual men and women (n = 217) and found that the bisexual men had experienced greater stress related to their bisexual identity and that bisexual issues had played a more significant role in their decision to seek mental health services. Mathy (2002a,b) compared the mental health status of 73 transgender individuals and nonclinical samples of nontransgender women and men, either homosexual or heterosexual. The transgender individuals were more likely to report suicidal ideation and attempts, to take psychotropic medications, and to have a problem with alcohol relative to the nontransgender men and heterosexual women, but no such differences were found between the transgender and lesbian individuals. For the latter two groups, the author attributed the higher likelihood of mental health and substance use problems to their experiencing both heterosexism and sexism. Bockting and colleagues (Bockting et al., 2005a) compared baseline data from an intervention study of 207 transgender participants, 480 men who have sex with men, and 122 bisexually active women; the transgender individuals were most likely to report depression (52 percent versus 38 percent and 40 percent, respectively) and suicidal ideation (47 percent versus 31 percent and 32 percent, respectively). However, this study did not assess depression with a standardized instrument.

While more research has been conducted on mental health than on physical health conditions among LGBT adults, large gaps still remain in our understanding of mental health issues among LGBT people. There is conflicting evidence on the mental health status of LGB adults, and the existing research examining the mental health of transgender adults has limitations. It is clear, however, that deleterious effects on the mental health of lesbian, gay, and bisexual individuals result overwhelmingly from unique, chronic stressors due to the stigma they experience as a disadvantaged minority in American society (Meyer, 2003). Herek and Garnets (2007) note that sexual stigma leads to stress resulting from multiple types of "enacted stigma" (e.g., personal rejection and ostracism, discrimination, and criminal victimization), which can have serious and enduring psychological consequences. Beyond such direct manifestations of stigma, Herek and Garnets (2007) suggest there are pervasive effects of institutionalized stigma, or "heterosexism," among gay, lesbian, and bisexual populations, such as denial of the right to marriage in most states, negative economic effects in the workplace, and frequent disenfranchisement from religious and spiritual resources needed to ameliorate the effects of stress.

Herek and Garnets (2007) also identify two other sources of stress experienced by sexual minorities: "felt stigma" and "self-stigma." They contend that felt stigma—the subjective experience of stigma against one's group, even without direct experience of enacted stigma—may often occur as a consequence of societal events in which antigay hostility is demonstrated (e.g., antigay violence, antigay political campaigns). Likewise, these authors suggest that self-stigma may occur among some sexual minorities as a result of accepting society's negative attitudes toward them (e.g., internalized homophobia, internalized heterosexism, and internalized homonegativity). These negative feelings about one's own homosexual desires can have negative impacts on mental and physical health and heighten the stress experienced by sexual minorities.

Mood/Anxiety Disorders

Some population studies have compared rates of anxiety disorders in homosexually and heterosexually active men and women. Using data from the 1996 National Household Survey of Drug Abuse, Cochran and Mays (2000b) examined differences in the prevalence of psychiatric syndromes among sexually active individuals. Behavioral sexual orientation was compared between respondents who reported exclusively other-sex sex partners (n = 9,714) and those who reported any same-sex sex partners (n = 194) in the prior year. While most homosexually active individuals did not meet criteria for any of the syndromes assessed, multivariate logistic regression analyses revealed that homosexually active men were more likely than other men to evidence a panic attack syndrome.

Cochran and Mays (2000a) also examined possible associations between homosexual/bisexual behavior patterns and lifetime prevalence of affective disorders, including mania, major depression, and dysthymia, among men (aged 17–39) using data from the National Health and Nutrition Examination Survey (NHANES) III. Sexual orientation was defined behaviorally based on self-reports of sexual partners and classified into three groups: any male sex partners (n = 108), only female partners (n = 3,208), and no sexual partners (n = 187). The results revealed that homosexually/bisexually experienced men were no more likely than exclusively heterosexual men to meet criteria for lifetime diagnoses of affective disorders.

Similarly, Gilman and colleagues (2001) examined the risk of psychiatric disorders among individuals with same-sex and different-sex sexual partners based on data from the National Comorbidity Survey. Respondents were asked two sexual behavior questions: the number of women and, separately, men with whom they had engaged in sexual intercourse in the prior 5 years. Based on these responses, the respondents were classified into three groups: any same-sex partners (n = 125), exclusively heterosexual partners (n = 4,785), and no sexual partners (n = 967). Respondents with same-sex sexual partners had a higher 12-month prevalence of anxiety and mood disorders than respondents with different-sex partners only. The authors note the limitation that using a behavioral definition of sexual orientation excludes those respondents not sexually active in the 5 years prior to the interview.

Cochran and colleagues (2003) later analyzed data from the MacArthur Foundation National Survey of Midlife Development in the United States (MIDUS) to examine possible sexual orientation–related differences in morbidity, distress, and use of mental health services. The sexual orientation of 2,917 adults (aged 25–74) was based on self-report as heterosexual (n = 2,844), homosexual (n = 41), or bisexual (n = 32). The samples of individuals who identified as homosexual and those who identified as bisexual were combined for analysis. The results revealed that gay/bisexual men had a higher prevalence of panic attacks than heterosexual men, while lesbian/bisexual women had a higher prevalence of generalized anxiety disorder than heterosexual women. However, the authors note the limited number of participants who reported a homosexual or bisexual orientation.

More recently, Bostwick and colleagues (2010) used data from the 2004–2005 National Epidemiologic Survey on Alcohol and Related Conditions (n = 34,653) to examine lifetime and past-year mood and anxiety disorders among different sexual orientation groups. Identity, attraction, and behavior measures were used to assess sexual orientation. The authors found mental health disparities among some sexual-minority groups. Self-identified lesbian, gay, or bisexual individuals had higher rates of mood and anxiety disorders than self-identified heterosexual individuals. Women who reported exclusively same-sex sexual behavior and women who reported exclusively same-sex attraction were found to have some of the lowest rates of mood and anxiety disorders. With the exception of these women, however, individuals reporting any same-sex sexual behavior or same-sex attraction were found to have higher rates of most mood and anxiety disorders than those reporting exclusively different-sex sexual behavior or exclusively different-sex attraction. Bisexual behavior was found to be associated with the highest incidence of mood or anxiety disorders.

There have been relatively few studies on the prevalence of mood and anxiety disorders among transgender adults. In a study previously mentioned, Derogatis and colleagues (1978) found significantly higher levels of anxiety and depression among a sample of male-to-female transsexuals in comparison with nontransgender men. More recent literature on depression among transgender adults is presented in the next section.

Depression

Some evidence is available from population studies on differences in rates of major depression between homosexually and heterosexually active men and women. Cochran and Mays (2000b) examined possible differences in psychiatric syndromes between homosexually active and heterosexually active men and women using data from the National Household Survey of Drug Abuse. Men who have sex with men were more likely than exclusively heterosexual men to be diagnosed with major depression. Homosexually active women were no more likely than exclusively heterosexual women to evidence major depression syndrome.

Cochran and colleagues (2003), using data from the MIDUS survey, found that the sample of self-identified gay and bisexual men (combined for analysis) showed a higher prevalence of depression than heterosexual men. Gilman and colleagues (2001), using data from the National Comorbidity Survey, found that women with any same-sex partner had a significantly higher 12-month prevalence of major depression than women with only different-sex partners. Conron and colleagues (2008), using data from the Massachusetts Behavioral Risk Factor Surveillance System survey of adults aged 18–64 (n = 38,910), found that bisexual adults were significantly more likely to report feeling "sad or blue" than either heterosexual or lesbian and gay adults.

Cochran and colleagues (2007c) also looked at differences in mental health disorders using data from the National Latino and Asian American Study (n = 4,488). Sexual orientation was defined based on self-identity and past-year history of sexual experiences. Those who identified as gay, lesbian, or bisexual and/or reported any same-sex sexual experiences in the past year (n = 245) were compared with the rest of the sample. Results showed that lesbian/bisexual women were significantly more likely than heterosexual women to meet criteria for depressive disorders, either in the past year or in lifetime histories. Similarly, gay/bisexual men were significantly more likely than heterosexual men to report a recent suicide attempt. The authors note that the prevalence of mental health disorders found in sexual-minority Latinos and Asian Americans was similar to or lower than that found in population-based studies of lesbian, gay, and bisexual adults in general.

Rates of depression among transgender people are far less well studied. In a convenience sample of 392 transgender women and 123 transgender men aged 18–67 in San Francisco, rates of depression ranged from 55 percent among transgender men to 62 percent among transgender women (Clements-Nolle et al., 2001). Among LGBT participants in a sexual health seminar intervention, 52 percent of transgender participants (n = 207) reported depression. This was a higher percentage than that among men who have sex with men (n = 480, 38 percent) or bisexually active women (n = 122, 40 percent) (Bockting et al., 2005a). In their meta-analysis of 29 transgender studies, Herbst and colleagues (2008) found that a large percentage (weighted mean 43.9 percent) of transgender respondents indicated a desire for mental health counseling to address transgender-specific issues.

Suicide/Suicidal Behavior

Some studies have found that nonheterosexual adults are more likely than heterosexual adults to report past suicidal ideation and attempts. Cochran and Mays (2000a), using data from a national probability sample of 3,503 participants (NHANES III), found that men who reported same-sex sexual behavior showed greater lifetime prevalence rates of suicidal ideation and suicide attempts than men who reported exclusively different-sex sexual behavior, even after adjustment for possible demographic confounding.

Using data from the National Comorbidity Survey in a study previously described, Gilman and colleagues (2001) observed differences in suicide symptoms between men and women participants with same-sex (n = 125) and different-sex (n = 4,785) sexual partners. They found no significant differences in the 12-month prevalence of suicidal thoughts, plans, and attempts between those with same-sex and different-sex partners overall. Among women, however, they found a higher prevalence of suicidal thoughts and plans in the any same-sex partner group than in the other-sex partner group, and among men, a higher prevalence of suicidal plans and attempts in the any same-sex partner group than in the other-sex partner group. Also, the lifetime risk of suicidal thoughts was significantly greater for both men and women in the same-sex partner group than in the different-sex partner group. Overall, the authors note that the effects of having same-sex versus different-sex partners appear to be stronger for women than for men.

Other studies have demonstrated that suicidal ideation and behavior vary by both sexual orientation and gender. Mathy and colleagues (2003) compared suicidal intent, mental health difficulties, and mental health treatment among bisexual and transgender individuals. They found that, relative to bisexual males (n = 1,457), bisexual females (n = 792) and transgender individuals (n = 73) had a higher prevalence of all three variables (Mathy et al., 2003). In a study of 1,304 women conducted at 33 health care sites across the United States, Koh and Ross (2006) found that differences in rates of suicidal ideation and attempts varied among bisexual women (n = 143), lesbians (n = 524), and heterosexual women (n = 637) and were also correlated with disclosure of sexual orientation. Bisexual women who had disclosed their sexual orientation to a majority of friends, family, and coworkers were twice as likely to have reported suicidal ideation relative to heterosexual women. Among sexual minorities who had not disclosed their sexual orientation to a majority of friends, family, and coworkers, lesbians were 90 percent more likely to have ever made a suicide attempt, and bisexual women were three times more likely than heterosexual women to have done so (Koh and Ross, 2006).

One study, based on a convenience sample, suggests that rates of suicide attempts vary by age among sexual minorities. In a sample of New York City lesbian, gay, and bisexual persons aged 18–59 (n = 388) recruited through direct solicitation and snowball techniques in a variety of venues, Meyer and colleagues (2008) found that 15.6 percent of those aged 45–59 had made a serious suicide attempt, a higher percentage than that among those aged 18–29 or 30–44.

Other studies have found a relationship between race and suicide attempts. In a study of 388 black, white, and Latina/o lesbians, gay men, and bisexual individuals, Meyer and colleagues (2008) found that Latina/o sexual minorities reported a greater number of lifetime suicide attempts than white sexual minorities. Another study examined the lifetime prevalence of suicide attempts among men who have sex with men (n = 2,881) and found that the prevalence was higher among Native American respondents than among respondents reporting other racial/ethnic identities (Paul et al., 2002).

In a unique matched-control study, Herrell and colleagues (1999) provide evidence on suicidality from the Vietnam Era Twin Registry of 4,774 male–male twin pairs who responded to a mail and telephone survey. Most (103) of the 120 middle-aged twins in the analytical study sample who reported same-sex sexual behavior after age 18 had a twin who did not report such behavior. As defined by sexual behavior, same-sex sexual orientation was significantly associated with lifetime suicidal ideation and attempted suicide, even after adjustment for substance use and other depressive symptoms. However, the authors note limitations of the study due to their sampling design and selection criteria.

Other evidence on suicidal symptoms is available from a convenience sample of self-identified lesbian, gay, and bisexual individuals and their siblings (Balsam et al., 2005). The sample included 533 heterosexual, 558 lesbian or gay, and 163 bisexual participants who were compared on suicidal ideation and suicide attempts. Compared with heterosexuals, sexual minorities had a higher prevalence of suicidal ideation and suicide attempts, even after controlling for sibling variance. The authors also hypothesized that bisexual individuals would exhibit greater psychological distress than lesbians and gay men, but the results of their study did not support this hypothesis. Bisexual individuals reported engaging in more self-injurious behavior than lesbians and gay men, but did not have higher rates of suicidal ideation and suicidal attempts. The authors raise the caveat of their convenience sampling despite the possible benefits of their yoked sibling design.

Using convenience samples of the transgender population, researchers have found consistently high rates of suicidal ideation and attempts. In a sample of 392 transgender women and 123 transgender men in San Francisco, Clements-Nolle and colleagues (2001) found that 32 percent had attempted suicide; Mathy (2002b) found 37 percent ideation and 23 percent attempts among 73 North American self-identified transgender visitors to the MSNBC website; and among 248 transgender people of color in Washington, DC, 38 percent reported suicidal ideation during their lifetime (Xavier et al., 2005). The authors of the latter study further note that in their sample, transgender men were more likely than transgender women to report suicidal ideation (52 percent versus 33 percent), but transgender women were more likely than transgender men to attribute their suicidal ideation to their gender issues (79 percent versus 36 percent). Black participants were least likely of all racial/ethnic groups to report suicidal ideation (Xavier et al., 2005). In a study mentioned earlier involving participants in a sexual health seminar intervention, 47 percent of transgender persons reported suicidal ideation or attempts in the last 3 years, compared with 31 percent of men who have sex with men and 32 percent of behaviorally bisexual women (Bockting et al., 2005a).

Kenagy (2005b) reports on two surveys of 182 transgender adults ranging in age from 17 to 68 (with a mean age of 32). These respondents, primarily from the Philadelphia area, were recruited through snowball sampling and through organizations providing services to transgender persons. Black respondents made up more than 40 percent of the sample, representing the largest racial category, and more than 60 percent of the sample was male to female. Kenagy found that more than 30 percent of the respondents answered that they had "ever attempted suicide." Subsequent questions about these attempts focused on whether being transgender was a factor; the majority (more than 60 percent) responded affirmatively. A survey of 350 transgender adults in Virginia, ranging in age from 18 to over 65, recruited through service providers, support groups, and informal peer networks, found comparable results (Xavier et al., 2007).

Nuttbrock and colleagues (2010) conducted Life Chart Interviews with a convenience sample of 517 transgender women in New York City and compared data from younger (aged 19–39) and older (aged 40–59) participants. For the younger group, the lifetime prevalence of depression, suicidal ideation, and attempts was 54.7 percent, 53 percent, and 31.2 percent, respectively. For the older group, the corresponding figures were 52.4 percent, 53.5 percent, and 28 percent. Respondents were also asked to report on past symptoms of depression and suicidal ideation at five different stages of their life course. For the younger group, the authors found a significant decline in the prevalence of depression from earlier to later stages of the life course. While 38.4 percent had evidenced depression during ages 10–14, 19.1 percent had done so during ages 30–39. A similar trend was observed for suicide attempts, with 15.6 percent reporting an attempt during ages 10–14 and 8.7 percent reporting an attempt during ages 30–39. Of interest, for the older group, the prevalence of depression remained relatively constant through the life course: 23.5 percent evidenced depression during ages 10–14, 24.8 percent during ages 30–39, and 26.1 percent during ages 40–49. The authors interpret this difference between older and younger respondents as an indication of generational differences in adaptation due to the increased visibility of transgender identity.

Eating Disorders/Body Image

Some research, using small samples, suggests that sexual-minority status may be a risk factor for eating disorders among men. Far less research has been conducted among lesbians and bisexual women to determine whether there is an association—either positive or negative—between sexual orientation and eating disorders or body image.

Russell and Keel (2002), for example, conducted a study to examine eating disorders in a convenience sample (n = 122) of gay and heterosexual men, based on their self-identified sexual orientation and sexual behavior (past 2 years); bisexual men were excluded. They observed higher levels of body dissatisfaction and bulimic and anorexic symptoms in gay compared with heterosexual men, even after controlling for depression, self-esteem, and comfort with sexual orientation. Kaminski and colleagues (2005) examined body image in a convenience sample (n = 50) of self-identified gay and heterosexual men. They found that, compared with the heterosexual men, the gay men were more dissatisfied with their bodies even though they were no more likely to be heavier than their perceived ideal weight. In an earlier study, Beren and colleagues (1996) examined differences in body dissatisfaction in a convenience sample (n = 257) of lesbian, gay, and heterosexual adults. Sexual orientation was based on self-reports of attraction to the same or other sex. The authors found that, compared with heterosexual men, gay men reported more body dissatisfaction, even though they were not significantly further from their body ideal. No significant difference was found in body dissatisfaction between lesbians and heterosexual women. Feldman and Meyer (2007b) compared the prevalence of eating disorders in a venue-based sample of 126 white heterosexuals and 388 white, black, and Latino LGB men and women and found that, compared with the heterosexual men, the gay and bisexual men had a higher lifetime prevalence of such disorders. The authors did not find a significant difference in the lifetime prevalence of eating disorders among lesbians and heterosexual and bisexual women. In the previously mentioned study by Koh and Ross (2006), the authors found that bisexual women were more than twice as likely to have had an eating disorder than lesbians. If a bisexual woman reported that she was out, she was twice as likely to have had an eating disorder than a heterosexual woman. These studies demonstrate that further research is needed to elucidate the relationship between sexual orientation and eating disorders.

Transgender-Specific Mental Health Status

To alleviate gender dysphoria, some transgender individuals change gender roles (either part time or full time), take feminizing or masculinizing hormones, or have surgery (breast/chest, facial, or genital reconstructive surgery). The aim of these interventions is to affirm gender identity and find a gender role and expression that are consistent with that identity.

The clinical management of gender dysphoria has been guided largely by the *Standards of Care for Gender Identity Disorders* set forth by the World Professional Association for Transgender Health, now in its sixth revision (Meyer et al., 2001). Within the context of a holistic, flexible approach to helping individuals explore their identity and make informed decisions about available treatment options, the *Standards of Care* include minimal criteria for access to medical interventions to alleviate dysphoria. For adults, these include the following:

- **For hormone therapy**—Evaluation and recommendation by a mental health professional with competency in the assessment and treatment of sexual and gender identity disorders; a period of psychotherapy of a duration specified by the mental health professional (usually a minimum of 3 months) or 3 months of living full time in the preferred gender role (referred to as real life experience); and demonstrable knowledge of what hormones medically can or cannot do and their social benefits and risks.
- **For breast/chest surgery**—For female-to-males, the criteria are the same as for hormone therapy. For male-to-females desiring breast surgery, there is an additional requirement for documentation by both the physician prescribing hormones and the surgeon. The documentation must confirm that after undergoing at least 18 months of hormone therapy, the patient has not achieved sufficient breast enlargement to alleviate dysphoria.
- **For genital reconstructive surgery**—Evaluation and recommendation by two mental health professionals with competency in the assessment and treatment of sexual and gender identity disorders; 12 months of continuous hormone therapy (if applicable); 12 months of living full time in the preferred gender role (referred to as real life experience); if required by the mental health professional, regular participation in psychotherapy; demonstrable knowledge of the cost, required lengths of hospitalizations, likely complications, and

postsurgical rehabilitation requirements of various surgical approaches; and awareness of different competent surgeons.

The *Standards of Care* are based on the best available scientific knowledge and clinical consensus among professionals specializing in the assessment and treatment of gender dysphoria, although a rigorous empirical evaluation of the criteria has not been conducted. Nonetheless, the standards have been criticized by transgender community members with respect to the stigmatizing effect of a diagnosis of gender identity disorder, whether psychotherapy should be required before hormone therapy or surgery, whether a period of real life experience before hormone therapy is helpful or potentially harmful, and the value and length of the real life experience before surgery (see Bockting et al., 2009b, for a critical review). Indeed, hormone use (and to a lesser extent surgery) without adherence to the *Standards of Care* is not uncommon; reports of illicit hormone use in needs assessment studies range from 29 to 71 percent (Clements-Nolle et al., 1999; Nemoto et al., 2005; Xavier, 2000). In addition, a growing number of health providers with varying levels of competence in transgender-specific health care may prescribe hormones and provide access to surgery while making exceptions to or altogether ignoring the *Standards of Care* (Dean et al., 2000; Lombardi, 2001).

In recent years, alternative approaches have been formalized in written guidelines and protocols by individual community-based health care centers (Callen-Lorde Community Health Center, 2004; Howard Brown Health Center, 2010; Tom Waddell Health Center, 2006). These approaches, characterized as the "informed consent model," respond to the common criticism of the requirement in the *Standards of Care* for a mental health provider's evaluation and recommendation for hormone therapy. Instead, under the "informed consent model," the first contact is typically with a medical provider, followed by an appointment with an advocate to review one's transition plan or a psychosocial assessment, education, and counseling (as opposed to the other way around as is the case in the *Standards of Care*). This approach is aimed at giving transgender individuals greater autonomy in making their own, fully informed health care decision and allows for greater latitude in providing harm-reduction care. The feasibility, acceptability, and effectiveness of this alternative approach have not been systematically evaluated, however.

Only one published study has specifically attempted to evaluate whether adherence to the eligibility criteria of the *Standards of Care* predicted postoperative satisfaction (Lawrence, 2003). Of 232 male-to-female transsexuals, 51 (22 percent) reported having undergone surgery without meeting one or more of the criteria, 36 (16 percent) having had less than 12 months of real life experience, 14 (6 percent) having undergone less than 12 hours of psychotherapy, and 13 (6 percent) having undergone less than 12 months of hormone therapy before genital surgery. Of all the criteria, only the duration of real life experience was positively associated with satisfaction. This study was severely limited by a response rate of only 32 percent and did not include mental health as an outcome measure. Thus, while follow-up research has shown that the vast majority of reassigned transsexuals are satisfied (see below), no published study has examined specifically whether and to what degree psychotherapy and the real life experience predict mental health outcomes. The *Standards of Care* are currently being revised again, and the relevant research and recommendations for change have been published in volume 11 of the *International Journal of Transgenderism* (Bockting et al., 2009b).

Until recently, hormone therapy, the real life experience, and surgery were considered three steps in a linear process of sex reassignment. Various follow-up studies over the years have evaluated the outcomes of this process by assessing how well adjusted participants were as members of the other sex and their perceived satisfaction. This body of research shows that the vast majority of those who undergo sex reassignment are satisfied, and reversal to the original gender role and regrets are extremely rare (Green and Fleming, 1990; Kuiper and Cohen-Kettenis, 1988; Lawrence, 2006; Murad et al., 2010). Predictors of a good outcome include good prereassignment psychological adjustment, family support, psychological treatment, and good surgical outcomes (Carroll, 1999; Lawrence, 2003). While most of these studies have been retrospective, Mate-Kole and colleagues (1990) used a control group and found that transsexuals who had surgery relatively soon after diagnosis were socially more active and showed less neuroticism than those who were kept on a waiting list for at least 2 years.

Over the last 15 years, there has been a paradigm shift in the conceptualization of transgender identities toward recognition of greater diversity in gender identity and expression (Bockting, 2008). As a result, hormones, changes in gender role, and surgery each have become options in their own right, used either alone or in various combinations and no longer necessarily as three steps in a linear process of reassignment. Rather, clinical management of gender dysphoria now focuses largely on facilitating a transgender coming out process that may or may not include any of these medical interventions (Bockting and Coleman, 2007). Thus, individuals may explore and find a comfortable gender role and expression accompanied by hormones but no surgery, surgery but no hormones, neither, or both. Individuals may or may not change gender roles from male to female or female to male completely and permanently, may adopt both roles part time, or may grow up with a gender-variant or transgender identity without ever conforming to one role only to have to consider transitioning to another. In other words, greater acceptance and visibility of gender variance have contributed to an environment in which there is greater room to explore and define one's gender within or outside of a binary conceptualization of gender as either man or woman, masculine or feminine, including the adoption of such identity labels as gender variant or gender queer (Bockting, 2008).

No research to date, however, has systematically and empirically studied the natural history of transgender identity development; the clinical management of gender dysphoria under the new paradigm of a greater diversity of gender identities, roles, and expressions; or the outcomes of the interventions of hormone therapy, a change in gender role, and the various surgical options in their own right. Thus while data from a substantial number of follow-up studies show that the vast majority of transgender individuals who complete all three of the latter options are satisfied with the outcome, no studies have examined the current widespread practice of offering each as an option in its own right outside of a linear process of sex reassignment. Research on what predicts satisfaction and psychosocial adjustment in this new landscape of various interventions leading to various outcomes in terms of identity, role, and expression is entirely absent and sorely needed to inform both providers and consumers of transgender-specific health care.

PHYSICAL HEALTH STATUS

While LGBT adults have all of the same health concerns as the general population, there are some areas of physical health that are known to be distinct for sexual and gender minorities.

Sexual/Reproductive Health

Very little research has been conducted on the sexual health of LGBT people, and most of it has focused on sexual dysfunction among gay and bisexual men. Evidence indicates a high rate of sexual dysfunction among all HIV-infected men (homosexual and heterosexual) (Ende et al., 2006; Lallemand et al., 2002). Very limited evidence suggests that gay men experience erectile dysfunction more than heterosexual men. In a study using a convenience sample of self-identified gay men (n = 1,196) and a matched sample of heterosexual men (n = 1,558), none of whom were HIV-positive, Bancroft and colleagues (2005) found that the gay men reported erectile dysfunction more frequently than the heterosexual men. While the authors posit that "erectile dysfunction" may mean different things to gay and heterosexual men, they also suggest that the discrepancy may be associated with anxiety or other factors.

Men who have sex with men and take medication for erectile dysfunction (either through a physician or through other sources) may demonstrate higher rates of sexual risk taking. In a study of 342 self-identified gay men attending a pride event in Denver, Nettles and colleagues (2009) found that more than 25 percent (n = 89) reported having ever used medication for erectile dysfunction. Among this group, there were significantly more acts of sexual risk taking. Likewise, a study involving a convenience sample of 1,186 HIV-positive gay and bisexual men in New York and San Francisco demonstrated that using medication for erectile dysfunction (n = 144) was associated with unprotected insertive anal intercourse (Purcell et al., 2005). It is important to note that these studies did not determine whether respondents who used erectile dysfunction medication actually suffered from underlying problems with sexual function. The association between the use of erectile dysfunction medication and risky behaviors may be attributable to recreational use of the drugs.

A study that used primarily the Internet to recruit participants (139 married heterosexual women and 114 lesbian/bisexual women in relationships) applied a proposed ecological model to examine sexual satisfaction among women (Henderson et al., 2009). The survey results indicated that sexual satisfaction was influenced in both groups by similar factors, including relationship satisfaction and sexual functioning, suggesting that gender may play a greater role than sexual orientation in sexual satisfaction.

Transgender people may struggle with sexual functioning problems. For example, among 181 transgender-identified participants in a sexual health seminar in Minnesota aged 20–73 (141 transgender women and 34 transgender men), 38 percent reported difficulty becoming sexually aroused, 34 percent reported low sexual desire, 28 percent had difficulty reaching orgasm with a partner, and 35 percent had difficulty reaching orgasm alone (Bockting et al., 2005b). In a sample of 50 transsexual women in Belgium who had had sex reassignment surgery at least 6 months prior to the study, concerns about sexual function were reported, related in particular to arousal, lubrication, and pain (Weyers et al., 2009). While feminizing hormones would be expected to lower sexual desire, this expectation has not been unequivocally supported by empirical research (see Klein and Gorzalka, 2009, for a review). Research on the effects of masculinizing hormone therapy on sexual functioning among transgender men is limited; however, findings to date show increased sexual arousal and orgasmic ability (Klein and Gorzalka, 2009). Orgasmic ability after male-to-female genital reconstructive surgery appears to have improved with advances in surgical technique over the years; 85 percent of a sample of 232 patients of a U.S. surgeon reported achieving orgasm, with 67 percent reporting it as pleasurable or more pleasurable than before surgery (Lawrence, 2005).

Apart from studies of sexually transmitted infections (STIs) that are relevant to reproductive capabilities, very little research has focused specifically on reproductive health among LGBT adults. Reproductive health (as distinct from sexual health) can be defined as the ability to have or not have children at a time and with a partner of one's choosing. A few studies based on small, nonrepresentative samples suggest that pregnancy loss may be particularly difficult for lesbian women (Peel, 2010; Wojnar, 2007) and that lesbian and bisexual women may be at higher risk than heterosexual women for postpartum depression (Ross et al., 2007; see also Trettin et al., 2006). Among transgender individuals, hormone therapy may have an effect on fertility, although little research has been conducted on the reproductive health needs of this population.

Little research exists on patterns of motherhood or access to assisted reproductive technology among sexual-minority women. The American Society for Reproductive Medicine explicitly states that programs should treat all requests for assisted reproduction equally without regard to marital status or sexual orientation, and the American College of Obstetricians and Gynecologists states that sexual orientation should not be a barrier to fertility services for achieving pregnancy (American College of Obstetricians and Gynecologists, 2005; Ethics Committee of the American Society for Reproductive Medicine, 2009). In a study examining 2,431 self-identified lesbians and bisexual women and the coming out process, Morris and colleagues (2002) found that younger mothers were more likely than older mothers (those over 50) to have used nontraditional methods to conceive (e.g., donor insemination). They also found that, compared with mothers who had children before coming out, mothers who had children after coming out were more likely to have done so through insemination by a donor, through adoption, or through foster placement.

Unfortunately, many areas of reproductive health among LGBT adults remain entirely unstudied. These include the effects of hormone therapy on the fertility of transgender individuals and its implications for family planning in terms of both contraception and reproductive options (De Sutter, 2001, 2009). A survey of an international convenience sample of 121 transgender women demonstrated the desire for gamete banking prior to the onset of hormone therapy to allow for future insemination (De Sutter et al., 2002).

Cancer

The most comprehensive repository for cancer statistics in the United States is the National Cancer Institute's Surveillance Epidemiology and End Results database. Information is collected on incidence, prevalence, and survival for specific geographic areas, and mortality data are collected for the entire country. Demographic data, including age, race/ethnicity, sex, education, income, and geographic location also are collected. However, no data are collected on sexual orientation and gender identity, making it impossible for researchers to use this database to estimate the incidence and prevalence of cancer among sexual and gender minorities.

In 1999, when the Institute of Medicine report *Lesbian Health* was published, insufficient research had been conducted to determine whether lesbians were at greater risk for breast cancer than heterosexual women. Unfortunately, 12 years later the same is true. While the relative risk of breast cancer for lesbians and heterosexual women is the topic of much discussion, a definitive answer is still unavailable. It is believed that lesbians may be at higher risk for breast cancer because there is some evidence that they have a higher prevalence of certain risk factors, including nulliparity, alcohol consumption, smoking, and obesity. The evidence comes from a number of studies. Using cohort data from the Nurses' Health Study II (NHSII), Case and colleagues (2004) compared women from the cohort who identified as lesbian (n = 694) or bisexual (n = 317) with the cohort's heterosexual women (n = 89,812). They found that the lesbian and bisexual women were more likely to be nulliparous, were more likely to be overweight and obese (lesbians more so than bisexual women), had higher smoking rates, and were more likely to report having 60 or more alcohol-containing drinks a month. Diamant and colleagues (2000c) used data from the Los Angeles County Health Survey on 4,610 women who self-identified as heterosexual, 51 who self-identified as lesbian, and 36 who self-identified as bisexual. They found that the lesbians and bisexual women were significantly more likely to report tobacco use and were more likely to report drinking alcohol frequently and in greater quantities compared with the heterosexual women. Another study, using data from the California Health Interview Survey, a population-based telephone survey, found a significantly higher prevalence of cigarette smoking among self-identified lesbians (n = 343) and bisexual women (n = 511) than among heterosexual women (n = 24,830) (Tang et al., 2004). A more recent population-based study used aggregated data from the 2001–2008 Massachusetts Behavioral Risk Factor Surveillance System surveys. The authors found that lesbians (n = 719) were more likely to be obese but not more likely to be overweight than heterosexual women (n = 39,701), while there were no significant weight differences between bisexual (n = 432) and heterosexual women (Conron et al., 2010). Although binge drinking was not defined in this study, it was found that lesbians and bisexual women were more likely to binge drink and be current smokers than their heterosexual peers. As some of these risk factors are associated with other cancers, most notably lung cancer (smoking), it is likely that women who have sex with women may be at greater risk for some cancers than heterosexual women.

It has long been established that men who have sex with men have a greater risk for anal cancer (Koblin et al., 1996). Anal cancer is associated with infection by the human papillomavirus (HPV), which is often sexually transmitted (Ryan et al., 2000), and individuals practicing receptive anal intercourse are at a higher risk for this infection (Daling et al., 2004). People with AIDS are at an increased risk for HPV-associated cancers, including anal cancer (Chaturvedi et al., 2009), although it is not known whether this greater risk is associated with AIDS-related immunosuppression or other cofactors for such cancers. In a study involving four cities, 1,218 HIV-negative men who have sex with men were tested for anal HPV, which was detected in 57 percent of the sample (Chin-Hong et al., 2004). In this study, a history of receptive anal intercourse and five or more male sex partners in the preceding 6 months appeared to be predictive of HPV infection. Other studies have shown prevalence rates of HPV infection in HIV-negative gay and bisexual men ranging from 61 to 78 percent (Friedman et al., 1998; Palefsky et al., 1998). Among HIV-positive homosexual and bisexual men, the prevalence of anal HPV infection may be as high as 93 percent (Palefsky et al., 1998). Unlike the prevalence of cervical HPV infection, which peaks during the third decade of life in women, the prevalence of anal HPV infection is steady throughout the life course of men who have sex with men, well into the sixth decade of life (Chin-Hong et al., 2004).

Similar to screening for cervical cancer, screening for anal cancer may be performed with cytology to detect HPV-associated disease (Palefsky, 2009). Currently, there exist no guidelines recommending routine anal cancer screening and no consensus on the optimal method or frequency of such screening (Palefsky, 2009). Some studies have recommended screening HIV-negative homosexual and bisexual men every 2 or 3 years (Goldie et al., 2000) and screening HIV-positive homosexual and bisexual men annually (Goldie et al., 1999). To date, however, there have been no randomized clinical trials evaluating many aspects of anal cancer screening, and the natural history of progression from precursor lesion to cancer is unknown (Wong et al., 2010).

Research on cancer among the transgender population has been extremely limited. For example, there have been no long-term prospective studies of breast cancer among transgender women. However, case reports have been published of breast cancer among transgender women who have taken feminizing hormones (Ganly and Taylory, 1995; Pritchard et al., 1988; Symmers, 1968) and transgender men who have taken masculinizing hormones and undergone chest surgery, as some breast tissue remains after such surgery (Burcombe et al., 2003; Eyler and Whittle, 2001). Transgender men on testosterone therapy may be at increased risk for ovarian cancer (Hage et al., 2000; Pache et al., 1991), and cases of prostate cancer have been reported among transgender women taking feminizing hormones (Markland, 1975; van Haarst et al., 1998).

Cardiovascular Disease

Much of the research on cardiovascular disease in LGBT populations has focused on the increased risk of such disease among those infected with HIV and among transgender individuals taking masculinizing hormones. However, not enough research has been conducted to firmly establish these risks. One prospective observational study involving male (n = 17,816) and female (n = 5,652) participants from previously established cohorts in Europe, Australia, and the United States suggests that antiretroviral treatment may be associated with cardiovascular events, such as myocardial infarction (Friis-Moller et al., 2003). Gooren and colleagues (2008) analyzed the effects of hormone therapy on a number of known risk factors for cardiovascular disease among male-to-female and female-to-male transgender patients at a clinic in the Netherlands. They found that patients receiving hormone treatment experienced both positive and negative changes in relation to certain risk factors but were unable to conclude whether the treatment had a significant effect on the risk of cardiovascular disease. More recently, Elamin and colleagues (2010) conducted a meta-analysis to examine the cardiovascular effects of hormone treatment on transsexuals. While they did not find significant effects of hormones on cardiovascular events, the authors note that the quality of the evidence was very low, and in many cases the data were insufficient to permit drawing conclusions. Their meta-analysis does suggest that hormone therapy may increase serum triglycerides in transsexuals.

One study of 4,135 women aged 18–64 in Los Angeles County examined cardiovascular health among self-identified lesbian, bisexual, and heterosexual women. Results showed that lesbians were significantly more likely than heterosexuals to receive a diagnosis of heart disease. For bisexual women, the risk for heart disease, although less than that of lesbians, was also elevated relative to heterosexual women, even though bisexual women were the youngest group in the sample (Diamant and Wold, 2003).

Obesity

Some research suggests that lesbians and bisexual women have a higher risk of obesity than heterosexual females. As discussed previously, Case and colleagues (2004) found that lesbians and bisexual women were more likely to be overweight or obese than heterosexual women (and lesbians were more likely to be overweight or obese than bisexual women). In the study conducted by Cochran and colleagues (2001), also discussed previously, a greater prevalence of obesity was found among lesbians/bisexual women than in national estimates for women generally. For purposes of the study, the authors grouped lesbians and bisexual women together. Boehmer and colleagues (2007) used population-based data from the National Survey of Family Growth to compare lesbians' rates of obesity and being overweight with those of bisexual and heterosexual women. They found that lesbians were more likely to be obese or overweight than bisexual women, heterosexual women, and women who identified as "something else." These data, in conjunction with findings of earlier studies, suggest that lesbians may be at greater risk for obesity and the health problems it may cause.

A number of studies have examined why lesbians, and in some cases bisexual women, are more obese and overweight than heterosexual women. Suggested theories include an association with the impact of minority stress, more positive body images, different exercise patterns, and childhood sexual abuse; however, insufficient research has been conducted to understand these associations.

HIV/AIDS and Other Sexually Transmitted Infections

Despite substantial changes over three decades, the HIV epidemic still exacts a severe toll on men who have sex with men in the United States (CDC, 2009a). However, rates of HIV diagnosis among all age groups are higher in black men who have sex with men than in other racial or ethnic groups of men who have sex with men in the United States (Hall et al., 2007). Given the magnitude and distribution of unrecognized HIV infection among young men who have sex with men, especially black men who have sex with men, the HIV epidemic continues at a rapid pace in this population, at least in part because many young HIV-infected men who have sex with men are unaware of their infection and unknowingly expose their partners to HIV (MacKellar et al., 2005). Studies also have found HIV prevalence to be substantially greater among male-to-female than among female-to-male transgender persons (Clements-Nolle et al., 2001) and the prevalence of HIV/STIs to be low among white and very high among Latino and black male-to-female transgender persons (Nuttbrock et al., 2009b).

Numerous risk factors for HIV transmission among gay and bisexual men have been identified, including lack of knowledge of HIV serostatus (Marks et al., 2009), nonsupportive peer norms (Hart et al., 2004), optimistic beliefs about HIV treatment (Ostrow et al., 2002; Sullivan et al., 2007), greater numbers of male sexual partners, unprotected intercourse with HIV-positive partners, and amphetamine or heavy alcohol or drug use before sex (Koblin et al., 2006). While use of the Internet to obtain partners has been increasing among men who have sex with men, the evidence appears to be inconclusive as to whether Internet use encourages or discourages risky sexual behavior (Carballo-Dieguez et al., 2006; Garofalo et al., 2007).

Notably, there is conflicting evidence on risk behavior in men who have sex with both men and women, regardless of whether they identify as bisexual. In one study examining data from the 2002 Urban Latino Men's Health Survey, such men appear to be more likely to practice unprotected intercourse with their male partners (Munoz-Laboy and Dodge, 2007). Another study examining behavioral bisexuality and condom use based on data from the 2002 cycle of the National Survey of Family Growth found that bisexually active men, when reporting on their most recent same-sex encounter, cited the same condom use as heterosexual or homosexual men. Of interest, when condom use was based on most recent female partner, bisexually active men appeared to exhibit higher rates of condom use than either homosexually active or heterosexually active men (Jeffries and Dodge, 2007). Another study comparing men who have sex with men only (n = 97) with men who have sex with both men and women (n = 175) and men who have sex with women only (n = 775) found that the men who have sex with both men and women were less likely than the men who have sex with men only to be HIV-positive or to engage in unprotected receptive anal intercourse, but more likely than the men who have sex with women only to be HIV-positive and to engage in anal intercourse with female partners. However, compared with the men who have sex with men only, the men who have sex with both men and women were not significantly more likely to report unprotected anal intercourse with female partners (Zule et al., 2009). Spikes and colleagues (2009) found that HIV-positive black men with both male and female sexual partners engaged in more sexual and drug risk behaviors than their heterosexual and gay peers.

In a systematic review of 29 studies presenting data on HIV and transgender populations, Herbst and colleagues (2008) identified a number of risk factors for transgender women. Specifically, they found that transgender women in these studies had multiple sex partners who were predominantly male, had casual sex, and had sex while they were intoxicated or high. The percentage of transgender women who engaged in sex work ranged from 24 to 75 percent across 17 studies, with the weighted mean being 41.5 percent. No data on transgender men's risk factors were included in the meta-analysis because the findings from the handful of studies that addressed these factors were too limited. It is important to note the limitations on the generalizability of these findings. The studies included in this review used small samples, ranging from 19 to 515 participants; nearly half included fewer than 100 transgender individuals. Studies also were restricted in their geographic diversity, with some places, such as San Francisco, being oversampled and most studies being limited to urban areas. Further, since most of the studies used convenience sampling methods, participants engaging in HIV risk behaviors may have been overrepresented.

Another meta-analytic study (Crepaz et al., 2009) suggests that most HIV-positive men who have sex with men protect their partners during sexual activity, but a sizable percentage continue to engage in sexual behaviors that place others at risk for HIV infection and place themselves at risk for other STIs. Still other evidence (Parsons et al., 2005) suggests that some HIV-positive men who have sex with men appear to engage more in harm reduction strategies—for example, serosorting (selecting sexual partners based on HIV serostatus) and strategic positioning (assuming the receptive or insertive position during sexual intercourse according to HIV serostatus, with the receptive position posing the greater risk of transmission)—than in withdrawal before ejaculation during anal intercourse.

While studies with racial and ethnic minority men are urgently needed, strong evidence from a meta-analysis suggests that individual-, group-, and community-level behavioral interventions are effective in reducing the risk of acquiring sexually transmitted HIV in adult men who have sex with men (Herbst et al., 2007). As this analysis shows, and the social ecology model predicts, there are multiple levels at which interventions can have an impact on individual behavior.

Far less research on HIV has been conducted with women who have sex with women. According to *Lesbian Health* (IOM, 1999), prevalence rates of HIV among women who have sex with both women and men were higher than those among exclusively heterosexual or exclusively homosexual women. More recently, it has been noted that while female-to-female transmission of HIV appears to be possible, there have been no confirmed cases (CDC, 2008).

Although HIV has overwhelmed the field of STIs, there are other STIs of concern. In 2009, 42 clinics at 12 sites across the United States submitted STI and HIV data to the Centers for Disease Control and Prevention (CDC). Results from these clinical sites showed a median prevalence of 14.9 percent for gonorrhea overall among men who have sex with men (with a range of 6.5 to 27.9 percent). The median prevalence of chlamydia among men who have sex with men was 11.2 percent (with a range of 4.5 to 18.5 percent). Primary and secondary syphilis increased between 2005 and 2009, with men who have sex with men accounting for 62 percent of all primary and secondary syphilis cases in the United States (CDC, 2010). Median clinic syphilis seroreactivity (used as a proxy for syphilis prevalence) among men who have sex with men tested for syphilis increased from 4 percent in 1999 (range of 3 to 13 percent) to 11 percent in 2008 (range of 8 to 17 percent) (CDC, 2009b). STI (including HIV) positivity varied by race and ethnicity but tended to be highest among black men who have sex with men. Median positivity for STIs was higher among HIV-positive than among HIV-negative men who have sex with men (CDC, 2009b). In a recent study of 212 HIV-infected men who have sex with men, the baseline prevalence of asymptomatic STIs was found to be 14 percent (Rieg et al., 2008). Studies also suggest that gonorrhea and syphilis rates have been increasing among men who have sex with men in recent years (Fox et al., 2001; Heffelfinger et al., 2007).

While less research has been conducted on STIs among women who have sex with women, Diamant and colleagues (2000a) note that self-identified lesbians participate in a variety of sexual activities that may put them at risk for acquiring STIs. Drawing on a convenience sample of 1,200 self-identified lesbian and bisexual women, Stevens and Hall (2001) found that 20 percent of the women who were sexually active with men reported having unprotected anal, oral, and vaginal sex. Of the women who were sexually active only with women, 56 percent reported having unprotected oral, vaginal, and anal sex, as well as sharing uncovered dildos and sex toys. Lack of knowledge about risk behavior and disease transmission was also notable in this population.

Transgender-Specific Physical Health Status

As mentioned in the discussion of mental health status, some research has been conducted on the impact of hormone therapy and surgery on gender dysphoria. However, limited research has examined the effects and side effects of hormone therapy on physical health (e.g., Gooren et al., 2008; Moore et al., 2003), and no clinical trials on the subject have been conducted. This research, conducted mainly abroad, indicated a risk of venous thromboembolic disease and elevated levels of prolactin associated with feminizing hormone therapy, and elevations in liver enzymes, loss of bone mineral density, and increased risk for ovarian cancer associated with masculinizing hormone therapy (Dizon et al., 2006; Hage et al., 2000; Van Kesteren et al., 1997, 1998). Research on increased risk for cardiovascular disease remains inconclusive, in part because of methodological limitations of studies conducted to date (Elamin et al., 2010; Gooren and Giltay, 2008). Little research, beyond case studies, has examined the cosmetic and functional outcomes of genital reconstructive surgery (Klein and Gorzalka, 2009; Lawrence, 2006).

RISK AND PROTECTIVE FACTORS

The literature addresses a number of risk factors that affect the health of LGBT adults. Conversely, research on protective factors is largely lacking.

Risk Factors

The primary risk factors for LGBT adults examined in the literature are stigma, discrimination, and victimization; violence; substance use; and childhood abuse.

Stigma, Discrimination, and Victimization

Lesbians, gay men, and bisexual people are often the targets of stigma and discrimination because of their sexual orientation. In a 2005 national survey with a probability sample of self-identified lesbian, gay, and bisexual adults (n = 662), approximately 16 percent of lesbians and 18 percent of gay men reported they had experienced discrimination in employment or housing because of their sexual orientation (Herek, 2009a). Other studies with nonprobability samples also have shown that lesbian, gay, and bisexual adults are at risk for victimization because of their sexual orientation (Herek et al., 1999; Huebner et al., 2004; Otis and Skinner, 1996). Some evidence suggests that lesbians, gay men, and bisexual people have both lifetime and day-to-day experiences with bias and discrimination more frequently than heterosexual people. An analysis of data from the MIDUS survey, mentioned earlier in the chapter, found that self-identified homosexual and bisexual adults reported both lifetime and day-to-day experiences with discrimination more frequently than heterosexuals, and 42 percent attributed the discrimination partially or entirely to their sexual orientation (Mays and Cochran, 2001).

Not surprisingly, experiences with discrimination and victimization have negative effects on psychological well-being. In the MIDUS study, perceived discrimination was positively associated with indicators of psychiatric morbidity as well as harmful effects on quality of life (Mays and Cochran, 2001). Swim and colleagues (2009) found that everyday experiences with relatively minor incidents of prejudice based on sexual orientation were associated with elevations in negative mood (Swim et al., 2009). Szymanski (2005) examined the effects of external and internalized heterosexism and sexism on mental health in a study of 143 women who self-identified as lesbian (92 percent), bisexual (6 percent), and unsure (2 percent) and found that all three variables were related to psychological distress in the lesbians. Similarly, based on an Internet survey (n = 210), gay and bisexual men's experiences of sexual stigma—including harassment, rejection, and discrimination—appear to be associated with psychological distress (Szymanski, 2009).

While little research has examined the additive effects of various forms of social discrimination—including antigay violence, discrimination, and harassment—one study found higher levels of psychological distress in gay and bisexual Latino men. Such experiences were also associated with social isolation and low self-esteem (Diaz et al., 2001).

Because of the unique discrimination faced by bisexual men and women from both heterosexual and homosexual people, some studies using small samples have examined bisexual people's perception of their own identity. Results of a study comparing bisexual and lesbian/gay adults (n = 613) showed that the bisexual adults reported higher levels of identity confusion (uncertainty about one's sexual orientation) and lower levels of self-disclosure and community connectedness than the lesbian and gay adults (Balsam and Mohr, 2007). Another, smaller study (n = 43) using qualitative methods to explore minority stress among bisexual men and women, gay men, and lesbians showed that the bisexual men and women felt that both heterosexual and homosexual individuals can have biased opinions of bisexual people. Bisexual participants felt that some members of the gay and lesbian community perceived bisexuality as an inauthentic identity and viewed bisexuals as promiscuous (Hequembourg and Brallier, 2009). Bisexual participants reported feeling invisible and indicated that they lacked comfortable social spaces catering to bisexual people. Bisexual participants also reported concealing their bisexual identity to blend in better in gay/lesbian or heterosexual social spaces (Hequembourg and Brallier, 2009).

Research with convenience samples of transgender people in various communities across the United States highlights a high prevalence of enacted stigma and discrimination based on gender identity. In a study of 402 transgender people, 56 percent reported verbal harassment, 37 percent employment discrimination, and 19 percent physical violence (see below) (Lombardi et al., 2001). Among a sample of 248 transgender people of color in Washington, DC, 43 percent reported having been a victim of violence or crime and 13 percent of sexual abuse; 43 percent attributed this victimization to homophobia and 35 percent to transphobia (Xavier et al., 2005).

The extent to which transgender individuals are accepted within the LGB community has not been adequately studied. Qualitative data from a convenience sample of transsexual men with a gay or bisexual identity revealed mixed acceptance (Bockting et al., 2009a). Among a convenience sample of lesbian and feminist women, attitudes toward transsexuals were generally positive, particularly for those who knew a transgender person personally (Kendal et al., 1997).

Violence

Sexual minorities are at particular risk for hate or bias crimes based on their minority status; they may also be at risk for intimate partner violence. While the vast majority of studies focus on male victims, females in gay populations also frequently experience antigay violence. Convenience samples have revealed a high level of violence against transgender people as well (Lombardi, 2001; Xavier et al., 2005). As a result of hate crimes based on sexual orientation, lesbian and gay survivors have been found to manifest significantly more symptoms of depression, anger, anxiety, and posttraumatic stress compared with lesbian and gay victims of comparable crimes unrelated to their sexual orientation (Herek et al., 1999; see also Huebner et al., 2004; Otis and Skinner, 1996).

Data from the Federal Bureau of Investigation (2010), as well as some studies based on probability samples, suggest that hate crimes based on sexual orientation are prevalent in the United States. Using a probability sample of 912 Latino self-identified gay and bisexual men living in New York City, Miami, and Los Angeles, Diaz and colleagues (2001) found that 10 percent of this sample reported experiencing violence as an adult due to their sexual orientation. Similarly, a report by the Kaiser Family Foundation (2001), based on a probability sample of 405 lesbian, gay, and bisexual adults, found that 32 percent of the sample had ever been targeted for violence because of their sexual orientation. In a study using data from the Knowledge Networks panel (n = 662), Herek (2009b) provides prevalence estimates of hate crimes among self-identified lesbian, gay, and bisexual adults. Approximately 20 percent of respondents reported they had experienced a crime against their person or property based on their sexual orientation, with gay men being more likely than lesbians or bisexuals to have had such experiences. More than one-third of gay men (38 percent) reported experiencing hate crimes against their person or property, compared with 11–13 percent of lesbians, bisexual men, and bisexual women (Herek, 2009b).

Beyond hate crimes, couples with same-sex partners may also be at risk for intimate partner violence. Few studies have examined intimate partner violence in probability samples of same-sex partners. Tjaden and colleagues (1999), using data from the National Violence Against Women Survey, examined intimate partner violence in same- and different-sex cohabitating relationships (n = 8,000 men, 8,000 women), although sexual orientation was not assessed. Among the 1 percent of respondents (65 men, 79 women) in a current or past same-sex cohabitating relationship, rates of physical and sexual assault by a same-sex partner were similar for men and women. However, men experienced violence from a male partner at a rate similar to that of women with a male partner but more often than men or women with a female partner (Tjaden et al., 1999). Greenwood and colleagues (2002) examined battering victimization in intimate relationships in a probability sample (n = 2,881) of men who have sex with men from San Francisco, Los Angeles, Chicago, and New York. More than a third of the men reported at least one form of abuse.

Substance Use

Much research has focused on substance use among LGB adults, most of it suggesting that substance use is a problem for these populations. However, the most definitive evidence is available from population-based studies of substance use in heterosexual and nonheterosexual samples.

Studies have shown that nonheterosexuals have higher rates of smoking than heterosexuals, although typically in comparisons among women. Burgard and colleagues (2005) examined tobacco use among heterosexually and homosexually experienced women in the California Women's Health Survey (1998–2000), a large, annual statewide health surveillance survey of women in the state. Sexual orientation was based on self-reports of same-gender behavior. The authors found that the homosexually experienced women were more likely than the exclusively heterosexually experienced women to currently smoke.

Case and colleagues (2004) examined differences in health risk factors and physical functioning between heterosexual and self-identified lesbian/bisexual registered nurses in a prospective cohort (n = 116,671) recruited from 14 U.S. states for the NHSII. Compared with the heterosexual nurses, the lesbian and bisexual nurses had a higher prevalence of current and past smoking. Similarly, Conron and colleagues (2010) provide evidence of differences in smoking and drug use between heterosexuals and gays/lesbians from the Massachusetts Behavioral Risk Factor Surveillance System surveys (n = 67,359), an annual stratified household sample of adults in Massachusetts. Sexual orientation was based on self-reported sexual identity, which included gay or lesbian (2 percent), bisexual (1 percent), and heterosexual (97 percent). For purposes of analysis, respondents identifying as gay or lesbian were combined. Compared with the heterosexual adults, the sexual-minority respondents were more likely to report current and past smoking and any 30-day drug use.

Gruskin and colleagues (2007) compared prevalence rates of tobacco use among LGB individuals and the general population in California. Data on LGB individuals (n = 1,950) were collected using a large-scale population-based survey of tobacco use, while data on the general population (n = 20,525) were taken from the California Tobacco Survey; sexual orientation was determined by sexual self-identity and sexual behavior. Results showed that lesbians, bisexual women, and women who have sex with women were more likely to be daily, nondaily, or former smokers than women in the general California population. In the case of men, the prevalence of tobacco use was higher among gay men than among men in the general population; no significant differences in smoking were observed between bisexual men and men in the general population. Disparities in tobacco use between the LGB populations and the general population were still evident after controlling for key demographic variables.

Drabble and Trocki (2005) examined patterns of use of smoked substances (cigarettes and marijuana) using data from the 2000 National Alcohol Survey, a population-based telephone survey of adults aged 18 and older in the United States. Sexual orientation was defined as lesbian or gay self-identified (n = 36), bisexual self-identified (n = 50), heterosexual self-identified with same-sex partners in the past 5 years (n = 71), and exclusively heterosexual self-identified reporting no same-sex partners (n = 3,723). The authors found that, relative to the exclusively heterosexual women, the odds of past-year tobacco use were more than three times greater in the bisexual women and two times greater in the heterosexual women reporting same-sex partners. There was no significant difference in past-year tobacco use between the lesbians and exclusively heterosexual women. Using the same data set, Trocki and colleagues (2009) examined tobacco and marijuana use among lesbians (n = 36), gay men (n = 57), heterosexual men (n = 3,201) and women (n = 3,723) with only different-sex partners, bisexual men (n = 27) and women (n = 50), and heterosexual self-identified men (n = 83) and women (n = 71) with same-sex partners. They found that the bisexual and heterosexual women reporting same-sex partners had higher rates of cigarette smoking than the exclusively heterosexual women. They also found significantly higher rates of marijuana use among the bisexual women, lesbians, and heterosexual women with same-sex partners than among the exclusively heterosexual women. Among the gay men, marijuana use was significantly greater and tobacco use was elevated compared with the heterosexual men. These findings suggest that marijuana and tobacco use differ by sexual identity, particularly among women.

With regard to alcohol use, several population-based studies suggest that nonheterosexual women consume alcohol in greater amounts and more frequently and may be at greater risk of alcohol dependency than heterosexual women. Cochran and Mays (2000b) examined differences in psychiatric syndromes among homosexually and heterosexually active women and men in the 1996 National Household Survey of Drug Abuse. Homosexually active women were more likely than other women to be classified as having alcohol or drug dependency syndromes. Other evidence (Gilman et al., 2001), based on the previously mentioned National Comorbidity Survey, provides support for similar differences in alcohol use between women with same-sex and different-sex partners. Women with same-sex partners had a significantly earlier onset of alcohol use disorders than women with different-sex partners.

Burgard and colleagues (2005) examined alcohol use among heterosexually and homosexually experienced women using data from the California Women's Health Survey, described above. Sexual orientation was based on self-reports of same-gender behavior. Findings revealed that the homosexually experienced women were more likely than the exclusively heterosexually experienced women to consume alcohol more frequently and in greater quantities. Also, recently bisexually active women were more likely than women who were exclusively heterosexually active to report consuming alcohol in the past month, had more drinks per drinking day, and exhibited drinking patterns indicative of being binge drinkers.

Similar findings are available from comparisons of alcohol consumption among women who identified their sexual orientation as heterosexual, lesbian, or bisexual in a prospective cohort from the NHSII (Case et al., 2004). The authors found that lesbians and bisexual women were significantly more likely than heterosexual women to report having engaged in heavy drinking, defined as consuming 60 or more alcohol-containing drinks a month.

Drabble and colleagues (2005) examined the prevalence of drinking and alcohol-related problems among homosexual, bisexual, and heterosexual respondents in the 2000 National Alcohol Survey (n = 7,248). Sexual orientation was based on both self-identity and behavior, which yielded four categories of participants: homosexual, bisexual, heterosexual with same-sex partners, and exclusively heterosexual. Few significant differences were found among men by sexual orientation, with the only significant finding being that the gay men had lower abstention rates than the exclusively heterosexual men. By contrast, both the heterosexual women with same-sex partners and the bisexual women had significantly lower abstention rates than the exclusively heterosexual women. The lesbians and bisexual women also had significantly greater odds of reporting alcohol-related social consequences and alcohol dependence (according to criteria of the *Diagnostic and Statistical Manual of Mental Disorders*, fourth revision [DSM-IV]) than the exclusively heterosexual women.

In the previously mentioned study by Drabble and Trocki (2005), other differences in alcohol use were found among the four groups of female participants. Compared with the exclusively heterosexual women, the mean number of drinks per year was elevated among the lesbians, bisexual women, and women who self-identified as heterosexual but reported same-sex partners. When demographic variables were controlled, however, the only significant difference was between the exclusively heterosexual women and the heterosexual self-identified women with same-sex partners. When looking at alcohol consumption in different contexts, the authors found that the heterosexual self-identified women who reported same-sex partners were more likely both to frequent bars and to drink heavily in bars relative to the exclusively heterosexual women. The bisexual self-identified women were less likely to frequent bars, but were more likely to drink heavily in both bars and party contexts compared with the exclusively heterosexual women (Drabble and Trocki, 2005).

In a study using survey data from 1996–1998, Scheer and colleagues (2002) examined sexual and drug use behaviors among women who have sex with women who resided in low-income neighborhoods in Northern California. Based on sexual behavior, the respondents, aged 18–29, included women who had sex exclusively with men (n = 2,229), women who had sex with both men and women (n = 189), and women who had sex exclusively with women (n = 16). Compared with the women who had sex exclusively with men, the women who had sex with both men and women were more likely to report past and recent injection drug use.

Stall and colleagues (2001) examined alcohol and recreational drug use among urban men who have sex with men (n = 2,172) using data from the Urban Men's Health Study. The study sample included self-identified gay and bisexual men as well as men who reported a sexual encounter with another man in the past 5 years. Fifty-two percent of the sample reported recreational drug use and 85 percent reported alcohol use in the past 6 months. Further, 8 percent of the men who have sex with men engaged in frequent/heavy drinking (five or more drinks at a sitting at least once a week), 18 percent used three or more recreational drugs, and 19 percent used recreational drugs at least once a week.

Harawa and colleagues (2008) examined the role of drug use and addiction in sexual behavior by conducting focus groups with 46 nongay self-identified black men of predominantly low socioeconomic status. The authors identified drug use as playing a central role in same-sex sexuality, with participants describing alcohol and drug use and addiction and sex–drug transactions as being closely linked to same-sex sexual behavior (Harawa et al., 2008).

Many studies have found an association between nonheterosexual orientation and increased risk of substance use. However, McCabe and colleagues (2009) found significant variation in substance use outcomes across gender and sexual orientation definitions. Using data from the National Epidemiologic Survey on Alcohol and Related Conditions (n = 34,653 participants aged 20 and older), the authors found that most sexual-minority respondents did not report substance use or meet criteria for substance dependence. However, they also found that the effects of sexual-minority status on substance use and dependence were greater for sexual-minority women than for sexual-minority men, although this finding may be a result of the overall higher rates of substance use and dependence among men in the general population (McCabe et al., 2009).

While a meta-analysis of prior mental health research found that lesbian, gay, and bisexual individuals had a 1.5 times higher risk of alcohol and other substance dependence over 12 months compared with heterosexual individuals (King et al., 2008), data from convenience samples suggest that substance use may be a major concern among transgender people as well. Eighteen percent of 392 transgender women and 4 percent of 123 transgender men in San Francisco and 23 percent of 332 transgender women of color in San Francisco reported injection drug use. Fully 48 percent of 248 transgender people of color in Washington, DC, reported a problem with alcohol and drugs (Xavier et al., 2005). A previously mentioned study of 207 transgender individuals, 480 men who have sex with men, and 122 behaviorally bisexual women participating in a sexual health seminar assessed substance use among these three groups. Among transgender participants, 20 percent reported abusing alcohol, compared with 30 percent of men who have sex with men and 16 percent of bisexual women; 16 percent of transgender participants used marijuana, compared with 26 percent of men who have sex with men and 24 percent of bisexual women; and 3 percent of transgender participants used other drugs, compared with 9 percent of men who have sex with men and 2 percent of bisexual women (Bockting et al., 2005a).

Childhood Abuse

A small amount of research has documented higher rates of childhood abuse among sexual-minority men and women. Using data from the NHSII, Austin and colleagues (2008) compared rates of childhood abuse among self-identified lesbian, bisexual, and heterosexual women. They found that, compared with heterosexual women, lesbians and bisexual women were more likely to report physical and sexual abuse during childhood and adolescence. In a newer study using the same data set, Austin and Irwin (2010) showed that increased physical and sexual abuse among self-identified lesbian and bisexual women was positively associated with risk of tobacco and alcohol use as well as greater use in adolescence. Another study examining data from the National Survey of Midlife Development in the United States compared childhood maltreatment experiences among 2,917 self-identified heterosexual (n = 2,844), homosexual (n = 41), and bisexual (n = 32) individuals aged 25–74. For the purposes of analysis, homosexual and bisexual respondents were grouped together. The authors found that, compared with the heterosexual respondents, the homosexual/bisexual respondents reported higher rates of major physical maltreatment by their parents.

While little is known about experiences of childhood sexual abuse among sexual minorities, some evidence, derived from a probability sample of urban men who have sex with men (n = 1,078), suggests that such abuse may be common (20 percent) among sexual-minority men (Catania et al., 2008). Moreover, a few studies suggest that childhood sexual abuse may be linked with negative health outcomes in adulthood. In a study examining risk factors for obesity among a community sample of lesbians (n = 416), childhood sexual abuse was associated with obesity even after adjusting for age, race/ethnicity, and education (Aaron and Hughes, 2007). Similarly, high rates of childhood sexual abuse among a probability sample of Latino gay and bisexual men (n = 912) predicted HIV and mental health outcomes (Arreola et al., 2009). Feldman and Meyer (2007a) examined the relationship between childhood sexual abuse and eating disorders in a community sample of 193 self-identified white, black, and Latino gay and bisexual men and found that 33 percent of the sample had experienced childhood physical abuse, and 34 percent had experienced childhood sexual abuse. They also found that childhood sexual abuse was a predictor of subclinical or full-syndrome eating disorders. Little is known about racial and ethnic variation in the prevalence of childhood sexual abuse, but a recent study of 669 LGB men and women found that black and Latino participants reported the highest rates of childhood sexual abuse, while Latinos and Asian Americans reported the highest rates of childhood physical abuse (Balsam et al., 2010). In a nonprobability sample of 181 transgender seminar participants in Minnesota, 23 percent of participants reported childhood sexual abuse and 38 percent childhood physical abuse (Bockting et al., 2005b).

Protective Factors

Although research on protective factors is sparse, small studies suggest the possibility of a few factors that may be protective, all of which require more research. For example, one protective factor may be living and/or working in supportive environments. Hatzenbuehler and colleagues (2010) examined the psychological impact on sexual minorities of living in states with constitutional amendments banning marriage among same-sex couples and found a statistically significant increase in the rates of generalized anxiety disorder and mood and alcohol use disorders among LGB participants over a 3-year period. Sexual minorities who lived in states that did not have such amendments showed no significant increases in psychiatric morbidities. Similarly, a national study of lesbians, gay men, and bisexual people explored the antecedents affecting the degree to which they disclosed their LGB identities in the workplace. The authors found that employees had less fear of disclosing and disclosed more often when they worked in a group that seemed supportive and shared their stigma (Ragins et al., 2007). An earlier study that focused on workplace discrimination found that organizational policies and practices were strongly associated with perceived discrimination (Ragins and Cornwell, 2001).

Support from family and friends may be another protective factor. A study found that perceived social support for romantic relationships predicted greater relationship well-being and, in turn, more positive mental and physical health outcomes; this was true for both same-sex and mixed-sex partners (Blair and Holmberg, 2008). In surveying 340 self-identified gay men aged 18–78, Willoughby and colleagues (2008) found that social networks of adult gay men may play important roles in both the promotion and prevention of health risk. Similarly, in a study of 106 self-identified Latino lesbians and gay men aged 20–53, social support, active coping, and identification with the Latino gay and lesbian community were all associated with psychological well-being (Zea et al., 1999).

Studies have shown that positive health effects are associated with marriage (Herdt and Kertzner, 2006; Herek, 2006). These positive effects derive in part from the economic impact of the benefits, rights, and privileges available to married couples, as well as the increased social support and relative stability associated with a legally recognized commitment (Herek, 2006). Preliminary research has indicated that same-sex couples in legally recognized relationships experience greater psychological benefits than those in similar long-term relationships that lack legal recognition (Riggle et al., 2010).

Using survey data collected in 1994, Luhtanen (2003) measured self-esteem, life satisfaction, and depression among groups of lesbians/bisexual women (n = 168) and gay/bisexual men (n = 152) aged 19–73. For purposes of the study, lesbians and bisexual women were combined and analyzed as a group, as were gay and bisexual men. The most robust predictor of psychological well-being in both groups was having a positive LGB identity (Luhtanen, 2003). In a study of 182 lesbian and bisexual women, Singh and colleagues (2006) found that participants with higher levels of social ease (defined as the level of comfort with others in social situations) or higher levels of self-disclosure (defined as communication of a personal nature with others) had less internalized homophobia. Of interest, the authors did not find a significant relationship between levels of internalized homophobia and social support or financial freedom (Singh et al., 2006).

Many of the protective factors of health among sexual minorities may be considered to contribute to their resiliency. Definitions of resilience vary, ranging from a risk factor that has been averted or unrealized (Keyes, 2004), to a phenomenon that involves a relatively good outcome despite one's suffering risk experiences (Rutter, 2007), to a class of phenomena characterized by patterns of positive adaptation in the context of significant adversity or risk (Masten and Reed, 2002). Despite these differing definitions, studies typically focus on the capacity to recover from psychological trauma or to adapt successfully to adversity. Indeed, resilience per se is not directly observable and can only be inferred by observing a person's adaptation (Masten, 2007). Minority stress theory (Meyer, 2003), discussed briefly in Chapter 1, posits that individuals from stigmatized social groups experience excess stress and negative life events due to their minority status in addition to the general stressors experienced by all people, and consequently must have greater capacity for adaptation. Moreover, various social structures, institutions, and processes beyond the individual contribute further to the experience of minority stress. Meyer (2003) contends that minority stress includes both internalized and external stress processes that can cause negative mental health outcomes. Resilience represents one category of variables, in addition to social support and coping, that can affect the association between minority stress and distress. Most research on resiliency factors involves studies with heterosexual children, adolescents, and adults. The studies cited in this section include the few notable exceptions that have examined resiliency factors associated with health among gay and lesbian adults. More research on the impact of resilience on the association between risk factors and health outcomes in sexual-minority populations is warranted.

The limited amount of research on transgender people has focused less on protective factors than on the factors associated with positive outcomes of sex reassignment. These factors, mentioned earlier in this chapter, include psychological adjustment, family support, psychological treatment, and good surgical outcomes (Carroll, 1999; Lawrence, 2003).

HEALTH SERVICES

Most of the available research on the interactions of LGBT adults with various aspects of the health system tends to focus on the different patterns of access to and utilization of health care services by the LGBT community. Very few studies have examined how lack of access and utilization affects the health status of LGBT populations, an area that requires more research. Similarly, the literature tends to focus on processes of care rather than on the outcomes of the delivery or quality of care.

Access and Utilization

The limited research available suggests that LGBT adults have different patterns of access and utilization of health care services than heterosexual adults. For example, Sanchez and colleagues (2007) compared 360 self-identified LGB individuals and 10,000 adults in New York City and found that the former had higher rates of emergency department use than the general population. In another example, Kerker and colleagues (2006) conducted a multilingual population-based survey in New York City to determine the use of Pap tests and mammograms among women who have sex with women (n = 269). They found that these women were significantly less likely than other women to have had a Pap test in the past 36 months or a mammogram in the past 24 months. Earlier research had yielded similar findings (Cochran et al., 2001; Diamant et al., 2000b; Marrazzo et al., 2001).

Much of the research that specifically examines access issues for sexual minorities relates to the use of mental health services. One study, examining data from the MIDUS survey, found that individuals who self-identified as either homosexual or bisexual used mental health services more than did self-identified heterosexual individuals (Cochran et al., 2003). In a comparison of a convenience sample of self-identified lesbians (n = 63) and a matched sample of self-identified heterosexual women (n = 57), Razzano and colleagues (2002) found that lesbians in their sample used mental health services, as well as alcohol and drug-related services, significantly more than heterosexual women. Specifically among black women, Matthews and Hughes (2001) compared a convenience sample of lesbians, defined by behavior and attraction measures (n = 70), with a sample of heterosexual women (n = 40) and found that the lesbians attended counseling or therapy at significantly higher rates than their heterosexual counterparts. In a previously mentioned study, Page (2004) found that bisexual men and women were less likely to seek help for sexual orientation issues and rated services as less helpful relative to lesbian and gay respondents in comparable research.

Some research suggests that use of preventive screening may be less frequent among lesbians and bisexual women than among heterosexual women. In a study using pooled data from seven separate surveys conducted between 1987 and 1996, Cochran and colleagues (2001) compared data on approximately 12,000 women who have sex with women against national estimates for women. Of the surveyed women in the pooled data, most self-identified as lesbian, with a much smaller percentage self-identifying as bisexual and an even smaller percentage self-identifying as other/heterosexual. The authors found that self-identified lesbians/bisexual women were less likely to have had a pelvic examination in the last 5 years than women in the general population and that lesbians/bisexual women in their 40s were less likely to have received a mammogram. It should be noted that when pooling the data, the authors combined the samples of lesbians and bisexual women. Another study examining use of preventive services among lesbians (n = 524), bisexual women (n = 143), and heterosexual women (n = 637) found that the bisexual women were the least likely to undergo mammography (Koh, 2000).

In a study conducted by Diamant and colleagues (2000c), described above, self-identified lesbians, but not bisexual women, were significantly less likely than heterosexual women to have had a Pap test or a clinical breast exam within the previous 2 years. However, the authors found that for women aged 50 and older, there was no difference in receiving mammograms between heterosexual women and lesbians, nor were there differences between bisexual and heterosexual women in receiving Pap tests, clinical breast exams, or mammograms. More recently, Buchmueller and Carpenter (2010) used data from the 2000–2007 Behavioral Risk Factor Surveillance System to compare women in same-sex and different-sex relationships. They found that women in same-sex relationships were significantly less likely than women in different-sex relationships to have had recommended mammograms or Pap tests in the last 3 years. Even when insurance coverage was equalized across the groups, the gap in preventive care services remained.

The literature also points to a number of barriers that may influence LGBT individuals' interactions with health services. Such barriers include lack of health insurance, fear of discrimination from providers, lack of knowledge on the part of providers, lack of perceived severity of medical conditions, and dissatisfaction with services (Heck et al., 2006; Nemoto et al., 2005; Newman et al., 2008; Owens et al., 2007; Rhodes and Diclemente, 2003; van Dam et al., 2001).

Perceived discrimination by health care providers may be a significant barrier to access to and utilization of health care services. A few studies have examined different providers and their attitudes toward sexual-minority patients. Javaherian and colleagues (2008) collected qualitative and quantitative data from a questionnaire administered to occupational therapy practitioners (n = 1,051) to assess comfort levels in working with lesbian, gay, or bisexual patients. They found that while most of the providers felt comfortable and prepared to work with sexual-minority patients, less than 20 percent of the sample had received education in this area. A study based on a convenience sample of providers of substance abuse treatment (n = 46) showed wide variability in their attitudes toward sexual-minority patients (Cochran et al., 2007a). While this range of attitudes is likely to exist in the general population, provider attitudes could affect the success of treatment in the context of a substance abuse treatment program. In a qualitative assessment of training needs among providers of HIV-related care to transgender people (n = 13), providers admitted discomfort with interviewing such patients, stated a need for more standards and guidelines for their care, and acknowledged a lack of understanding of distinct transgender identities and the nuances of transgender-specific care (Lurie, 2005). Using qualitative interviews, Simpson and Helfrich (2007) asked providers to identify barriers that prevented lesbians from accessing services for intimate partner violence. The providers identified systemic barriers that reflect cultural attitudes, institutional barriers that originate in the policies of service agencies, and individual barriers that emerge from individual attitudes. Training and education interventions to impact the attitudes of providers, such as that described by Kelley and colleagues (2008) for medical students, hold promise for addressing these issues.

An earlier study (Smith et al., 1985) of 424 bisexuals and 1,921 lesbians found that 40 percent of each group believed that disclosing information to physicians about their sexual preference would hinder the quality of their medical care. About one-third of each group had not disclosed their sexual behavior, although they wanted to, because physicians had not asked. Another study examined LGB people's (n = 88) disclosure of sexual identity to health care providers and found that many respondents reported previous negative interactions with providers and avoided discussing sexuality with providers (Eliason and Schope, 2001). While many of these studies had sampling limitations, they highlight potential barriers that deserve further scrutiny.

Research with convenience samples of transgender people indicates that lack of access to health care is an important concern for this segment of the LGBT community. Access to transgender-specific health care in accordance with the *Standards of Care* varies across the United States (Rachlin et al., 2008). One major barrier is that, with some notable exceptions, health insurance and other third-party payers (Medicare, Medical Assistance) exclude coverage of transgender-specific health care, particularly surgery. The cost of medical care, lack of access to specialists, and a paucity of transgender-friendly and -knowledgeable providers are perceived barriers to care. On the other hand, being under the care of a physician is associated with reduced high-risk behavior, such as smoking cessation, medically supervised hormone therapy, and access to clean needles for hormone injection (Sanchez et al., 2009).

The recently conducted National Transgender Discrimination Survey (n = 6,456), described in detail in Chapter 3, reported that 28 percent of transgender respondents experienced verbal harassment in a medical setting, and 50 percent encountered providers that lacked knowledge of some aspect of their health needs (Grant et al., 2010). Qualitative research supports the finding that transgender people often have negative experiences when interacting with health care providers who lack the cultural competence to respond sensitively to their health concerns (Bockting et al., 1998; Clements-Nolle et al., 1999; Sperber et al., 2005). In a survey using a convenience sample of 248 transgender people of color in Washington, DC, 33 percent reported insensitivity or hostility from health care providers; 11 percent reported difficulty accessing transgender-specific health care procedures (counseling, hormone therapy, or surgery to alleviate gender dysphoria), and 70 percent of those taking hormones had acquired them from friends or on the street (Xavier et al., 2005). Participants in this survey indicated multiple needs for general and transgender-specific health care services not currently met. Among 332 transgender women of color in San Francisco, needs for general health care services were high and generally met; however, this was often not the case for social services, substance use treatment, psychological counseling, and transition-related medical services. Further focus group findings (n = 48) indicated that this population was generally dissatisfied with the quality of available health and social services (Nemoto et al., 2005). Similarly, a survey of transgender people in Philadelphia (n = 81) found high levels of need for health and social services that were largely unmet, especially among female-to-males (Kenagy, 2005a).

Quality of Care

Very little research has been conducted on the quality of care experienced by sexual and gender minorities. A limited amount of research has explored the preferences of lesbian, gay, and bisexual patients with respect to receiving care. Findings indicate that satisfaction among sexual-minority patients is associated with a number of factors, including the provider's LGB-specific knowledge, the competency of care, and sensitivity to areas of concern for sexual minorities (Burckell and Goldfried, 2006; Saulnier, 2002; Seaver et al., 2008). Page (2007) explored self-identified bisexual men and women's (n = 217) experiences with psychotherapy and found that respondents viewed knowledge of bisexual-specific issues and validation of bisexual identity as important to a positive patient–provider relationship. As mentioned above, some research suggests that the quality of care received by transgender people is affected by a lack of culturally competent providers (Bockting et al., 1998; Clements-Nolle et al., 1999; Sperber et al., 2005). In a convenience sample of 122 female-to-male transgender persons ranging in age from 18 to 60, Rachlin and colleagues (2008) found mixed reviews of health care services. About one-third of respondents rated the care they received as either poor or fair; about one-quarter rated their health care provider's sensitivity to their needs as "a trans person" as either "horrible" or poor or fair.

Some literature examines specific care environments for LGBT populations. For example, Brown and McDuffie (2009) surveyed prison systems in the United States regarding the care provided to transgender inmates. They found wide variability in terms of access to sex hormones, with some systems allowing continuation of treatment, some requiring that hormone treatment be stopped, and others allowing the initiation of treatment. In a survey of substance abuse services specializing in LGBT clients, Cochran and colleagues (2007b) found no difference between the specialized services offered to LGBT clients and those offered to the general population. These studies are limited by their lack of generalizability, however.

At the University of Minnesota, results from five consecutive patient satisfaction surveys over a 10-year period showed that satisfaction with transgender-specific health care services was high (Bockting et al., 2004). Few significant differences were found between transgender patients (n = 180) and other sexual health patients (n = 837), except that in one year, transgender patients reported higher satisfaction on their perceived ability to handle the problems that originally had led them to seek services. This is one of the very few studies examining patient satisfaction with the delivery of transgender-specific health care, and it indicates that, despite the challenges associated with the gate-keeping role (i.e., the requirement for evaluation and recommendation from a mental health professional to access hormone therapy and surgery), high satisfaction can be achieved.

CONTEXTUAL INFLUENCES

Several salient contextual influences, including sociodemographic and familial factors, influence the health of sexual- and gender-minority adults.

Sociodemographic Factors

One prominent contextual influence on LGBT individuals is race/ethnicity and its intersection with low socioeconomic status. While few studies have examined racial/ethnic differences in health outcomes across sexual- and gender-minority populations, some studies suggest that racial/ethnic variability in mental disorders may exist. Using a sample of 388 New York City residents who identified as lesbian, gay, or bisexual, Meyer and colleagues (2008) found that black LGB individuals experienced a lower prevalence of all psychiatric disorders than Latino and white LGB individuals (Meyer et al., 2008). The same study also found that Latino sexual minorities attempted suicide more often than white sexual minorities. Using survey data to examine health indicators among racial and ethnic minorities, Mays and colleagues (2002) compared a sample of self-identified black and Latino lesbians obtained from a non-population-based survey (n = 365) with a sample of self-identified heterosexual black and Latino women drawn from a population-based survey. She found that black and Latino lesbians and bisexual women had some negative health outcomes compared with heterosexual women, including higher rates of obesity and increased rates of tobacco and alcohol use; they also had lower rates of health insurance coverage.

While few studies have looked at racial/ethnic differences in health outcomes in LGBT populations, even fewer have explored the effect of geography. Some small qualitative studies suggest that social isolation exists among rural LGB populations (McCarthy, 2000; Williams et al., 2005). To evaluate the health status of lesbians living in southern states, Austin and Irwin (2010) compared findings from a convenience sample of self-identified lesbians living in the south (n = 1,141) with results from CDC's Behavioral Risk Factor Surveillance System. They found that the lesbians residing in southern states were more likely to have experienced recent depression and more likely to have engaged in risky health behaviors than women in the general U.S. population (in both southern and nonsouthern states).

Socioeconomic status is another relevant contextual factor that may affect sexual minorities. One study, examining a sample of men who have sex with men (n = 2,605) derived from the Urban Men's Health Study, found that as income and level of education decreased, the men who have sex with men were less likely to identify as gay, more likely to have sex with women, and less likely to be involved in the gay community (Barrett and Pollack, 2005). As mentioned in Chapter 2, evidence also suggests that there are income differences based on sexual orientation.

Cultural context based on one's country of origin can influence the health of LGBT populations as well. Cultural norms of the home country and the ways in which they are modified by migration/immigration have been shown to affect the sexual health of Asian/Pacific Islander men who have sex with men (Chng and Geliga-Vargas, 2000). Other research suggests less tolerance toward LGB individuals in some Latin American countries than in the United States (Bianchi et al., 2007; Nierman et al., 2007). It should be noted, however, that laws in both Argentina and Mexico City allow marriage between same-sex couples. Research on the sexuality of Asian and Latino people in the United States has been sparse, and many of the studies that have been conducted suffer from sampling problems and other methodological limitations. However, some data are available from probability samples and are discussed elsewhere in this report (e.g., Chae and Ayala, 2010; Cochran et al., 2007c; Diaz et al., 2001).

Familial Factors

Some research, discussed below, examines gay men and lesbians in terms of families, and a very small amount of research looks at transgender family life. However, the committee could find no research on the family lives of bisexual people. Studies of partnering relationships typically refer to same-sex or different-sex couples. The experiences of bisexual people in these relationships do not appear to be reflected in research.

As noted in Chapter 2, gay men and lesbians are less likely to become parents than their heterosexual peers (Gates et al., 2007; Patterson, 2004; Patterson and Riskind, 2010). Results from the 2002 National Survey of Family Growth (NSFG) revealed that 35 percent of self-identified lesbians (aged 15–44) reported having given birth to at least one child, compared with 65 percent of same-aged heterosexual women. In the 2002 NSFG, only 16 percent of self-identified gay men reported having a biological or adoptive child, compared with 48 percent of same-aged heterosexual men (Gates et al., 2007; Patterson and Riskind, 2010). Thus, available data suggest that while fewer lesbian and gay than heterosexual adults become parents, many lesbian and gay adults do become parents.

Why are there fewer lesbian and gay than heterosexual parents? Lesbian and gay adults may be less likely to become parents in part because they have fewer unplanned pregnancies. However, data from the 2002

NSFG reveal that both gay men and lesbians endorse the value of parenthood as strongly as their heterosexual peers and that many childless gay and lesbian adults express the desire to become parents (Riskind and Patterson, 2010). Among gay men in particular, however, there appears to be a sizable gap between the desire for parenthood and actual intentions, such that many who want to have children do not actually intend to become fathers (Riskind and Patterson, 2010). The psychological burden of infertility among heterosexual individuals is acknowledged to be great, but it has not been studied among lesbian, gay, or bisexual populations.

The health implications of greater childlessness among lesbian and gay populations across the life course, although potentially sizable, have gone essentially unstudied. As discussed earlier, for example, nulliparity is an established risk factor for some cancers. For this reason, lesbians' reduced likelihood of childbearing may place them at higher risk than their heterosexual peers for certain diseases.

When lesbian and gay individuals do become parents, they may do so through multiple pathways (Goldberg, 2009; Patterson and Riskind, 2010). Some marry different-sex partners and have biological, adoptive, or foster children before coming out. Others have children after coming out through the use of donor insemination, surrogacy, heterosexual intercourse, adoption, and/or foster parenting. Increasing numbers of same-sex partners live in jurisdictions that provide legal recognition of their relationship, but the implications of this for parenting have not yet been studied. The increasing availability of assisted reproductive technology to nonheterosexual adults has opened up new possibilities for family formation among members of sexual minorities, but research likewise has not yet fully explored these issues. In short, modes of family formation among lesbian and gay adults are diverse; however, the life-course consequences of different choices for the adults who make them have not yet received much systematic study.

The parenting abilities and competencies of lesbian and gay adults have been explored in a number of small-scale studies (Goldberg, 2009; Golombok and Badger, 2010; Patterson, 2004), a few of which have identified special strengths or difficulties. For example, one study, based on a convenience sample of 256 families, found lesbian and gay parents to be less likely than others to report using physical punishment as a discipline technique (Johnson and O'Connor, 2002); this type of difference would be expected to have positive consequences for children of lesbian and gay parents. On the other hand, a study based on a convenience sample of 87 lesbian mothers in the United States and Canada revealed that those in the United States (who lived in states that did not provide legal recognition of marriage between same-sex couples) expressed more anxiety about legal problems and discrimination based on sexual orientation than those in Canada, whose family relationships enjoyed the protection of law (Shapiro et al., 2009). In general, research has shown lesbian mothers and gay fathers to be very similar to matched groups of heterosexual parents with respect to their parenting attitudes and practices, although studies based on representative samples generally are not available (Golombok and Badger, 2010).

Considerable research has focused on development among the children of lesbian and gay parents, and some of these studies have been based on representative or near-representative samples. In a study of 7-year-olds drawing on the Avon Longitudinal Study of Parents and Children, conducted in the United Kingdom, Golombok and colleagues (2003) found that children of lesbian mothers were well adjusted on a series of standardized assessments of socioemotional development, and similar in this regard to the offspring of heterosexual mothers. In a study based on U.S. census data, Rosenfeld (2010) found that, once demographic characteristics of families had been taken into account, children of same-sex and different-sex couples were making progress through school at about the same rates (i.e., were no more and no less likely to have been held back a grade in school), and that both groups of children were making more rapid progress through school than children living in group quarters. In studies based on data from Wave I of the National Longitudinal Study of Adolescent Health (a near-representative sample of adolescents in the United States), Wainright and colleagues (2004) found that adolescents living with same-sex parents did not differ from those living with different-sex parents on measures of psychosocial adjustment, school outcomes, peer relations, romantic relationships, delinquency, victimization, or substance use (Wainright and Patterson, 2006, 2008; Wainright et al., 2004).

Findings of studies of representative samples of the children of lesbian and gay parents have been consistent with those of studies based on smaller and/or convenience samples. The findings show similar patterns of adjustment among children and adolescents growing up with lesbian, gay, and heterosexual parents across a broad spectrum of measures, including overall adjustment, gender development, peer relationships, and social and academic competence (Biblarz and Stacey, 2010; Goldberg, 2010a; Patterson, 2009). Especially notable among recent reports are extensions of these findings to samples of adoptive children and adolescents, as well as to samples of those with gay fathers in addition to lesbian mothers (Erich et al., 2009; Farr et al., 2010). In a study based on a convenience sample of 78 17-year-old offspring of lesbian mothers, Gartrell and Bos (2010) found that the adolescents were developing in positive ways, such as showing greater social and academic competence than a normative sample of same-aged adolescents with heterosexual parents. Overall, the results of research to date suggest that the offspring of lesbian and gay parents are generally well adjusted.

There has been relatively little research on parenting among transgender adults or on development among the children of transgender parents.

What research has been reported suggests that substantial proportions of transgender adults are parents (Erich et al., 2008). Moreover, research on children of transgender parents has found them to be developing in normal ways (Green, 1978, 1998). This is a nascent area of research, however, and any conclusions must be viewed as preliminary.

The results of research to date on lesbian and gay parents and on their children, although clear, are nevertheless subject to a number of limitations (Goldberg, 2010b; Tasker and Patterson, 2007). In large part because of the absence of sexual orientation assessments in national survey data sets, large representative samples of these populations have rarely been studied. Longitudinal or observational studies are still uncommon. Moreover, research on low-income families, as well as on ethnic, racial, or religious minorities, has remained relatively scarce. There are only a handful of studies on children of transgender parents, and these are based on small convenience samples.

Among adults, family support and acceptance play an important role in psychological adjustment. For transgender adults, higher perceptions of the quality of their family's relationship have been shown to be associated with healthier levels of life satisfaction and self-esteem (Erich et al., 2008). This study involved 91 self-identified transsexuals gathered by a snowball technique from a convenience sample. However, not all transgender individuals receive sufficient family support. In a study involving 20 transwomen of color, the majority of respondents reported hostility and aggression from their families (Koken et al., 2009).

When families do not provide adequate support, many LGBT individuals create families of choice composed of friends. Research shows mixed levels of support from families of choice and families of origin for lesbians who choose to become mothers. Using a convenience sample of self-identified lesbians, DeMino and colleagues (2007) found that, compared with lesbians without children (n = 42), lesbian mothers (n = 47) felt that they received less support from their friends, including their gay and lesbian friends, and more support from their families of origin. A study of couples becoming parents through adoption found that lesbian couples (n = 36) perceived less support from their families than heterosexual couples (n = 39). Levels of support from friends and general well-being were similar for both groups (Goldberg and Smith, 2008).

SUMMARY OF KEY FINDINGS AND RESEARCH OPPORTUNITIES

Findings

Given the length of the phase of life represented by early/middle adulthood, it is not surprising that more data are available for this cohort than for the other phases of the life course discussed in Chapters 4 and 6. These data provide some key insights into the health status of LGBT adults, which are presented below.

Mental Health Status

- As a group, LGB adults, largely behaviorally defined, appear to experience more mood and anxiety disorders than heterosexual adults. Little research has examined the prevalence of mood and anxiety disorders among transgender people.
- LGB adults appear to be more likely than heterosexual adults to experience depression both over a period of 12 months and over a lifetime. Very limited research on transgender adults and depression has been undertaken, but studies conducted with convenience samples suggest elevated rates of risk in this population.
- Studies suggest that LGB people are more likely than heterosexual people to report suicidal ideation and behavior. Some evidence indicates that suicidal ideation and behavior may vary by sexual orientation and gender. Studies of transgender people suggest their rates of suicidal ideation and behavior may be comparable to or higher than those in LGB populations.
- Limited research has explored the prevalence of eating disorders within the LGBT community. These studies indicate that gay and bisexual men may be at higher risk for eating disorders compared with heterosexual men. Far less research has explored rates of eating disorders among lesbians, bisexual women, and transgender people.
- Results of older studies suggest that the vast majority of individuals who underwent sex reassignment surgery are satisfied with the results. More recent research on this subject has not been conducted.

Physical Health Status

- Very limited research suggests that gay men have higher rates of erectile dysfunction than heterosexual men. Little research has focused on reproductive health among LGBT people.
- Lesbians and bisexual women may be at higher risk for breast cancer than heterosexual women. Some research suggests that lesbians and bisexuals have higher rates of risk factors associated with breast cancer, although the data are not clear.
- Men who have sex with men, particularly those who are HIV-positive, are at increased risk for anal cancer. Currently, there exist no guidelines recommending routine anal cancer screenings and no consensus on the optimal method or frequency of such screening.

- Research on health outcomes for transgender people is very limited, although some studies suggest that long-term hormone use may increase the risk for cancer. Similarly, very little research, particularly in the United States, has examined the effects and side effects of hormone treatment on physical health (including reproductive health), and no clinical trials on this subject have been conducted.
- Lesbians and bisexual women may be at greater risk for obesity, although the data on bisexual women are less clear. Insufficient research has been conducted to elucidate the mechanisms of risk.
- HIV continues to exact a severe toll on adult men who have sex with men, with black and Latino men being disproportionately affected. Among transgender people, little HIV research has been conducted, but small studies suggest that transgender females are at high risk.
- Little research on HIV has been conducted among women who have sex with women. The few studies that exist suggest higher HIV prevalence among women who have sex with both men and women compared with exclusively heterosexual or homosexual women.

Risk and Protective Factors

- LGBT people are frequently the targets of stigma and discrimination because of their sexual- and gender-minority status.
- LGB adults experience violent victimization because of their sexual-minority status. Convenience samples of transgender people have yielded similar results.
- Like heterosexual adults, LGB adults experience intimate partner violence. Data on the frequency and extent of such violence are extremely limited.
- LGB adults appear to have higher rates of substance use (including smoking and alcohol consumption) than heterosexual adults. Most of the research on this subject has been conducted among women, with much less being known about gay and bisexual men. Limited research among transgender adults indicates that substance use is a major concern for this population.
- Although the research on protective factors for LGBT adults is limited, there is some indication that such factors as supportive living/working environments, support from family and friends, and a positive LGB identity may be protective. The limited amount of research on transgender people has focused less on protective factors and more on the factors associated with positive outcomes of sex reassignment (psychological adjustment, family support, psychological treatment, and good surgical outcomes).

Health Services

- Very little research has been done on health outcomes resulting from LGBT people's lack of access to and utilization of health care services.
- With respect to health services, LGBT adults appear to have different access and utilization patterns. Some research suggests that sexual-minority adults access mental health services more than their heterosexual counterparts.
- Some studies indicate that lesbians and bisexual women use preventive services less than heterosexual women, but these studies are not conclusive.
- Lack of health insurance (including the exclusion of some services, such as sex reassignment surgery, by third-party payers), fear of discrimination from providers, and dissatisfaction with services may act as barriers to accessing all health services for LGBT adults.
- Very little research has been conducted on the quality of care experienced by sexual and gender minorities.
- Limited data suggest high satisfaction rates with transgender-specific health care services among transgender patients when those services are accessible from knowledgeable providers.

Contextual Influences

- While limited research suggests there are racial/ethnic differences in the health of LGBT adults, very little research has examined differences based on geographic or other sociodemographic factors.
- Gay men and lesbians are less likely to be parents than their heterosexual peers. The health implications of this have been largely unstudied.
- Development among the children of lesbian and gay parents has received a great deal of attention. Studies show that these children are well adjusted and developmentally similar to the children of different-sex parents. Limited research suggests that substantial numbers of transgender people are parents, and their children appear to be developing in healthy ways.

Research Opportunities

Although a number of studies provide useful information on the health status of LGBT adults, very limited data exist in some areas. The research that has been conducted has been uneven in that it has been much less likely to focus on bisexual and transgender people, and within-group differences have seldom been examined. In addition, many of the available studies have relied on small convenience samples. There are many opportunities for additional research. Both cross-sectional and longitudinal research is needed on the intersection of contextual factors (e.g., race, geography, socioeconomic status), attending to multiple levels of consideration (e.g., community, structural, biomedical), with respect to sexual- and gender-minority status. Similarly, research is needed to address the risk and protective factors associated with, as well as interventions to promote, health and well-being in LGBT populations. The following topics in LGBT health research would benefit from additional study:

- **Demographic and descriptive information**, including the percentage of adults who are LGBT and how that percentage varies by demographic characteristics such as race, ethnicity, socioeconomic status, geography, and religion; also, the percentage of LGBT adults who are parents, as well as the general experiences and health status of LGBT adults and how these vary by demographic characteristics.
- **Family and interpersonal relations**, including the effect of the greater likelihood of childlessness in LGBT populations and their experience of parenting (with a particular focus on the experience of gay, bisexual, and transgender parents, which is largely absent from the research literature); the experience and prevalence of "chosen families"; and the experience of intrafamily and domestic violence (such as intimate partner violence), as well as anti-LGBT victimization.
- **Health services**, including barriers to access (particularly related to identity disclosure and interactions with providers), utilization rates, and quality of care received.
- **Mental health**, including eating disorders, the prevalence of depression and suicidality (particularly unknown among transgender adults), and the effects of stigma and discrimination (particularly unknown among bisexual adults).
- **Physical health**, including substance use (particularly among transgender individuals); cancer rates, risks, and treatment (e.g., breast cancer among lesbians and bisexual women; anal cancer rates and evaluations of the effectiveness of screening among men who have sex with men; cancer among transgender adults in general, about which very little is known); cardiovascular disease among all LGBT adults; and obesity (particularly among lesbian and bisexual women).
- **Sexual and reproductive health**, including HIV rates and interventions (particularly addressing racial disparities); fertility, infertility, and reproductive health issues; and reproductive technology and its use.

REFERENCES

Aaron, D. J., and T. L. Hughes. 2007. Association of childhood sexual abuse with obesity in a community sample of lesbians. *Obesity* 15(4):1023–1028.

American College of Obstetricians and Gynecologists. 2005. *Special populations*. Washington, DC: American College of Obstetricians and Gynecologists.

Arreola, S. G., T. B. Neilands, and R. Diaz. 2009. Childhood sexual abuse and the sociocultural context of sexual risk among adult Latino gay and bisexual men. *American Journal of Public Health* 99(Suppl. 2):S432–S438.

Austin, E. L., and J. A. Irwin. 2010. Health behaviors and health care utilization of southern lesbians. *Women's Health Issues* 20(3):178–184.

Austin, S. B., H. J. Jun, B. Jackson, D. Spiegelman, J. Rich-Edwards, H. L. Corliss, and R. J. Wright. 2008. Disparities in child abuse victimization in lesbian, bisexual, and heterosexual women in the Nurses' Health Study II. *Journal of Womens Health* 17(4):597–606.

Balsam, K. F., and J. J. Mohr. 2007. Adaptation to sexual orientation stigma: A comparison of bisexual and lesbian/gay adults. *Journal of Counseling Psychology* 54(3):306–319.

Balsam, K. F., T. P. Beauchaine, R. M. Mickey, and E. D. Rothblum. 2005. Mental health of lesbian, gay, bisexual, and heterosexual siblings: Effects of gender, sexual orientation, and family. *Journal of Abnormal Psychology* 114(3):471–476.

Balsam, K. F., K. Lehavot, B. Beadnell, and E. Circo. 2010. Childhood abuse and mental health indicators among ethnically diverse lesbian, gay, and bisexual adults. *Journal of Consulting and Clinical Psychology* 78(4):459–468.

Bancroft, J., L. Carnes, E. Janssen, D. Goodrich, and J. S. Long. 2005. Erectile and ejaculatory problems in gay and heterosexual men. *Archives of Sexual Behavior* 34(3):285–297.

Barrett, D. C., and L. M. Pollack. 2005. Whose gay community? Social class, sexual self-expression, and gay community involvement. *The Sociological Quarterly* 46(3):437–456.

Battle, J., C. J. Cohen, D. Warren, G. Fergerson, and S. Audam. 2002. *Say it loud: I'm black and I'm proud; black pride survey 2000*. New York: The Policy Institute of the National Gay & Lesbian Task Force.

Beren, S. E., H. A. Hayden, D. E. Wilfley, and C. M. Grilo. 1996. The influence of sexual orientation on body dissatisfaction in adult men and women. *International Journal of Eating Disorders* 20(2):135–141.

Bianchi, F. T., C. A. Reisen, M. C. Zea, P. J. Poppen, M. G. Shedlin, and M. M. Penha. 2007. The sexual experiences of Latino men who have sex with men who migrated to a gay epicentre in the USA. *Culture, Health & Sexuality* 9(5):505–518.

Biblarz, T. J., and J. Stacey. 2010. How does the gender of parents matter? *Journal of Marriage and Family* 72:3–22.

Blair, K. L., and D. Holmberg. 2008. Perceived social network support and well-being in same-sex versus mixed-sex romantic relationships. *Journal of Social and Personal Relationships* 25(5):769–791.

Bockting, W. O. 2008. Psychotherapy and the real-life experience: From gender dichotomy to gender diversity. *Sexologies* 17(4):211–224.

Bockting, W. O., and E. Coleman. 2007. Developmental stages of the transgender coming out process: Toward an integrated identity. In *Handbook of transgender medicine and surgery*, edited by R. Ettner, S. Monstrey, and E. Evan. New York: Haworth Press.

Bockting, W. O., B. E. Robinson, and B. R. Rosser. 1998. Transgender HIV prevention: A qualitative needs assessment. *AIDS Care* 10(4):505–525.

Bockting, W. O., B. Robinson, A. Benner, and K. Scheltema. 2004. Patient satisfaction with transgender health services. *Journal of Sex & Marital Therapy* 30(4):277–294.

Bockting, W. O., C.-Y. Huang, H. Ding, B. B. Robinson, and B. R. S. Rosser. 2005a. Are transgender persons at higher risk for HIV than other sexual minorities? A comparison of HIV prevalence and risks. *International Journal of Transgenderism* 8(2):123–131.

Bockting, W. O., B. E. Robinson, J. Forberg, and K. Scheltema. 2005b. Evaluation of a sexual health approach to reducing HIV/STD risk in the transgender community. *AIDS Care* 17(3):289–303.

Bockting, W. O, A. Benner, and E. Coleman. 2009a. Gay and bisexual identity development among female-to-male transsexuals in North America: Emergence of a transgender sexuality. *Archives of Sexual Behavior* 38(5):688–701.

Bockting, W. O., D. King, and R. Ekins, eds. 2009b. Special issue: Toward version 7 of the world professional association for transgender health's standards of care. *International Journal of Transgenderism* 11.

Boehmer, U., D. J. Bowen, and G. R. Bauer. 2007. Overweight and obesity in sexual-minority women: Evidence from population-based data. *American Journal of Public Health* 97(6): 1134–1140.

Bostwick, W. B., C. J. Boyd, T. L. Hughes, and S. E. McCabe. 2010. Dimensions of sexual orientation and the prevalence of mood and anxiety disorders in the United States. *American Journal of Public Health* 100(3):468–475.

Brown, G. R., and E. McDuffie. 2009. Health care policies addressing transgender inmates in prison systems in the United States. *Journal of Correctional Health Care* 15(4):280–291.

Buchmueller, T., and C. S. Carpenter. 2010. Disparities in health insurance coverage, access, and outcomes for individuals in same-sex versus different-sex relationships, 2000–2007. *American Journal of Public Health* 100(3):489–495.

Burckell, L. A., and M. R. Goldfried. 2006. Therapist qualities preferred by sexual-minority individuals. *Psychotherapy* 43(1):32–49.

Burcombe, R. J., A. Makris, M. Pittam, and N. Finer. 2003. Breast cancer after bilateral subcutaneous mastectomy in a female-to-male trans-sexual. *Breast* 12(4):290–293.

Burgard, S. A., S. D. Cochran, and V. M. Mays. 2005. Alcohol and tobacco use patterns among heterosexually and homosexually experienced California women. *Drug & Alcohol Dependence* 77(1):61–70.

Callen-Lorde Community Health Center. 2004. *Transgender health program protocols*. New York: Callen-Lorde Community Health Center.

Carballo-Dieguez, A., M. Miner, C. Dolezal, B. Rosser, and S. Jacoby. 2006. Sexual negotiation, HIV-status disclosure, and sexual risk behavior among Latino men who use the internet to seek sex with other men. *Archives of Sexual Behavior* 35(4):473–481.

Carroll, R. A. 1999. Outcomes of treatment for gender dysphoria. *Journal of Sex Education & Therapy* 24(3):128–136.

Case, P., S. B. Austin, D. J. Hunter, J. E. Manson, S. Malspeis, W. C. Willett, and D. Spiegelman. 2004. Sexual orientation, health risk factors, and physical functioning in the Nurses' Health Study II. *Journal of Women's Health* 13(9):1033–1047.

Catania, J. A., J. Paul, D. Osmond, S. Folkman, L. Pollack, J. Canchola, J. Chang, and T. Neilands. 2008. Mediators of childhood sexual abuse and high-risk sex among men-who-have-sex-with-men. *Child Abuse & Neglect* 32(10):925–940.

CDC (Centers for Disease Control and Prevention). 2008. *Cases of HIV infection and AIDS in the United States and dependent areas, 2007*. Atlanta, GA: CDC.

CDC. 2009a. *HIV/AIDS surveillance report: Cases of HIV infection and AIDS in the United States and dependent areas, 2007*. Atlanta, GA: CDC.

CDC. 2009b. *Sexually transmitted disease surveillance, 2008*. Atlanta, GA: CDC.

CDC. 2010. *STDs in men who have sex with men*. Atlanta, GA: CDC.

Chae, D. H., and G. Ayala. 2010. Sexual orientation and sexual behavior among Latino and Asian Americans: Implications for unfair treatment and psychological distress. *Journal of Sex Research* 47(5):451–459.

Chaturvedi, A. K., M. M. Madeleine, R. J. Biggar, and E. A. Engels. 2009. Risk of human papillomavirus-associated cancers among persons with AIDS. *Journal of the National Cancer Institute* 101(16):1120–1130.

Chin-Hong, P. V., E. Vittinghoff, R. D. Cranston, S. Buchbinder, D. Cohen, G. Colfax, M. da Costa, T. Darragh, E. Hess, F. Judson, B. Koblin, M. Madison, and J. M. Palefsky. 2004. Age-specific prevalence of anal human papillomavirus infection in HIV-negative sexually active men who have sex with men: The EXPLORE Study. *Journal of Infectious Diseases* 190(12):2070–2076.

Chng, C. L., and J. Geliga-Vargas. 2000. Ethnic identity, gay identity, sexual sensation seeking and HIV risk taking among multiethnic men who have sex with men. *AIDS Education & Prevention* 12(4):326–339.

Clements-Nolle, K., K. Kitano, W. Wilkinson, and R. Marx. 1999. HIV prevention and health service needs of the transgender community in San Francisco. *International Journal of Transgenderism* 3(1/2):1.

Clements-Nolle, K., R. Marx, R. Guzman, and M. Katz. 2001. HIV prevalence, risk behaviors, health care use, and mental health status of transgender persons: Implications for public health intervention. *American Journal of Public Health* 91(6):915–921.

Cochran, B. N., K. M. Peavy, and A. M. Cauce. 2007a. Substance abuse treatment providers' explicit and implicit attitudes regarding sexual minorities. *Journal of Homosexuality* 53(3):181–207.

Cochran, B. N., K. M. Peavy, and J. S. Robohm. 2007b. Do specialized services exist for LGBT individuals seeking treatment for substance misuse? A study of available treatment programs. *Substance Use & Misuse* 42(1):161–176.

Cochran, S. D., and V. M. Mays. 2000a. Lifetime prevalence of suicide symptoms and affective disorders among men reporting same-sex sexual partners: Results from NHANES III. *American Journal of Public Health* 90(4):573–578.

Cochran, S. D., and V. M. Mays. 2000b. Relation between psychiatric syndromes and behaviorally defined sexual orientation in a sample of the US population. *American Journal of Epidemiology* 151(5):516–523.

Cochran, S. D., and V. M. Mays. 2006. Estimating prevalence of mental and substance-using disorders among lesbians and gay men from existing national health data. In *Sexual orientation and mental health*, edited by A. M. Omoto and H.S. Kurtzman. Washington, DC: American Psychological Association. Pp. 143–165.

Cochran, S. D., V. M. Mays, M. Alegria, A. N. Ortega, and D. Takeuchi. 2007c. Mental health and substance use disorders among Latino and Asian American lesbian, gay, and bisexual adults. *Journal of Consulting and Clinical Psychology* 75(5):785–794.

Cochran, S. D., V. M. Mays, D. Bowen, S. Gage, D. Bybee, S. J. Roberts, R. S. Goldstein, A. Robison, E. J. Rankow, and J. White. 2001. Cancer-related risk indicators and preventive screening behaviors among lesbians and bisexual women. *American Journal of Public Health* 91(4):591–597.

Cochran, S. D., J. G. Sullivan, and V. M. Mays. 2003. Prevalence of mental disorders, psychological distress, and mental health services use among lesbian, gay, and bisexual adults in the United States. *Journal of Consulting and Clinical Psychology* 71(1):53–61.

Conron, K. J., M. J. Mimiaga, and S. J. Landers. 2008. *A health profile of Massachusetts adults by sexual orientation identity: Results from the 2001–2006 Behavioral Risk Factor Surveillance System Surveys*. Boston, MA: Massachusetts Department of Public Health.

Conron, K. J., M. J. Mimiaga, and S. J. Landers. 2010. A population-based study of sexual orientation identity and gender differences in adult health. *American Journal of Public Health* 100(10):1953–1960.

Corliss, H. L., S. D. Cochran, V. M. Mays, S. Greenland, and T. E. Seeman. 2009. Age of minority sexual orientation development and risk of childhood maltreatment and suicide attempts in women. *American Journal of Orthopsychiatry* 79(4):511–521.

Crepaz, N., G. Marks, A. Liau, M. M. Mullins, L. W. Aupont, K. J. Marshall, E. D. Jacobs, R. J. Wolitski, and HIV/AIDS Prevention Research Synthesis Team. 2009. Prevalence of unprotected anal intercourse among HIV-diagnosed MSM in the United States: A meta-analysis. *AIDS* 23(13):1617–1629.

Daling, J. R., M. M. Madeleine, L. G. Johnson, S. M. Schwartz, K. A. Shera, M. A. Wurscher, J. J. Carter, P. L. Porter, D. A. Galloway, and J. K. McDougall. 2004. Human papillomavirus, smoking, and sexual practices in the etiology of anal cancer. *Cancer* 101(2):270–280.

De Sutter, P. 2001. Gender reassignment and assisted reproduction: Present and future reproductive options for transsexual people. *Human Reproduction* 16(4):612–614.

De Sutter, P. 2009. Reproductive options for transpeople: Recommendations for revision of the WPATH's standards of care. *International Journal of Transgenderism* 11(3):183–185.

De Sutter, P., K. Kira, A. Verschoor, and A. Hotimsky. 2002. The desire to have children and the preservation of fertility in transsexual women: A survey. *International Journal of Transgenderism* 6(3):1–1. http://www.iiav.nl/ezines/web/IJT/97-03/numbers/symposion/ijtvo06no03_02.htm (accessed February 14, 2011).

Dean, L., I. H. Meyer, K. Robinson, R. L. Sell, R. Sember, V. M. Silenzio, D. J. Bowen, J. Bradford, E. Rothblum, J. White, P. Dunn, A. Lawrence, D. Wolfe, and J. Xavier. 2000. Lesbian, gay, bisexual, and trangender health: Findings and concerns. *Journal of the Gay & Lesbian Medical Association* 4(3):102–151.

DeMino, K. A., G. Appleby, and D. Fisk. 2007. Lesbian mothers with planned families: A comparative study of internalized homophobia and social support. *American Journal of Orthopsychiatry* 77(1):165–173.

Derogatis, L. R., J. K. Meyer, and E. Vazquez. 1978. A psychological profile of the transsexual. I. The male. *The Journal of Nervous and Mental Disease* 166(4):234–254.

Derogatis, L. R., J. K. Meyer, and P. Boland. 1981. A psychological profile of the transsexual. II. The female. *Journal of Nervous and Mental Disease* 169(3):157–168.

Devor, A. H. 2004. Witnessing and mirroring: A fourteen stage model of transsexual identity formation. *Journal of Gay & Lesbian Psychotherapy* 8(1):41–67.

Diamant, A. L., and C. Wold. 2003. Sexual orientation and variation in physical and mental health status among women. *Journal of Women's Health* 12(1):41–49.

Diamant, A. L., J. Lever, and M. A. Schuster. 2000a. Lesbians' sexual activities and efforts to reduce risks for sexually transmitted diseases. *Journal of the Gay & Lesbian Medical Association* 4(2):41–48.

Diamant, A. L., M. A. Schuster, and J. Lever. 2000b. Receipt of preventive health care services by lesbians. *American Journal of Preventive Medicine* 19(3):141–148.

Diamant, A. L., C. Wold, K. Spritzer, and L. Gelberg. 2000c. Health behaviors, health status, and access to and use of health care: A population-based study of lesbian, bisexual, and heterosexual women. *Archives of Family Medicine* 9(10):1043–1051.

Diaz, R. M., G. Ayala, E. Bein, J. Henne, and B. V. Marin. 2001. The impact of homophobia, poverty, and racism on the mental health of gay and bisexual Latino men: Findings from 3 US cities. *American Journal of Public Health* 91(6):927–932.

Dizon, D. S., T. Tejada-Berges, S. Koelliker, M. Steinhoff, and C. O. Granai. 2006. Ovarian cancer associated with testosterone supplementation in a female-to-male transsexual patient. *Gynecologic & Obstetric Investigation* 62(4):226–228.

Drabble, L., and K. Trocki. 2005. Alcohol consumption, alcohol-related problems, and other substance use among lesbian and bisexual women. *Journal of Lesbian Studies* 9(3):19–30.

Drabble, L., L. T. Midanik, and K. Trocki. 2005. Reports of alcohol consumption and alcohol-related problems among homosexual, bisexual and heterosexual respondents: Results from the 2000 National Alcohol Survey. *Journal of Studies on Alcohol* 66(1):111–120.

Drasin, H., K. P. Beals, M. N. Elliott, J. Lever, D. J. Klein, and M. A. Schuster. 2008. Age cohort differences in the developmental milestones of gay men. *Journal of Homosexuality* 54(4):381–399.

Elamin, M. B., M. Z. Garcia, M. H. Murad, P. J. Erwin, and V. M. Montori. 2010. Effect of sex steroid use on cardiovascular risk in transsexual individuals: A systematic review and meta-analyses. *Clinical Endocrinology* 72(1):1–10.

Eliason, M. J., and R. D. Schope. 2001. Does "don't ask don't tell" apply to health care? Lesbian, gay, and bisexual people's disclosure to health care providers. *Journal of the Gay and Lesbian Medical Association* 5(4):125–134.

Ende, A. R., V. Lo Re, 3rd, M. J. DiNubile, and K. Mounzer. 2006. Erectile dysfunction in an urban HIV-positive population. *AIDS Patient Care & STDs* 20(2):75–78.

Erich, S., J. Tittsworth, J. Dykes, and C. Cabuses. 2008. Family relationships and their correlations with transsexual well-being. *Journal of GLBT Family Studies* 4(4):419–432.

Erich, S., H. Kanenberg, K. Case, T. Allen, and T. Bogdanos. 2009. An empirical analysis of factors affecting adolescent attachment in adoptive families with homosexual and straight parents. *Children and Youth Services Review* 31(3):398–404.

Erickson, E. H. 1950. Eight stages of man. In *Childhood and society*, edited by E. H. Erickson. New York: Norton. Pp. 67–77.

Ethics Committee of the American Society for Reproductive Medicine. 2009. Access to fertility treatment by gays, lesbians, and unmarried persons. *Fertility & Sterility* 92(4):1190–1193.

Eyler, A. E., and S. Whittle. 2001. *FTM breast cancer: Community awareness and illustrative cases*. Paper presented at XVII Harry Benjamin International Gender Dysphoria Association Symposium, Galveston, TX, October 31-November 4.

Farr, R. H., S. L. Forssell, and C. J. Patterson. 2010. Gay, lesbian, and heterosexual adoptive parents: Couple and relationship issues. *Journal of GLBT Family Studies* 6(2):199–213.

Federal Bureau of Investigation. 2010. *About hate crime statistics*. http://www2.fbi.gov/ucr/hc2009/abouthcs.html (accessed December 7, 2010).

Feldman, M. B., and I. H. Meyer. 2007a. Childhood abuse and eating disorders in gay and bisexual men. *International Journal of Eating Disorders* 40(5):418–423.

Feldman, M. B., and I. H. Meyer. 2007b. Eating disorders in diverse lesbian, gay, and bisexual populations. *International Journal of Eating Disorders* 40(3):218–226.

Fox, K. K., C. del Rio, K. K. Holmes, E. W. Hook, 3rd, F. N. Judson, J. S. Knapp, G. W. Procop, S. A. Wang, W. L. Whittington, and W. C. Levine. 2001. Gonorrhea in the HIV era: A reversal in trends among men who have sex with men. *American Journal of Public Health* 91(6):959–964.

Friedman, H. B., A. J. Saah, M. E. Sherman, A. E. Busseniers, W. C. Blackwelder, R. A. Kaslow, A. M. Ghaffari, R. W. Daniel, and K. V. Shah. 1998. Human papillomavirus, anal squamous intraepithelial lesions, and human immunodeficiency virus in a cohort of gay men. *Journal of Infectious Diseases* 178(1):45–52.

Friis-Moller, N., C. A. Sabin, R. Weber, A. d'Arminio Monforte, W. M. El-Sadr, P. Reiss, R. Thiebaut, L. Morfeldt, S. De Wit, C. Pradier, G. Calvo, M. G. Law, O. Kirk, A. N. Phillips, and J. D. Lundgren. 2003. Combination antiretroviral therapy and the risk of myocardial infarction. *New England Journal of Medicine* 349(21):1993–2003.

Gagne, P., R. Tewksbury, and D. McGaughey. 1997. Coming out and crossing over. *Gender & Society* 11(4):478–508.

Ganly, I., and E. W. Taylory. 1995. Breast cancer in a transsexual man receiving hormone replacement therapy. *British Journal of Surgery* 82(3):341.

Garofalo, R., A. Herrick, B. S. Mustanski, and G. R. Donenberg. 2007. Tip of the iceberg: Young men who have sex with men, the Internet, and HIV risk. *American Journal of Public Health* 97(6):1113–1117.

Gartrell, N., and H. Bos. 2010. US National Longitudinal Lesbian Family Study: Psychological adjustment of 17-year-old adolescents. *Pediatrics* 726(1):28–36.

Gates, G. J. 2010. *Sexual minorities in the 2008 General Social Survey: Coming out and demographic characteristics*. Los Angeles, CA: The Williams Institute.

Gates, G. J., M. V. L. Badgett, J. E. Macomber, and K. Chambers. 2007. *Adoption and foster care by gay and lesbian parents in the United States*. Los Angeles, CA: The Williams Institute.

Gilman, S. E., S. D. Cochran, V. M. Mays, M. Hughes, D. Ostrow, and R. C. Kessler. 2001. Risk of psychiatric disorders among individuals reporting same-sex sexual partners in the national comorbidity survey. *American Journal of Public Health* 91(6):933–939.

Goldberg, A. E. 2009. Lesbian and heterosexual preadoptive couples' openness to transracial adoption. *American Journal of Orthopsychiatry* 79(1):103–117.

Goldberg, A. E. 2010a. *Children of lesbian and gay parents: Adjustment and experiences*. Washington, DC: American Psychological Association.

Goldberg, A. E. 2010b. *Lesbian and gay parents and their children: Research on the family life cycle*. Washington, DC: American Psychological Association.

Goldberg, A. E., and J. Z. Smith. 2008. Social support and psychological well-being in lesbian and heterosexual preadoptive couples. *Family Relations* 57(3):281–294.

Goldie, S. J., K. M. Kuntz, M. C. Weinstein, K. A. Freedberg, M. L. Welton, and J. M. Palefsky. 1999. The clinical effectiveness and cost-effectiveness of screening for anal squamous intraepithelial lesions in homosexual and bisexual HIV-positive men. *Journal of the American Medical Association* 281(19):1822–1829.

Goldie, S. J., K. M. Kuntz, M. C. Weinstein, K. A. Freedberg, and J. M. Palefsky. 2000. Cost-effectiveness of screening for anal squamous intraepithelial lesions and anal cancer in human immunodeficiency virus-negative homosexual and bisexual men. *American Journal of Medicine* 108(8):634–641.

Golombok, S., and S. Badger. 2010. Children raised in mother-headed families from infancy: A follow-up of children of lesbian and single heterosexual mothers, at early adulthood. *Human Reproduction* 25(1):150–157.

Golombok, S., B. Perry, A. Burston, C. Murray, J. Mooney-Somers, M. Stevens, and J. Golding. 2003. Children with lesbian parents: A community study. *Developmental Psychology* 39(1):20–33.

Gooren, L. J., and E. J. Giltay. 2008. Review of studies of androgen treatment of female-to-male transsexuals: Effects and risks of administration of androgens to females. *Journal of Sexual Medicine* 5(4):765–776.

Gooren, L. J., E. J. Giltay, and M. C. Bunck. 2008. Long-term treatment of transsexuals with cross-sex hormones: Extensive personal experience. *Journal of Clinical Endocrinology & Metabolism* 93(1):19–25.

Grant, J. M., L. A. Mottet, J. Tanis, D. Min, J. L. Herman, J. Harrison, and M. Keisling. 2010. *National transgender discrimination survey report on health and health care*. Washington, DC: National Center for Transgender Equality and the National Gay and Lesbian Task Force.

Green, R. 1978. Sexual identity of 37 children raised by homosexual or transsexual parents. *American Journal of Psychiatry* 135(6):692–697.

Green, R. 1998. Transexuals' children. *International Journal of Transgenderism* 2(3). http://www.iiav.nl/ezines/web/IJT/97-03/numbers/symposion/ijtc0601.htm (accessed December 16, 2010).

Green, R., and D. T. Fleming. 1990. Transsexual surgery follow-up: Status in the 1990s. *Annual Review of Sex Research* 1:163–174.

Greenwood, G. L., M. V. Relf, B. Huang, L. M. Pollack, J. A. Canchola, and J. A. Catania. 2002. Battering victimization among a probability-based sample of men who have sex with men. *American Journal of Public Health* 92(12):1964–1969.

Gruskin, E. P., G. L. Greenwood, M. Matevia, L. M. Pollack, L. L. Bye, and V. Albright. 2007. Cigar and smokeless tobacco use in the lesbian, gay, and bisexual population. *Nicotine & Tobacco Research* 9(9):937–940.

Hage, J. J., J. J. Dekker, R. B. Karim, R. H. Verheijen, and E. Bloemena. 2000. Ovarian cancer in female-to-male transsexuals: Report of two cases. *Gynecologic Oncology* 76(3):413–415.

Hall, H. I., R. H. Byers, Q. Ling, and L. Espinoza. 2007. Racial/ethnic and age disparities in HIV prevalence and disease progression among men who have sex with men in the United States. *American Journal of Public Health* 97(6):1060–1066.

Harawa, N. T., J. K. Williams, H. C. Ramamurthi, C. Manago, S. Avina, and M. Jones. 2008. Sexual behavior, sexual identity, and substance abuse among low-income bisexual and non-gay-identifying African American men who have sex with men. *Archives of Sexual Behavior* 37(5):748–762.

Hart, T., J. L. Peterson, and Community Intervention Trial for Youth Study. 2004. Predictors of risky sexual behavior among young African American men who have sex with men. *American Journal of Public Health* 94(7):1122–1124.

Hatzenbuehler, M. L., K. A. McLaughlin, K. M. Keyes, and D. S. Hasin. 2010. The impact of institutional discrimination on psychiatric disorders in lesbian, gay, and bisexual populations: A prospective study. *American Journal of Public Health* 100(3):452–459.

Heck, J. E., R. L. Sell, and S. S. Gorin. 2006. Health care access among individuals involved in same-sex relationships. *American Journal of Public Health* 96(6):1111–1118.

Heffelfinger, J. D., E. B. Swint, S. M. Berman, and H. S. Weinstock. 2007. Trends in primary and secondary syphilis among men who have sex with men in the United States. *American Journal of Public Health* 97(6):1076–1083.

Henderson, A. W., K. Lehavot, and J. M. Simoni. 2009. Ecological models of sexual satisfaction among lesbian/bisexual and heterosexual women. *Archives of Sexual Behavior* 38(1):50–65.

Hequembourg, A. L., and S. A. Brallier. 2009. An exploration of sexual minority stress across the lines of gender and sexual identity. *Journal of Homosexuality* 56(3):273–298.

Herbst, J. H., C. Beeker, A. Mathew, T. McNally, W. F. Passin, L. S. Kay, N. Crepaz, C. M. Lyles, P. Briss, S. Chattopadhyay, R. L. Johnson, and Task Force on Community Preventive Services. 2007. The effectiveness of individual-, group-, and community-level HIV behavioral risk-reduction interventions for adult men who have sex with men: A systematic review. *American Journal of Preventive Medicine* 32(Suppl. 4):S38–S67.

Herbst, J. H., E. D. Jacobs, T. J. Finlayson, V. S. McKleroy, M. S. Neumann, N. Crepaz, and HIV/AIDS Prevention Research Synthesis Team. 2008. Estimating HIV prevalence and risk behaviors of transgender persons in the United States: A systematic review. *AIDS & Behavior* 12(1):1–17.

Herdt, G., and R. Kertzner. 2006. I do, but I can't: The impact of marriage denial on the mental health and sexual citizenship of lesbians and gay men in the United States. *Sexuality Research and Social Policy* 3(1):33–49.

Herek, G. M. 2006. Legal recognition of same-sex relationships in the United States—a social science perspective. *American Psychologist* 61(6):607–621.

Herek, G. M. 2009a. Hate crimes and stigma-related experiences among sexual minority adults in the United States. *Journal of Interpersonal Violence* 24(1):54–74.

Herek, G. M. 2009b. Hate crimes and stigma-related experiences among sexual minority adults in the United States: Prevalence estimates from a national probability sample. *Journal of Interpersonal Violence* 24(1):54–74.

Herek, G. M., and L. D. Garnets. 2007. Sexual orientation and mental health. *Annual Review of Clinical Psychology* 3:353–375.

Herek, G. M., J. R. Gillis, and J. C. Cogan. 1999. Psychological sequelae of hate-crime victimization among lesbian, gay, and bisexual adults. *Journal of Consulting and Clinical Psychology* 67(6):945–951.

Herrell, R., J. Goldberg, W. R. True, V. Ramakrishnan, M. Lyons, S. Eisen, and M. T. Tsuang. 1999. Sexual orientation and suicidality: A co-twin control study in adult men. *Archives of General Psychiatry* 56(10):867–874.

Horowitz, S. M., D. L. Weis, and M. T. Laflin. 2003. Bisexuality, quality of life, lifestyle, and health indicators. *Journal of Bisexuality* 3:5–28.

Howard Brown Health Center. 2010. *Trans hormone informed consent protocol.* Chicago, IL: Howard Brown Health Center.

Huebner, D. M., G. M. Rebchook, and S. M. Kegeles. 2004. Experiences of harassment, discrimination, and physical violence among young gay and bisexual men. *American Journal of Public Health* 94(7):1200–1203.

IOM (Institute of Medicine). 1999. *Lesbian health: Current assessment and directions for the future.* Washington, DC: National Academy Press.

Javaherian, H., A. B. Christy, and M. Boehringer. 2008. Occupational therapy practitioners' comfort level and preparedness in working with individuals who are gay, lesbian, or bisexual. *Journal of Allied Health* 37(3):150–155.

Jeffries, W. L. I. V., and B. Dodge. 2007. Male bisexuality and condom use at last sexual encounter: Results from a national survey. *Journal of Sex Research* 44(3):278–289.

Johnson, S. M., and E. O'Connor. 2002. *The gay baby boom: The psychology of gay parenthood.* New York: New York University Press.

Kaiser Family Foundation. 2001. *Inside-out: A report on the experiences of lesbians, gays, and bisexuals in America and the public's view on issues and policies related to sexual orientation.* Washington, DC: The Henry J. Kaiser Family Foundation.

Kaminski, P. L., B. P. Chapman, S. D. Haynes, and L. Own. 2005. Body image, eating behaviors, and attitudes toward exercise among gay and straight men. *Eating Behaviors* 6(3):179–187.

Kelley, L., C. L. Chou, S. L. Dibble, and P. A. Robertson. 2008. A critical intervention in lesbian, gay, bisexual, and transgender health: Knowledge and attitude outcomes among second-year medical students. *Teaching & Learning in Medicine* 20(3):248–253.

Kenagy, G. P. 2005a. The health and social service needs of transgender people in Philadelphia. *International Journal of Transgenderism* 8(2–3):49–56.

Kenagy, G. P. 2005b. Transgender health: Findings from two needs assessment studies in Philadelphia. *Health & Social Work* 30(1):19–26.

Kendal, M., H. Devor, and N. Strapko. 1997. Feminist and lesbian opinions about transsexuals. In *Gender blending*, edited by B. Bullough and V. Bullough. Amherst, NY: Prometheus. Pp. 146–159.

Kerker, B. D., F. Mostashari, and L. Thorpe. 2006. Health care access and utilization among women who have sex with women: Sexual behavior and identity. *Journal of Urban Health* 83(5):970–979.

Keyes, C. L. M. 2004. Risk and resilience in human development: An introduction. *Research in Human Development* 1(4):223–227.

King, M., J. Semlyen, S. S. Tai, H. Killaspy, D. Osborn, D. Popelyuk, and I. Nazareth. 2008. A systematic review of mental disorder, suicide, and deliberate self harm in lesbian, gay and bisexual people. *BMC Psychiatry* 8:70.

Klein, C., and B. B. Gorzalka. 2009. Sexual functioning in transsexuals following hormone therapy and genital surgery: A review (CME). *Journal of Sexual Medicine* 6(11):2922–2939.

Koblin, B. A., N. A. Hessol, A. G. Zauber, P. E. Taylor, S. P. Buchbinder, M. H. Katz, and C. E. Stevens. 1996. Increased incidence of cancer among homosexual men, New York City and San Francisco, 1978–1990. *American Journal of Epidemiology* 144(10):916–923.

Koblin, B. A., M. J. Husnik, G. Colfax, Y. Huang, M. Madison, K. Mayer, P. J. Barresi, T. J. Coates, M. A. Chesney, and S. Buchbinder. 2006. Risk factors for HIV infection among men who have sex with men. *AIDS* 20(5):731–739.

Koh, A. S. 2000. Use of preventive health behaviors by lesbian, bisexual, and heterosexual women: Questionnaire survey. *Western Journal of Medicine* 172(6):379–384.

Koh, A. S., and L. K. Ross. 2006. Mental health issues: A comparison of lesbian, bisexual and heterosexual women. *Journal of Homosexuality* 51(1):33–57.

Koken, J. A., D. S. Bimbi, and J. T. Parsons. 2009. Experiences of familial acceptance-rejection among transwomen of color. *Journal of Family Psychology* 23(6):853–860.

Kuiper, B., and P. Cohen-Kettenis. 1988. Sex reassignment surgery: A study of 141 Dutch transsexuals. *Archives of Sexual Behavior* 17(5):439–457.

Lallemand, F., Y. Salhi, F. Linard, A. Giami, and W. Rozenbaum. 2002. Sexual dysfunction in 156 ambulatory HIV-infected men receiving highly active antiretroviral therapy combinations with and without protease inhibitors. *Journal of Acquired Immune Deficiency Syndromes: JAIDS* 30(2):187–190.

Lawrence, A. A. 2003. Factors associated with satisfaction or regret following male-to-female sex reassignment surgery. *Archives of Sexual Behavior* 32(4):299–315.

Lawrence, A. A. 2005. Sexuality before and after male-to-female sex reassignment surgery. *Archives of Sexual Behavior* 34(2):147–166.

Lawrence, A. A. 2006. Patient-reported complications and functional outcomes of male-to-female sex reassignment surgery. *Archives of Sexual Behavior* 35(6):717–727.

Lawrence, A. A. 2010. Sexual orientation versus age of onset as bases for typologies (subtypes) for gender identity disorder in adolescents and adults. *Archives of Sexual Behavior* 39(2):514–545.

Lev, A. I. 2004. *Transgender emergence: Therapeutic guidelines for working with gender*. New York: Haworth Press.

Lewins, F. 1995. *Transsexualism in society: A sociology of male-to-female transsexuals*. South Melbourne, Australia: MacMillan Education Australia.

Lombardi, E. 2001. Enhancing transgender health care. *American Journal of Public Health* 91(6):869–872.

Lombardi, E. L., R. A. Wilchins, D. Priesing, and D. Malouf. 2001. Gender violence: Transgender experiences with violence and discrimination. *Journal of Homosexuality* 42(1):89–101.

Luhtanen, R. K. 2003. Identity, stigma management, and well-being: A comparison of lesbians/bisexual women and gay/bisexual men. *Journal of Lesbian Studies* 7(1):85–100.

Lurie, S. 2005. Identifying training needs of health-care providers related to treatment and care of transgendered patients: A qualitative needs assessment conducted in New England. *International Journal of Transgenderism* 8(2–3):93–112.

MacKellar, D. A., L. A. Valleroy, G. M. Secura, S. Behel, T. Bingham, D. D. Celentano, B. A. Koblin, M. Lalota, W. McFarland, D. Shehan, H. Thiede, L. V. Torian, R. S. Janssen, and G. Young Men's Survey Study. 2005. Unrecognized HIV infection, risk behaviors, and perceptions of risk among young men who have sex with men: Opportunities for advancing HIV prevention in the third decade of HIV/AIDS. *Journal of Acquired Immune Deficiency Syndromes: JAIDS* 38(5):603–614.

Makadon, H. J., K. H. Mayer, J. Potter, and H. Goldhammer, eds. 2007. *The Fenway guide to lesbian, gay, bisexual, and transgender health*. Philadelphia, PA: American College of Physicians Press.

Markland, C. 1975. Transexual surgery. *Obstetrics and Gynecology Annual* 4:309–330.

Marks, G., G. A. Millett, T. Bingham, L. Bond, J. Lauby, A. Liau, C. S. Murrill, and A. Stueve. 2009. Understanding differences in HIV sexual transmission among Latino and black men who have sex with men: The brothers y hermanos study. *AIDS & Behavior* 13(4):682–690.

Marrazzo, J. M., L. A. Koutsky, N. B. Kiviat, J. M. Kuypers, and K. Stine. 2001. Papanicolaou test screening and prevalence of genital human papillomavirus among women who have sex with women. *American Journal of Public Health* 91(6):947–952.

Masten, A. S., ed. 2007. *Adolescent psychopathology and the developing brain: Integrating brain and prevention science*, edited by D. Romer and E. Walker. New York: Oxford University Press.

Masten, A. S., and M. G. Reed. 2002. Resilience in development. In *The handbook of positive psychology*, edited by S. R. Snyder and S. J. Lopez. Oxford, England: Oxford University Press.

Mate-Kole, C., M. Freschi, and A. Robin. 1990. A controlled study of psychological and social change after surgical gender reassignment in selected male transsexuals. *The British Journal of Psychiatry* 157(2):261–264.

Mathy, R. M. 2002a. A nonclinical comparison of transgender identity and sexual orientation—a framework for multicultural competence. *Journal of Psychology & Human Sexuality* 13(1):31–54.

Mathy, R. M. 2002b. Transgender identity and suicidality in a nonclinical sample—sexual orientation, psychiatric history, and compulsive behaviors. *Journal of Psychology & Human Sexuality* 14(4):47–65.

Mathy, R. M. 2003. Transgender identity and suicidality in a nonclinical sample—sexual orientation, psychiatric history, and compulsive behaviors. *Journal of Psychology & Human Sexuality* 14(4):47–65.

Mathy, R. M., B. A. Lehmann, and D. L. Kerr. 2003. Bisexual and transgender identities in a nonclinical sample of north Americans: Suicidal intent, behavioral difficulties, and mental health treatment. *Journal of Bisexuality* 3(3–4):93–109.

Matthews, A. K., and T. L. Hughes. 2001. Mental health service use by African American women: Exploration of subpopulation differences. *Cultural Diversity and Ethnic Minority Psychology* 7(1):75–87.

Mays, V. M., and S. D. Cochran. 2001. Mental health correlates of perceived discrimination among lesbian, gay, and bisexual adults in the United States. *American Journal of Public Health* 91(11):1869–1876.

Mays, V. M., A. K. Yancey, S. D. Cochran, M. Weber, and J. E. Fielding. 2002. Heterogeneity of health disparities among African American, Hispanic, and Asian American women: Unrecognized influences of sexual orientation. *American Journal of Public Health* 92(4):632–639.

McCabe, S. E., T. L. Hughes, W. B. Bostwick, B. T. West, and C. J. Boyd. 2009. Sexual orientation, substance use behaviors and substance dependence in the United States. *Addiction* 104(8):1333–1345.

McCarthy, L. 2000. Poppies in a wheat field: Exploring the lives of rural lesbians. *Journal of Homosexuality* 39(1):75–94.

Meyer, I. H. 2003. Prejudice as stress: Conceptual and measurement problems. *American Journal of Public Health* 93(2):262–265.

Meyer, I. H. 2007. Prejudice and discrimination as social stressors. In *The health of sexual minorities: Public health perspectives on lesbian, gay, bisexual, and transgender populations*, edited by I. H. Meyer and M. E. Northridge. New York: Springer Science + Business Media. Pp. 242–267.

Meyer, I. H., J. Dietrich, and S. Schwartz. 2008. Lifetime prevalence of mental disorders and suicide attempts in diverse lesbian, gay, and bisexual populations. *American Journal of Public Health* 98(6):1004–1006.

Meyer, W. J. I., W. Bockting, P. Cohen-Kettenis, C. Coleman, D. DiCeglie, H. Devor, L. Gooren, J. J. Hage, S. Kirk, B. Kuiper, D. Laub, A. A. Lawrence, Y. Menard, S. Monstrey, J. Patton, L. Schaefer, A. Webb, and C. C. Wheeler. 2001. *Standards of care for gender identity disorders, sixth version.* http://www.wpath.org/Documents2/socv6.pdf (accessed March 25, 2011).

Minton, H. L., and G. J. McDonald. 1983. Homosexual identity formation as a developmental process. *Journal of Homosexuality* 9(2/3):91–104.

Moore, E., A. Wisniewski, and A. Dobs. 2003. Endocrine treatment of transsexual people: A review of treatment regimens, outcomes, and adverse effects. *Journal of Clinical Endocrinology & Metabolism* 88(8):3467–3473.

Morris, J. F., K. F. Balsam, and E. D. Rothblum. 2002. Lesbian and bisexual mothers and nonmothers: Demographics and the coming-out process. *Journal of Family Psychology* 16(2):144–156.

Munoz-Laboy, M., and B. Dodge. 2007. Bisexual Latino men and HIV and sexually transmitted infections risk: An exploratory analysis. *American Journal of Public Health* 97(6):1102–1106.

Murad, M. H., M. B. Elamin, M. Z. Garcia, R. J. Mullan, A. Murad, P. J. Erwin, and V. M. Montori. 2010. Hormonal therapy and sex reassignment: A systematic review and meta-analysis of quality of life and psychosocial outcomes. *Clinical Endocrinology* 72(2):214–231.

Nemoto, T., D. Operario, and J. Keatley. 2005. Health and social services for male-to-female transgender persons of color in San Francisco. *International Journal of Transgenderism* 8(2–3):5–19.

Nettles, C. D., E. G. Benotsch, and K. A. Uban. 2009. Sexual risk behaviors among men who have sex with men using erectile dysfunction medications. *AIDS Patient Care & STDs* 23(12):1017–1023.

Newman, P. A., K. J. Roberts, E. Masongsong, and D. Wiley. 2008. Anal cancer screening: Barriers and facilitators among ethnically diverse gay, bisexual, transgender, and other men who have sex with men. *Journal of Gay & Lesbian Social Services: Issues in Practice, Policy & Research* 20(4):328–353.

Nierman, A. J., S. C. Thompson, A. Bryan, and A. L. Mahaffey. 2007. Gender role beliefs and attitudes toward lesbians and gay men in chile and the U.S. *Sex Roles* 57(1–2):61–67.

Nuttbrock, L., W. Bockting, S. Hwahng, A. Rosenblum, M. Mason, M. Marci, and J. Becker. 2009a. Gender identity affirmation among male-to-female transgender persons: A life course analysis across types of relationships and cultural/lifestyle factors. *Sexual and Relationship Therapy* 24(2):108–125.

Nuttbrock, L., S. Hwahng, W. Bockting, A. Rosenblum, M. Mason, M. Macri, and J. Becker. 2009b. Lifetime risk factors for HIV/sexually transmitted infections among male-to-female transgender persons. *Journal of Acquired Immune Deficiency Syndromes: JAIDS* 52(3):417–421.

Nuttbrock, L., S. Hwahng, W. Bockting, A. Rosenblum, M. Mason, M. Macri, and J. Becker. 2010. Psychiatric impact of gender-related abuse across the life course of male-to-female transgender persons. *Journal of Sex Research* 47(1):12–23.

Ostrow, D. E., K. J. Fox, J. S. Chmiel, A. Silvestre, B. R. Visscher, P. A. Vanable, L. P. Jacobson, and S. A. Strathdee. 2002. Attitudes towards highly active antiretroviral therapy are associated with sexual risk taking among HIV-infected and uninfected homosexual men. *AIDS* 16(5):775–780.

Otis, M. D., and W. F. Skinner. 1996. The prevalence of victimization and its effect on mental. *Journal of Homosexuality* 30(3):93–121.

Owens, G. P., E. D. Riggle, and S. S. Rostosky. 2007. Mental health services access for sexual minority individuals. *Sexuality Research & Social Policy: A Journal of the NSRC* 4(3):92–99.

Pache, T. D., S. Chadha, L. J. G. Gooren, W. C. J. Hop, K. W. Jaarsma, H. B. R. Dommerholt, and B. C. J. M. Fauser. 1991. Ovarian morphology in long-term androgen-treated female to male transsexuals. A human model for the study of polycystic ovarian syndrome? *Histopathology* 19(5):445–452.

Page, E. H. 2004. Mental health services experiences of bisexual women and bisexual men: An empirical study. *Journal of Bisexuality* 4:137–160.

Page, E. H. 2007. Bisexual women's and men's experiences of psychotherapy. In *Becoming visible: Counseling bisexuals across the lifespan*, edited by B. A. Firestein. New York: Columbia University Press. Pp. 52–71.

Palefsky, J. 2009. Human papillomavirus-related disease in people with HIV. *Current Opinion in HIV & AIDS* 4(1):52–56.

Palefsky, J. M., E. A. Holly, M. L. Ralston, and N. Jay. 1998. Prevalence and risk factors for human papillomavirus infection of the anal canal in human immunodeficiency virus (HIV)-positive and HIV-negative homosexual men. *Journal of Infectious Diseases* 177(2):361–367.

Parsons, J. T., E. W. Schrimshaw, R. J. Wolitski, P. N. Halkitis, D. W. Purcell, C. C. Hoff, and C. A. Gomez. 2005. Sexual harm reduction practices of HIV-seropositive gay and bisexual men: Serosorting, strategic positioning, and withdrawal before ejaculation. *AIDS* 19(Suppl. 1):S13–S25.

Patterson, C. J. 2004. What difference does a civil union make? Changing public policies and the experiences of same-sex couples: Comment on solomon, rothblum, and balsam. *Journal of Family Psychology* 18(2):287–289.

Patterson, C. J. 2009. Lesbian and gay parents and their children: A social science perspective. *Nebraska Symposium on Motivation* 54:141–182.

Patterson, C. J., and R. G. Riskind. 2010. To be a parent: Issues in family formation among gay and lesbian adults. *Journal of GLBT Family Studies* 6(3):326–340.

Paul, J. P., J. Catania, L. Pollack, J. Moskowitz, J. Canchola, T. Mills, D. Binson, and R. Stall. 2002. Suicide attempts among gay and bisexual men: Lifetime prevalence and antecedents. *American Journal of Public Health* 92(8):1338–1345.

Peel, E. 2010. Pregnancy loss in lesbian and bisexual women: An online survey of experiences. *Human Reproduction* 25(3):721–727.

Peterson, J. L., and K. T. Jones. 2009. HIV prevention for black men who have sex with men in the United States. *American Journal of Public Health* 99(6):976–980.

Pritchard, T. J., D. A. Pankowsky, J. P. Crowe, and F. W. Abdul-Karim. 1988. Breast cancer in a male-to-female transsexual: A case report. *Journal of the American Medical Association* 259(15):2278–2280.

Purcell, D. W., R. J. Wolitski, C. C. Hoff, J. T. Parsons, W. J. Woods, and P. N. Halkitis. 2005. Predictors of the use of viagra, testosterone, and antidepressants among HIV-seropositive gay and bisexual men. *AIDS* 19(Suppl. 1):S57–S66.

Rachlin, K., J. Green, and E. Lombardi. 2008. Utilization of health care among female-to-male transgender individuals in the United States. *Journal of Homosexuality* 54(3):243–258.

Ragins, B. R., and J. M. Cornwell. 2001. Pink triangles: Antecedents and consequences of perceived workplace discrimination against gay and lesbian employees. *Journal of Applied Psychology* 86(6):1244–1261.

Ragins, B. R., R. Singh, and J. M. Cornwell. 2007. Making the invisible visible: Fear and disclosure of sexual orientation at work. *Journal of Applied Psychology* 92(4): 1103–1118.

Razzano, L. A., A. Matthews, and T. L. Hughes. 2002. Utilization of mental health services: A comparison of lesbian and heterosexual women. *Journal of Gay & Lesbian Social Services: Issues in Practice, Policy & Research* 14(1):51–66.

Rhodes, S. D., and R. J. Diclemente. 2003. Psychosocial predictors of hepatitis B vaccination among young African-American gay men in the deep south. *Sexually Transmitted Diseases* 30(5):449–454.

Rieg, G., R. J. Lewis, L. G. Miller, M. D. Witt, M. Guerrero, and E. S. Daar. 2008. Asymptomatic sexually transmitted infections in HIV-infected men who have sex with men: Prevalence, incidence, predictors, and screening strategies. *AIDS Patient Care & STDs* 22(12):947–954.

Riggle, E. D., S. S. Rostosky, and S. G. Horne. 2010. Psychological distress, well-being, and legal recognition in same-sex couple relationships. *Journal of Family Psychology* 24(1):82–86.

Riskind, R. G., and C. J. Patterson. 2010. Parenting intentions and desires among childless lesbian, gay, and heterosexual individuals. *Journal of Family Psychology* 24(1):78–81.

Rogers, T. L., K. Emanuel, and J. Bradford. 2003. Sexual minorities seeking services: A retrospective study of the mental health concerns of lesbian and bisexual women. *Journal of Lesbian Studies* 7(1):127.

Rosenfeld, M. J. 2010. Nontraditional families and childhood progress through school. *Demography* 47(3):755–775.

Ross, L. E., L. Steele, C. Goldfinger, and C. Strike. 2007. Perinatal depressive symptomatology among lesbian and bisexual women. *Archives of Women's Mental Health* 10(2):53–59.

Rothblum, E. D., and R. Factor. 2001. Lesbians and their sisters as a control group: Demographic and mental health factors. *Psychological Science* 12(1):63–69.

Russell, C. J., and P. K. Keel. 2002. Homosexuality as a specific risk factor for eating disorders in men. *International Journal of Eating Disorders* 31(3):300–306.

Rutter, M. 2007. Resilience, competence, and coping. *Child Abuse & Neglect* 31(3):205–209.

Ryan, D. P., C. C. Compton, and R. J. Mayer. 2000. Carcinoma of the anal canal. *New England Journal of Medicine* 342(11):792–800.

Sanchez, J. P., S. Hailpern, C. Lowe, and Y. Calderon. 2007. Factors associated with emergency department utilization by urban lesbian, gay, and bisexual individuals. *Journal of Community Health: The Publication for Health Promotion and Disease Prevention* 32(2):149–156.

Sanchez, N. F., J. P. Sanchez, and A. Danoff. 2009. Health care utilization, barriers to care, and hormone usage among male-to-female transgender persons in new york city. *American Journal of Public Health* 99(4):713–719.

Saulnier, C. F. 2002. Deciding who to see: Lesbians discuss their preferences in health and mental health care providers. *Social Work* 47(4):355–365.

Scheer, S., I. Peterson, K. Page-Shafer, V. Delgado, A. Gleghorn, J. Ruiz, F. Molitor, W. McFarland, and J. Klausner. 2002. Sexual and drug use behavior among women who have sex with both women and men: Results of a population-based survey. *American Journal of Public Health* 92(7):1110–1112.

Seaver, M. R., K. M. Freund, L. M. Wright, J. Tjia, and S. M. Frayne. 2008. Healthcare preferences among lesbians: A focus group analysis. *Journal of Women's Health* 17(2):215–225.

Shapiro, D. N., C. Peterson, and A. J. Stewart. 2009. Legal and social contexts and mental health among lesbian and heterosexual mothers. *Journal of Family Psychology* 23(2):255–262.

Simpson, E. K., and C. A. Helfrich. 2007. Lesbian survivors of intimate partner violence: Provider perspectives on barriers to accessing services. *Journal of Gay & Lesbian Social Services: Issues in Practice, Policy & Research* 18(2):39–59.

Singh, A., B. J. Dew, D. G. Hays, and A. Gailis. 2006. Relationships among internalized homophobia, sexual identity development, and coping resources of lesbian and bisexual women. *Journal of LGBT Issues in Counseling* 1:15–31.

Smith, E. M., S. R. Johnson, and S. M. Guenther. 1985. Health care attitudes and experiences during gynecologic care among lesbians and bisexuals. *American Journal of Public Health* 75:1085–1087.

Sperber, J., S. Landers, and S. Lawrence. 2005. Access to health care for transgendered persons: Results of a needs assessment in Noston. *International Journal of Transgenderism* 8(2–3):75–91.

Spikes, P. S., D. W. Purcell, K. M. Williams, Y. Chen, H. Ding, and P. S. Sullivan. 2009. Sexual risk behaviors among HIV-positive black men who have sex with women, with men, or with men and women: Implications for intervention development. *American Journal of Public Health* 99(6):1072–1078.

Stall, R., J. P. Paul, G. Greenwood, L. M. Pollack, E. Bein, G. M. Crosby, T. C. Mills, D. Binson, T. J. Coates, and J. A. Catania. 2001. Alcohol use, drug use and alcohol-related problems among men who have sex with men: The Urban Men's Health Study. *Addiction* 96(11):1589–1601.

Stevens, P. E., and J. M. Hall. 2001. Sexuality and safer sex: The issues for lesbians and bisexual women. *Journal of Obstetric, Gynecologic, & Neonatal Nursing* 30(4): 439–447.

Sullivan, P. S., A. J. Drake, and T. H. Sanchez. 2007. Prevalence of treatment optimism-related risk behavior and associated factors among men who have sex with men in 11 states, 2000–2001. *AIDS & Behavior* 11(1):123–129.

Swim, J. K., K. Johnston, and N. B. Pearson. 2009. Daily experiences with heterosexism: Relations between hetersexist hassles and psychological well-being. *Journal of Social and Clinical Psychology* 28(5):597–629.

Symmers, W. S. 1968. Carcinoma of breast in trans-sexual individuals after surgical and hormonal interference with the primary and secondary sex characteristics. *British Medical Journal* 2(5597):83–85.

Szymanski, D. M. 2005. Heterosexism and sexism as correlates of psychological distress in lesbians. *Journal of Counseling & Development* 83(3):355–360.

Szymanski, D. M. 2009. Examining potential moderators of the link between heterosexist events and gay and bisexual men's psychological distress. *Journal of Counseling Psychology* 56(1):142–151.

Tang, H., G. L. Greenwood, D. W. Cowling, J. C. Lloyd, A. G. Roeseler, and D. G. Bal. 2004. Cigarette smoking among lesbians, gays, and bisexuals: How serious a problem? (United States). *Cancer Causes & Control* 15(8):797–803.

Tasker, C., and C. J. Patterson. 2007. Research on gay and lesbian parenting: Retrospect and prospect. *Journal of Gay, Lesbian, Bisexual and Transgender Family Issues* 3:9–34.

Tjaden, P., N. Thoennes, and C. J. Allison. 1999. Comparing violence over the life span in samples of same-sex and opposite-sex cohabitants. *Violence & Victims* 14(4):413–425.

Tom Waddell Health Center. 2006. *Protocols for hormonal reassignment of gender.* San Francisco, CA.

Trettin, S., E. L. Moses-Kolko, and K. L. Wisner. 2006. Lesbian perinatal depression and the heterosexism that affects knowledge about this minority population. *Archives of Women's Mental Health* 9(2):67–73.

Trocki, K. F., L. A. Drabble, and L. T. Midanik. 2009. Tobacco, marijuana, and sensation seeking: Comparisons across gay, lesbian, bisexual, and heterosexual groups. *Psychology of Addictive Behaviors* 23(4):620–631.

van Dam, M. A. A., A. S. Koh, and S. L. Dibble. 2001. Lesbian disclosure to health care providers and delay of care. *Journal of the Gay & Lesbian Medical Association* 5(1):11–19.

van Haarst, E. P., D. W. Newling, L. J. Gooren, H. Asscheman, and D. M. Prenger. 1998. Metastatic prostatic carcinoma in a male-to-female transsexual. *British Journal of Urology* 81(5):776.

Van Kesteren, P. J., H. Asscheman, J. A. J. Megens, and L. J. G. Gooren. 1997. Mortality and morbidity in transsexual subjects treated with cross-sex hormones. *Clinical Endocrinology* 47(3):337–343.

Van Kesteren, P. J., P. Lips, L. J. G. Gooren, H. Asscheman, and J. Megens. 1998. Long-term follow-up of bone mineral density and bone metabolism in transsexuals treated with cross-sex hormones. *Clinical Endocrinology* 48(3):347–354.

Wainright, J. L., and C. J. Patterson. 2006. Delinquency, victimization, and substance use among adolescents with female same-sex parents. *Journal of Family Psychology* 20(3):526–530.

Wainright, J. L., and C. J. Patterson. 2008. Peer relations among adolescents with female same-sex parents. *Developmental Psychology* 44(1):117–126.

Wainright, J. L., S. T. Russell, and C. J. Patterson. 2004. Psychosocial adjustment, school outcomes, and romantic relationships of adolescents with same-sex parents. *Child Development* 75(6):1886–1898.

Weyers, S., E. Elaut, P. De Sutter, J. Gerris, G. T'Sjoen, G. Heylens, G. De Cuypere, and H. Verstraelen. 2009. Long-term assessment of the physical, mental, and sexual health among transsexual women. *Journal of Sexual Medicine* 6(3):752–760.

Williams, T., J. Connolly, D. Pepler, and W. Craig. 2005. Peer victimization, social support, and psychosocial adjustment of sexual minority adolescents. *Journal of Youth and Adolescence* 34(5):471–482.

Willoughby, B. L., B. S. Lai, N. D. Doty, E. R. Mackey, and N. M. Malik. 2008. Peer crowd affiliations of adult gay men: Linkages with health risk behaviors. *Psychology of Men & Masculinity* 9(4):235–247.

Wojnar, D. 2007. Miscarriage experiences of lesbian couples. *Journal of Midwifery & Women's Health* 52(5):479–485.

Wong, A. K., R. C. Chan, N. Aggarwal, M. K. Singh, W. S. Nichols, and S. Bose. 2010. Human papillomavirus genotypes in anal intraepithelial neoplasia and anal carcinoma as detected in tissue biopsies. *Modern Pathology* 23(1):144–150.

Xavier, J. M. 2000. *The Washington, DC transgender needs assessment survey: Final report for phase 2*. Washington, DC: Administration for HIV and AIDS, District of Columbia.

Xavier, J. M., M. Bobbin, B. Singer, and E. Budd. 2005. A needs assessment of transgendered people of color living in Washington, DC. *International Journal of Transgenderism* 8(2/3): 31–47.

Xavier, J. M., J. Bradford, and J. Honnold. 2007. *The health, health-related needs, and lifecourse experiences of transgender Virginians*. Richmond, VA: Virginia Department of Health.

Zea, M. C., C. A. Reisen, and P. J. Poppen. 1999. Psychological well-being among Latino lesbians and gay men. *Cultural Diversity and Ethnic Minority Psychology* 5(4):371–379.

Zucker, K. J., and A. A. Lawrence. 2009. Epidemiology of gender identity disorder: Recommendations for the standards of care of the world professional association for transgender health. *International Journal of Transgenderism* 11(1):8–18.

Zule, W. A., G. V. Bobashev, W. M. Wechsberg, E. C. Costenbader, and C. M. Coomes. 2009. Behaviorally bisexual men and their risk behaviors with men and women. *Journal of Urban Health* 86(Suppl. 1):48–62.

6

Later Adulthood

The cohort of LGBT people currently in later life grew up and moved into adulthood in much less supportive environments than those experienced by younger cohorts. Before entering adulthood, the oldest of this cohort would have seen, in 1952, the creation of an official diagnosis that listed homosexuality as a sociopathic personality disturbance (Bayer, 1987) and watched Senator McCarthy include gay men and lesbians on his blacklist. As adults, this cohort witnessed routine harassment by authorities, as well as the Stonewall Rebellion in 1969 and the American Psychiatric Association's removal of homosexuality from the *Diagnostic and Statistical Manual of Mental Disorders* in 1973 (see Chapter 2 for a full historical overview).

For all adults, later life is known as a period of both growth and decline (Baltes et al., 1999), with studies on the latter vastly outnumbering those on the former. Significant research effort has begun focusing on the diseases and disorders that accompany old age and the lifestyles of the elderly, including dementia; the living environments of later life; the need for and delivery of care from both interpersonal and institutional perspectives; the related social, and especially family, relations of older persons; end-of-life preparations; bereavement; and the personal and environmental characteristics of successful aging. These areas of research are certainly not restricted to heterosexual persons; the experiences of aging LGBT persons may be similarly characterized, with the addition of the legacies and experiences of stigma. In fact, studies of aging among LGBT elders will generate new knowledge about aging in general as questions are framed and concepts considered that fall outside of traditional "heteronormative" perspectives.

The committee chose to define the start of later life, while a vague and contested concept, as generally coinciding with retirement. The bulk of the empirical literature on LGBT aging, however, makes reference to a variety of (mostly younger) ages than this traditional cut-off point and is included in the discussion that follows. Ages younger than the traditional retirement age are included in this chapter in the context of preparations for later life, mainly as pertains to the well-known "baby boomer" cohort, the next in line to become seniors. This age issue is part of the recurring pattern noted throughout this report: much of the empirical literature on which the report draws either does not provide an age breakdown or uses a breakdown that does not match the age ranges used to organize the chapters of the report. Thus, the text that follows builds upon, and sometimes includes references to, studies and observations from the preceding chapter on early/middle adulthood. In so doing, it highlights the continuous nature of the life course while at the same time elucidating the particular circumstances of the later years.

In general, LGBT elders have not been the subject of extensive research; a recent publication reviews some of the extant literature and echoes this statement (see Fredriksen-Goldsen and Muraco, 2010). Just as aging is infrequently considered in LGBT research, the field of gerontology has infrequently considered LGBT aging issues (Scherrer, 2009). The studies in this area that have typically been reported have used small and mainly regional samples, often recruited from public venues, such as community centers, street fairs, and pride festivals. The vast majority of studies include self-identified LGBT persons; if studies describe samples of LGBT persons otherwise identified, they are highlighted below. The studies in this area also focus disproportionately on gay men and lesbians; few studies have focused on bisexual or transgender elders. Most studies, moreover, have a high representation of white individuals; very few articles have been written on racial/ethnic minorities. Although many samples include LGBT older persons of color, they are often in proportions insufficient for further analysis; thus, very little is known about these groups. The same is true for other metrics of diversity (such as rural residence, culture, or religion). Finally, almost no published research exists on the very later years of LGBT persons—ages 85 and older.

Given the limited research in this area, this chapter draws significantly on the few large-scale studies that have included older LGBT persons (and those approaching later life). It also includes a variety of more regional studies with less representative and smaller samples, as noted above. When possible, these restricted samples are described within the limiting parameters of the cited studies.

This chapter examines research that has been conducted on the health of LGBT elders and factors that influence their health outcomes. It begins by describing research on the development of sexual orientation and gender identity in this age group. The next two sections examine first mental health status and then physical health status. The chapter then addresses in turn risk and protective factors; health services; and contextual influences, including demographic characteristics, the role of the family, and end-of-life issues. The final section presents a summary of key findings and research opportunities.

DEVELOPMENT OF SEXUAL ORIENTATION AND GENDER IDENTITY

Although the age at which gay men and lesbians come out appears to be earlier today than in previous cohorts, there remains great variability in the time of coming out and evidence that the process may extend over the life course (Brown et al., 2001; de Vries and Blando, 2004). Grov and colleagues (2006) conducted a cross-sectional street-intercept survey with 2,733 participants at a series of LGB community events in New York City and Los Angeles. Their sample was broken down into five age cohorts, the oldest of which was 55 and older. The authors found that women and men in the youngest cohort (aged 18–24) reported coming out to themselves at younger ages than women and men in the oldest cohort. The average age of coming out to self and coming out to others for the youngest women was 15.88 and 16.87 years, respectively; the average comparable ages for the oldest cohort of women were 24.90 and 27.38, respectively. The average age of coming out to self and coming out to others for the youngest men was 15.01 and 16.94 years, respectively; the average comparable ages for the oldest cohort of men were 20.31 and 24.11, respectively. Uneven and smaller subsamples of racial and ethnic minority LGB persons prevented fuller analyses; however, within-cohort analyses revealed no racial differences in the age at which participants came out to themselves and others.

In the Still Out, Still Aging: The MetLife Study of Lesbian, Gay, Bisexual and Transgender Baby Boomers (MetLife, 2010) national survey of LGBT people aged 45–64 (n = 1,201), the extent to which LGBT respondents reported being out varied significantly. Transgender and bisexual respondents were far less likely to be out: only 39 percent of transgender and just 16 percent of bisexual people were completely or mostly out, compared with 74 percent of gay men and 76 percent of lesbians. The majority of gay men and lesbians reported having completely or very accepting families; for transgender and bisexual respondents, these percentages were lower (42 and 24 percent, respectively). Almost one-third (31 percent) of bisexuals said family members were not very or not at all accepting, a far higher percentage than the next least-accepted subpopulation of transgender people (12 percent).

LGBT respondents were also asked about the extent to which they disclosed their sexual orientation and/or gender identity with a variety of people. Although more than a quarter (29 percent) said they were open with anyone, many reported that they were guarded with some people. For example, 33 percent had not disclosed to their neighbors, and more than 30 percent had not disclosed at work (32 percent for coworkers and 30 percent for supervisors); 20 percent were guarded with their siblings and their parents, while 28 percent were guarded with other family members. There were also other groups of people to whom the participants had not come out—acquaintances (30 percent), people at the place where they attended religious services (16 percent), health care providers (16 percent), and even "closest friends" (12 percent). Bisexual people were less likely to disclose their sexual orientation than the other subpopulations; only 12 percent of bisexual people said they were open with anyone, compared with 30 percent of lesbians, 38 percent of gay men, and 28 percent of transgender respondents (MetLife, 2010).

In his secondary analysis of 372 men aged 50–85 in the Urban Men's Health Study—a probabilistic sample of men who have sex with men obtained in San Francisco, Los Angeles, Chicago, and New York using a modified random-digit dialing approach—Rawls (2004) found that almost 5 percent of the men in this sample had never told someone they were gay or bisexual; half of the men had not told someone else they were gay or bisexual until after the age of 21 and about one-quarter of the men until after age 26. Considered by current age, the proportion of men who reported that they had disclosed their orientation to many in their social environment significantly decreased over the three age groups in the sample—50–59, 60–69, and 70 and older. Of interest, among the older two groups, there were no significant differences between those with lower and higher levels of disclosure in their experience of distress and depression. This latter finding in particular is reminiscent of results of earlier research, particularly Lee's (1987) study of older Canadian gay men and Adelman's (1990) study of a small sample of gay men and lesbians over age 60 in the San Francisco Bay Area. In both of these studies, those with lower disclosure reported greater happiness and life satisfaction, leaving open questions about the time/cohort and/or life-course consequences of coming out.

Transgender persons who are visibly gender role nonconforming in childhood tend to come out at an early age (Bockting and Coleman, 2007). For the older generations, this was typically during adolescence or early adulthood; today's generation typically comes out in childhood or shortly after the onset of puberty (Möller et al., 2009; Wallien and Cohen-Kettenis, 2008). However, transgender persons who are not visibly gender role nonconforming in childhood typically do not come out until much later in life, during midlife or beyond. This is a particularly common developmental pathway among transgender women (as opposed to transgender men) (Doctor, 1988; Landen et al., 1998). Some transgender people who were not visibly gender role nonconforming in childhood do retrospectively report cross-gender feelings in childhood, whereas others do not. Most do, however, recall cross-dressing during adolescence. Initially, such cross-dressing is often sexually arousing, and may be restricted to particular articles of clothing (e.g., lingerie) and, possibly, compulsive (i.e., fetishistic). After many years of cross-dressing in private, the main motivation for cross-dressing may shift toward more fully doing so for comfort and, eventually, to express a cross-gender identity. This developmental pathway has been described as late onset (as opposed to early onset [Doorn et al., 1994]), secondary (as opposed to primary [Person and Ovesey, 1974]), marginal (as opposed to nuclear [Buhrich and McConaghy, 1978]), or autogynephilic (as opposed to homosexual) transsexualism[1] (Blanchard, 1989).

Thus, according to these typologies, most transsexual men and many transsexual women experience a strong cross-gender identity starting in childhood (primary transsexualism). For many transsexual women, however, the cross-gender identity develops more gradually over the life course and increases in intensity, and after years of compartmentalizing this identity privately, these transsexual women come out during midlife or beyond to transition and pursue hormone therapy and/or surgery to feminize. At a later age, however, hormone therapy is less effective at feminizing, either because it cannot reverse the long-term masculinizing effects of testosterone or because only lower doses of feminizing hormones can be prescribed given the higher prevalence of medical contraindications and chronic disease among older individuals (Dahl et al., 2006). For these individuals, years of being "in the closet" and in effect delaying experiences of felt stigma may have mental health implications, although research comparing the mental health of those who come out early versus later in life has yielded mixed findings (see Lawrence, 2010, for a review). What is clear is that the majority of transsexual individuals who come out later in life benefit from treatment of gender dysphoria and are satisfied with sex reassignment (Lawrence, 2003, 2010).

For transgender people, coming out later in life also means working through developmental events commonly experienced earlier in life, such as a kind of "second adolescence," first experiences in the other gender role (including dating and sexual experimentation), and exploration of

[1] As a reminder, *transgender* is an umbrella term that encompasses a diverse group of individuals who depart from traditional gender norms. *Transsexuals* are those who desire to feminize or masculinize their appearance through the use of hormone therapy and/or surgery (or have already done so), and they are included in the broader category of *transgender* people. This discussion refers to a specific type of transsexualism that involves a developmental process occurring later in life.

one's masculinity or femininity (Bockting and Coleman, 2007). Many who come out later in life are heterosexually married and have a family, whose members face their own process of coming to terms with their loved one's transgender identity (Emerson, 1996; Lev, 2004).

MENTAL HEALTH STATUS

Some significant literature examines the potential challenges faced by LGBT persons in later life; there have been few empirical studies in this area, however. Some of the many challenges reported include the present and past effects of stigma and discrimination and a greater reliance on nontraditional sources of support, such as friends and other non–family members, in an environment in which such support frequently is not recognized either formally (by policy, for example) or informally (by social organizations and family members, for example) (see Barker, 2002, for a discussion of "friend" caretakers to the elderly in general). Confronting these challenges is believed to tax the mental health of LGBT elders, as discussed below.

It is important to note, however, that LGBT people in later adulthood typically are well adjusted and mentally healthy. Studies using probability samples indicate that the majority of older LGB adults do not report mental health problems (Cochran and Mays, 2006; Herek and Garnets, 2007). While national probability samples of the transgender population are not available, studies based on nonprobability samples similarly show that the same is true for many if not most transgender adults (Clements-Nolle et al., 2001; Nuttbrock et al., 2010).

Mood/Anxiety Disorders

Limited data are available on mood or anxiety disorders among older LGBT individuals. The reports available in the literature typically are for an adult population undifferentiated by age, obscuring the particular experiences of older adults.

Depression

Among older adults in the general population, estimates of the prevalence of major depression range from less than 1 percent to approximately 5 percent, but can reach 13.5 percent for those who require home health care (NIMH, 2007). Compared with these estimates, studies of both older gay men and older lesbians have found elevated levels of depression. Shippy and colleagues (2004) found that 30 percent of a sample of 233 gay men aged 50–87 reported depression. Bradford and colleagues (1993), reporting on the National Lesbian Health Care Survey of 1,925 self-identified lesbians aged 17–80, found that among the approximately 3 percent of the sample over age 55, 24 percent reported having experienced depression at some point in their lives. Valanis and colleagues (2000), analyzing data from the Women's Health Initiative (n = 93,311), found that 15–17 percent of lesbians aged 50–79 had been depressed.

In a household probability sample of 2,881 men who have sex with men (analyzed by age decade), Mills and colleagues (2004) found a rate of depression of 17 percent among men aged 50–69 (n = 397) and 5 percent among men aged 70 and older (n = 41). Not having a domestic partner, a recent history of antigay threats or violence, not identifying as gay, and feeling highly alienated from the gay community were associated with both distress and depression. Based on data gathered from 416 self-identified lesbian, gay, and bisexual adults aged 60–91, Grossman (2006) found that most older LGB adults in the study appeared to have developed some resilience to the minority stress in their lives. However, signs of emotional distress were still present in their lives. For example, 27 percent reported feeling lonely, 10 percent reported sometimes or often considering suicide, and 17 percent still wished they were heterosexual. For 93 percent of participants, having known people who were HIV-positive or had died of AIDS was an additional factor that caused emotional distress.

Several authors have commented that older transgender adults have particularly high rates of depression (e.g., Cook-Daniels and Munson, 2010). Empirical evidence is sparse on this point, however. A recent study by Fredriksen-Goldsen and colleagues (2011) offers some data on this and other points of relevance. The study was based on an 11-site sample with a total of 2,560 self-identified LGBT persons between the ages of 50 and 95 (including 175 transgender persons) recruited through agency lists, respondent-driven sampling, and in-depth interviews. Thirty-one percent of the LGBT persons in this sample were depressed; transgender persons reported significantly higher levels of depression than nontransgender persons, although the exact percentages were not known.

Suicide/Suicidal Behavior

The National Institute of Mental Health (NIMH, 2007) identified a national average of 11 suicides per 100,000 in the general population; persons over age 65 died by suicide at a rate of 14.7 per 100,000. From another perspective, the proportion of older adults in the United States is about 12 percent, but the elderly account for 18 percent of the nation's suicides (Statewide Office of Suicide Prevention, 2009). These statistics differ dramatically by gender: men die by suicide at a rate five times that among women.

Even against this backdrop, the lifetime risk of suicide attempts appears particularly high among gay and bisexual men, as reported in a metareview by King and colleagues (2008), although this analysis had no age-specific focus. Others have reported an elevated risk of suicide attempts and suicidality in samples including older gay men and lesbians. For example, Paul and colleagues (2002) examined suicidality by age cohort using data from the Urban Men's Health Study—a household probability sample of 2,881 men who have sex with men in four major U.S. cities, 14 percent of whom were age 25 in 1970 (meaning they were 55 in 2000). The authors found that 12 percent of this group had attempted suicide (equivalent to the percentage in all other age cohorts), with the mean age of first attempt being 37.4 years (one-quarter of men in this cohort who had attempted suicide had done so before age 25).

In a study using the previously described data set of 416 self-identified lesbian, gay, and bisexual adults aged 60–91, D'Augelli and Grossman (2001) found that 13 percent of their sample had attempted suicide (an attempt was especially likely among those who had been victimized at some point in their lives, as described further below). Among the study participants, better mental health was correlated with higher self-esteem, less loneliness, and lower internalized homophobia. Compared with women, men reported significantly more internalized homophobia, alcohol abuse, and suicidality related to their sexual orientation. Less lifetime suicidal ideation was associated with lower internalized homophobia, less loneliness, and more people knowing about participants' sexual orientation (D'Augelli and Grossman, 2001).

Although some studies examining suicidal ideation and attempts among transgender adults include individuals in later adulthood, these studies typically do not provide analyses of their data according to the age of participants. Therefore, it is difficult to identify findings that are specifically pertinent to transgender individuals in later adulthood. These studies are discussed in the previous chapter on early/middle adulthood.

As noted frequently throughout this chapter, research on LGBT elders is sparse, an observation that is apparent in this section. It is also important to note that much of what is known about suicide attempts or ideation is for "any time in the lives" of these persons as currently assessed. Many of these behaviors and thoughts may well have occurred in much earlier years and thus are not related to experiences in later life (and perhaps even intimate particular resilience among older, surviving adults).

Transgender-Specific Mental Health Status

Studies on the mental health of transgender people include participants in later life, yet data for this age group typically are not presented separately. One recent study, however, does provide some insight into the mental health of older transgender individuals. While this study encompasses midlife participants, its focus on older in comparison with younger adults makes its inclusion appropriate. Nuttbrock and colleagues (2010) conducted Life Chart Interviews with a convenience sample of 571 transgender women in New York City and compared data from older (aged 40–59, n = 238) and younger (aged 19–39, n = 333) participants. Two-thirds (66.3 percent) of the older as opposed to 84.1 percent of the younger participants reported coming out in one or more interpersonal contexts (family, friends, work, school). Lifetime prevalence of depression was 52.4 percent for the older group and 54.7 percent for the younger group. Among the older group, 35.5 percent reported depression during two or more life stages (early adolescence, late adolescence, early/young adulthood, early middle age, later middle age); depression was high during early adolescence (23.5 percent) and remained relatively constant into early (24.8 percent) and later (26.1 percent) middle age. This pattern differed from that of the younger group, in whom depression was extremely high during early adolescence (38.4 percent) but then declined significantly into early middle age (19.1 percent). Lifetime prevalence of suicidal ideation, planning, and attempts among the older group was 53.5 percent, 34.9 percent, and 28.0 percent, respectively; 6.7 percent reported suicide attempts during two or more life stages. For both the older and younger groups, gender-related stigma (gender-related psychological and physical abuse) was associated with depression.

PHYSICAL HEALTH STATUS

The now well-known health concomitants of aging are similarly represented among heterosexual and LGBT older adults, although they may be exacerbated by factors associated with gender identity and sexual orientation. These factors are rarely studied, and thus are fertile ground for subsequent research. For example, data suggest that LGBT adults, including older persons, rate their health more poorly than heterosexual adults. The Massachusetts Department of Public Health issued a report in 2009 that included 1,598 LGBT and heterosexual adults (with mean ages in the range of middle adulthood). Among participants, 67.3 percent of transgender adults (n = 35), 73.5 percent of bisexual adults (n = 100), and 78 percent of gay and lesbian adults (n = 749) rated their overall health as "excellent" or "very good," compared with 82.5 percent of heterosexual adults (n = 371) (Massachusetts Department of Public Health, 2009).

In a national study comparing more than 1,200 LGBT people aged 45–64 with a group of just over 1,200 individuals aged 45–64 from the general population, the MetLife (2010) survey found that the percentage reporting recent receipt of (and need for) care was greatest (19 percent) among the 5 percent of the sample identifying as transgender—comparable to the percentage of lesbians, somewhat greater than the percentage of bisexual women and men (17 percent), and much higher than the percentage of gay men as well as women and men from the general population (9 percent).

Finally, Fredriksen-Goldsen and colleagues (2011) found that almost one in four (23 percent) of their sample of 2,560 LGBT adults aged 50 and older reported that their general health was poor.

Sexual/Reproductive Health

Although the study of sexuality has seen tremendous growth over the last 60–70 years, beginning with Kinsey's groundbreaking research in the 1940s and 1950s, research on sexuality and aging has lagged. It is likely that research in this field is largely undeveloped as a result of ageism and inaccurate beliefs about sexuality ending in later life. As Schlesinger (1996) has noted, myths surrounding older persons and sexuality (i.e., that older persons are sexually undesirable and are not desirous of or capable of sexual expression) continue to influence our culture's perspectives on sexuality and the elderly. Research has shown that these beliefs are false and that many adults continue to be sexually active throughout their lives (Lindau et al., 2007). While the very notion of a gay and lesbian gerontology raises the issue of sexuality directly (de Vries and Blando, 2004), limited research has explored sexual health among older LGBT people.

In contrast, there is some research on sexual dysfunction in these groups. Erectile dysfunction has been associated with aging among men, although no research has investigated the extent of the problem among men who have sex with men. Rawls (2004) reports on a reanalysis of existing data on men who have sex with men who either identified as gay or reported same-sex contact in the Urban Men's Health Study (Catania et al., 2001). Of the total sample of 2,881 men, 372 between the ages of 50 and 85 were included in the analysis. Among these men, 38.5 percent reported some "sexual difficulties" in the year prior to their interview. Of those reporting sexual difficulties, just under two-thirds cited health problems and/or medications as a contributing factor, and more than one-third cited psychological problems.

Some reference to sexual dysfunction is included in research on prostate cancer, as noted by Asencio and colleagues (2009) in their qualitative focus group study of 36 midlife and older gay men (the majority being aged 50–70). The authors found that the fear of sexual dysfunction would influence respondents' decisions about how to treat prostate cancer, with age, socioeconomic status, and race moderating this association.

Little empirical research has explored sexual functioning among older lesbians, bisexuals, and transgender persons. In terms of reproductive health, Moore and colleagues (2003) report high rates of polycystic ovarian disease in transgender men, with implications for the risk of endometrial cancer.

The literature includes some discussion (and controversy; see, e.g., Garnets and Peplau, 2006) about "lesbian bed death." Early research (e.g., Kehoe, 1989) on older lesbians found large numbers reporting no sexual experience in the previous year and low rates of sexual satisfaction. Kehoe's study was conducted with 100 self-identified lesbians over age 60 who responded to calls for participants posted in lesbian and feminist newsletters and bookstores, women's centers, and college and university campuses and associations. Little published research has followed this early, groundbreaking work to support or challenge its findings, and the concept remains in the lexicon of the literature.

Valanis and colleagues (2000) report on the Women's Health Initiative study, which included women aged 50–79 of postmenopausal status (n = 93,311). Women were placed into five sexual orientation groups based on their responses: heterosexual (n = 90,578), bisexual (n = 740), lifetime lesbian (sex only with women ever) (n = 264), adult lesbian (sex only with women after age 45) (n = 309), and never had adult sex (n = 1,420). The authors compared reproductive health outcomes and behaviors among the participants. Their results demonstrate similarities in oral contraceptive use and rates of pregnancy and hormone replacement therapy among the five sexual orientation groups. The rate of oral contraceptive use was highest for bisexual women (54.6 percent), and also high for adult lesbians (52.1 percent) and heterosexual women (45.4 percent). Heterosexual women had the highest rate of hysterectomy (41.5 percent), although the rates were similar for adult lesbians (35.0 percent) and bisexual women (39.6 percent). Adult lesbians, lifetime lesbians, bisexual women, and heterosexual women had similar rates of ever using hormone replacement therapy (HRT) (66–71 percent), higher than the rate among the no adult sex group (48 percent). These results reveal that, despite differences in sexual orientation, rates of hysterectomy, oral contraceptive use, and HRT use are extremely similar.

Valanis and colleagues also found high rates of ever being pregnant among the bisexuals (80.8 percent) and adult lesbians (63 percent) compared with the lifetime lesbians (35 percent). In the aggregate, these data indicate that pregnancy and parenting may play a significant role in the lives of many women who have sex with women, with relevance for psychosocial and physical well-being.

Cook-Daniels and Munson (2010) have been among the very few to study sexual practices and behaviors among transgender elders. They report on a sample comprising 272 transgender participants and/or their intimate partners aged 50–79, generated by means of an online survey in which participants were recruited through listservs directed to transgender adults and support groups. Gender identity was available for about one-third of these respondents. About half of these individuals identified as male-to-female and about one-third as female-to-male, with the remainder identifying as nontransgender male or female. About one-quarter of respondents to a question about sexual practices said they were celibate or not in a sexual relationship; sexual practices and behaviors were varied. Cook-Daniels and Munson (2010) also report on the particulars of sexual activities, including body parts that were "on" or "off limits"; the extent to which sexuality, including libido, was influenced by being transgender or by being the partner of a transgender person; negotiation of sex; and other areas not typically noted in the existing research but with relevance for populations beyond transgender persons.

In addition, Cook-Daniels and Munson (2010) report on the sexual violence experiences of transgender elders. Using the online survey and sampling methods described above, another sample of 53 transgender persons aged 50–64 was formed, 88 percent of whom were male-to-female. Almost two-thirds of these respondents reported "unwanted sexual touch," half having experienced this within the past 15 years. In the Virginia survey mentioned above, 27 percent of respondents (about one-third of female-to-males and one-quarter of male-to-females) reported having been forced to engage in unwanted sexual activity after age 12. In the Kenagy (2005) Philadelphia surveys, a higher proportion—58 percent—of a broad, undifferentiated age group had been forced to have sex; the proportion was significantly higher for male-to-females. Clearly, this is an area that merits greater examination with many issues being unaddressed, including, for example, sexual functioning after sex reassignment surgery and the impact of long-term hormone use on sexual functioning. This area takes on even greater importance in the context of abuse against transgender persons more generally, which is noted to be high (e.g., Witten and Whittle, 2004) and explored further below.

Cancer

Prostate cancer has the highest prevalence among men over age 60 (Altekruse et al., 2010) and has recently received significant public attention. Much of what is known about the impact of prostate cancer is based on older heterosexual men in long-term marital relationships (Blank, 2008) and focuses largely on erectile dysfunction. Blank and colleagues (2009) suggest that the experiences for gay men, who often lack long-term partners and may be participants in sexual behaviors that differ from those in traditional heterosexual encounters, may be quite different and largely understudied.

As previously mentioned, data from focus groups (a total of five groups comprising 36 participants with a mean age of 49.3 years, most aged

50–70) suggest that gay men have limited understanding of their prostate and the range of sexual challenges associated with prostate cancer and its treatment. The gay men in these groups, of varying socioeconomic status, addressed physician–patient relationships, including coming out to one's medical provider (an issue also noted in other research), as well the potential treatment-related sexual problems attributable to their sexual practices, sexual roles, and beliefs about gay relationships and the gay community (Asencio et al., 2009). There are no known data on incidence rates of prostate cancer among gay or bisexual men; information on sexual orientation is not collected in the Surveillance Epidemiology and End Results database. It is important to note that transgender women, even after reconstructive surgery, retain their prostate; there are also no data on prostate cancer in this population.

Some strains of the human papillomavirus (HPV) are causally linked to the development of anal cancer, although little is known of its prevalence among HIV-negative men. As discussed in Chapter 5, in a study of 1,218 HIV-negative men who have sex with men aged 18–89 (Chin-Hong et al., 2004), the overall prevalence of anal HPV infection was 57 percent and was similar across all age groups. The sample included men aged 55 and older (the oldest age group included in the study; the sample was self-selected and based on both HIV status and self-reported sexual behaviors). Significant predictors included a history of receptive anal intercourse (and age at first receptive anal intercourse) and the number of male sex partners during the preceding 6 months.

For women, breast cancer is the most prevalent form of cancer in later life; in fact, age is the greatest risk factor for the disease. In the Women's Health Initiative study mentioned earlier in this chapter, Valanis and colleagues (2000) found that 14 percent of the no adult sex group and lifetime lesbians and 17.6 percent of the bisexuals reported ever having had any cancer, compared with 11.9 percent of heterosexual women. The bisexual group also had the highest rate of breast cancer (8.4 percent). In fact, all of the nonheterosexual groups had higher rates of breast cancer than the heterosexual group, but were less likely than the heterosexual group to have recently had a Pap test or mammogram. Cervical cancer was highest among bisexual women (2.1 percent) and lifetime lesbians (2.2. percent). As noted in the previous chapter, health-related behaviors of lesbian and bisexual women (smoking, obesity, drinking) theoretically contribute to higher risks for breast, ovarian, and colon cancer.

Zaritsky and Dibble (2010) studied a sample of 370 self-identified lesbian and heterosexual sister pairs aged 40 or older who anonymously completed a survey about their health. The study used multiple methods, including respondent-driven sampling. For their secondary data analysis, the authors examined data on those sister pairs with at least one sister aged

50 or older (n = 42 pairs, or 84 women) and examined risk factors for reproductive cancers. They found that, compared with their sisters, older lesbians had greater risk factors for the major reproductive cancers (breast, ovarian, and endometrial) because they had higher rates of nulliparity, which resulted in less breastfeeding, as well as a trend toward obesity. On the other hand, the older lesbians had less risk for cervical cancer because obesity was the only risk factor for this form of cancer they were more likely to have than their sisters; the sisters were more likely to have used birth control pills and to have had more pregnancies, both of which are associated with a higher risk of cervical cancer. While the authors found no significant difference in rates of breast cancer between the groups, they note that this may have been due to the small sample.

Beyond case studies, little research exists on the risk for cancer among transgender elders, even though they may be at increased risk for breast, ovarian, uterine, or prostate cancer as a result of hormone therapy (Feldman and Goldberg, 2007; Van Kesteren et al., 1997).

Cardiovascular Disease

As mentioned in Chapter 5, lesbians may have higher rates of risk factors for cardiovascular disease—including smoking, drinking alcohol, and obesity—than heterosexual women. Roberts and colleagues (2003) surveyed 648 women, comparing various cardiovascular risk factors between 324 self-identified lesbians aged 40 and older residing in California and their self-identified heterosexual sisters closest in age. They found that lesbians, as a group and in comparison with their similarly aged heterosexual sisters, had significantly higher weights, body mass indexes, waist circumferences, and waist-to-hip ratios, which placed them at higher risk for cardiovascular disease.

In the sample from the Women's Health Initiative of women aged 50–79 described earlier, Valanis and colleagues (2000) found that the two lesbian groups had a slightly lower prevalence of stroke and hypertension than the other groups (bisexual, heterosexual, nonsexual), but had the highest rates of myocardial infarction. General health scores, however, were quite similar for the heterosexual, bisexual, and two lesbian groups. Eyler (2007) found that male-to-female transgender adults using estrogen had an increased risk for venous thromboembolism—a risk exacerbated by smoking, age, and inactive lifestyles.

There has been clinical concern about rates of diabetes, ovarian disease, and stroke among transgender elders (Feldman, 2007). An important health consideration for transgender elders is that Medicare generally does not cover transition-related care. This includes potentially long-term hormone treatments, the cessation of which may be both physically and emotionally traumatic. Among transgender individuals, there is some evidence of an association between poor hormonal therapies (e.g., outside of regular medical venues) and negative health outcomes in later life, including osteoporosis, cardiovascular disease, and poor oral health (Witten and Whittle, 2004). Williams and Freeman (2005) and Witten and Whittle (2004) suggest that many transgender elders may be at greater risk for health impairment than those who are younger because of the longer duration of hormone use, which may well exacerbate the effects of aging, such as cardiac or pulmonary problems. In addition, many transgender women start hormone therapy at older ages (middle age or later) and while having other aging-related health conditions, which may place them at risk for short- to medium-term adverse events (Feldman, 2007). Moreover, the options for lowering hormone doses or discontinuing hormone therapy are limited given the lack of access to sex reassignment surgery under Medicare and the health risks involved. Fredriksen-Goldsen and colleagues (2011) found that 45 percent of the older LGBT persons in their large study reported having high blood pressure; 43 percent reported high cholesterol and 6 percent reported having had a heart attack.

Obesity

A variety of studies, both qualitative and quantitative, have found that lesbians are more likely than heterosexual women to be overweight and obese, and research suggests this remains true into the later years (Clunis et al., 2005; Roberts et al., 2003; Valanis et al., 2000). This is an issue that has not been examined empirically for gay men and transgender persons in later life.

HIV/AIDS

HIV/AIDS remains a special and significant case for aging men and transgender women in particular. About 29 percent of people living with AIDS in the United States are currently aged 50 and over, but 70 percent of people with HIV in the United States are over age 40, suggesting that aging with the disease will be a significant health issue in years to come (CDC, 2007). The Centers for Disease Control and Prevention (CDC) estimates that the proportion of people living with HIV who are over age 50 is now more than double that of people under age 24, yet few (if any) HIV prevention programs target older adults, and it remains rare for physicians and other health care providers to talk with their older patients about HIV risk. While the percentage of gay and bisexual men included in these estimates is not clear, the percentage can be assumed to be large given that more than half of all new HIV infections in the United States occur among men who have sex with men (CDC, 2010).

Participants in an ethnographic study of older gay men (69 total participants representing a convenience sample, most aged 50–65) said they felt that HIV/AIDS has had a substantial effect on older gay men. Those who have been infected with the disease have had to face a disruption of their normal aging process, and those who have cared for others who have been infected have aged prematurely (Brown et al., 2001). One study of HIV/AIDS and aging (based on a sample of 914 HIV-positive persons aged 50 and older recruited from a network of New York City AIDS service organizations) found that more than half of the sample had depression, a proportion much larger than that in the general population (Karpiak et al., 2006). While sexual orientation was not used as a variable in that study, 33 percent of the sample identified as homosexual or bisexual. Although no published data address the risk and prevalence of HIV among transgender persons, a variety of community-based needs assessments suggest that they have a higher risk than (primarily white) gay men of comparable age.

There are similarities between the aging process and the course of HIV infection, with some evidence suggesting that HIV compresses the aging process, possibly accelerating the development of morbidities and frailty (see High et al., 2008). A funding opportunity announcement from the National Institutes of Health that calls for research on the medical management of older patients with HIV (Department of Health and Human Services, 2010) identifies nine areas of interest:

- age-related changes in immune function;
- age-related differences in response to treatment;
- age-related changes in pharmacokinetics, pharmacodynamics, and pharmacogenomics;
- metabolic complications of HIV/AIDS;
- neurologic complications of HIV/AIDS;
- neuropsychiatric complications of HIV/AIDS;
- HIV-related malignancies;
- frailty and functional status; and
- complexity of care.

Systematic research examining HIV among older transgender persons also is lacking in the literature, although several authors and reports have suggested a higher prevalence of HIV among transgender persons generally, in particular male-to-females (e.g., Kenagy and Hsieh, 2005).

Disability

The area of disability and aging among LGBT populations is rarely considered, empirically or theoretically; thus, there is little in this area on which to report. A few (mostly community) surveys on LGBT aging have asked about disability or chronic conditions. For example, almost 30 percent of a sample of 1,301 LGBT persons ranging in age from 18 to 92 reported some self-identified form of chronic illness or disability; these percentages increased to 36 percent of men and 38 percent of women aged 60 and older. This sample was drawn from community resources/organizations for a study conducted by a nonprofit LGBT senior housing agency. HIV/AIDS, discussed separately above, likely influences this reporting of illness and disability (Adelman et al., 2006). Cook-Daniels and Munson (2010), in their online survey of 272 transgender respondents described above, found that 36 percent had a physical or mental disability or challenge. In a recent report by Fredriksen-Goldsen and colleagues (2011), 47 percent of LGBT persons aged 50 and older reported a disability (significantly more women than men—53 and 43 percent, respectively).

In relative contrast, caregiving has been a productive area in gerontological research. A focus on older LGBT persons, however, is rare, although the study of AIDS caregiving, involving primarily younger gay men and lesbians, has been comparatively well represented. A qualitative study of caregiving conducted in Canada (Brotman et al., 2007) found that discrimination was salient in the lives of gay and lesbian elders and their caregivers. Similarly, in their study involving 36 chronically ill LGB adults aged 50 and over and their informal caregivers, Fredriksen-Goldsen and colleagues (2009) found that historical and current discrimination as experienced by chronically ill LGB adults and their caregivers appeared to manifest in higher levels of psychological distress, leading to cumulative mental and physical health problems, for both members of the caregiving dyad. No studies have specifically studied the issues transgender elders may face in terms of availability of appropriate caregivers. These issues are of particular concern as transgender individuals, even more so than LGB individuals (Bockting and Avery, 2005), face rejection from family and community members, who therefore may not be available or appropriate as caregivers (Witten, 2009; Witten and Eyler, 2007).

Transgender-Specific Physical Health Status

Witten and Eyler (2007) and others have commented on the paucity of research examining the physical health of transgender persons in later life. Witten notes, for example, that little is known about the risks associated with the use of "contragender" hormones and genital and other surgeries; similarly, little is known about age-related cancers (breast and prostate), heart disease (stroke, cardiovascular conditions), and cerebrovascular diseases among transgender people.

RISK AND PROTECTIVE FACTORS

In the MetLife (2010) survey, more than 1,200 LGBT participants were asked: "Some people have said that being LGBT has helped them prepare for aging. In what ways, if any, has being LGBT helped you prepare for aging?" Almost three-quarters of the sample felt that they were prepared for aging by their sexual-minority status, specifically the associated personal/interpersonal strengths and experience with overcoming adversity. Personal/interpersonal strengths cited included being more accepting of others, not taking anything for granted, being more resilient or having greater inner strength, having greater self-reliance, being more careful in legal and financial matters, and having a chosen family. Participants who had overcome adversity cited knowing how cruel society can be and being able to cope with discrimination.

When asked the opposite question—"In what ways, if any, has being LGBT made it more difficult for you to prepare for aging?"—about half responded affirmatively. They cited fewer opportunities to find a new relationship, fear of being doubly discriminated against as they age, feeling vulnerable with health care providers, and having fewer opportunities for social activities.

In an earlier review of almost 60 studies on gay men and aging, the authors found that happiness and successful adaptation to aging were commonly reported by older gay men, perhaps because of coping skills and competencies that are particularly well developed among aging homosexuals (Wahler and Gabbay, 1997).

Beyond these findings, the literature documents a number of risk and protective factors that influence the health of LGBT people throughout the life course. Stigma, discrimination, and victimization; violence; substance use; and childhood abuse have all been documented as risk factors for LGBT elders. Much less research has been conducted on protective factors, although crisis competence and social support have been identified. However, the dearth of literature in this area demonstrates the need for further research.

Risk Factors

Stigma, Discrimination, and Victimization

Discrimination plays a significant, recurring, and pervasive role in the lives of LGB persons, and perhaps in the lives of older LGB persons in particular, as suggested above.

In a recent study using data from the 2004–2005 National Epidemiologic Survey on Alcohol and Related Conditions, McLaughlin and colleagues (2010) examine associations between perceived discrimination and psychiatric disorders among individuals aged 20–90 (n = 34,653). LGB (n = 577) respondents were compared with black (n = 6,587), Latino (n = 6,359), and female (n = 20,089) respondents regarding self-reported experiences of past-year discrimination. Blacks reported the highest levels of discrimination (24.6 percent), followed by the LGB group (21.4 percent). Additionally, the authors found strong associations between self-reported discrimination and psychiatric disorders, although none of these associations were significant, likely because of the small LGB sample size. Unfortunately, the age of the respondents is not reported in this study, nor are subgroup analyses crossing racial and ethnic group membership with LGB status.

Fredriksen-Goldsen and colleagues (2011) found that older LGBT adults reported an average of four incidents of victimization and discrimination over the course of their lives due to their sexual orientation or gender identity; these experiences typically took the form of verbal insults (65 percent) and physical violence (40 percent). The rates were significantly higher for men than for women. For transgender adults aged 50 and older, the prevalence was even higher, with an average of about six incidents over the course of their lives.

Discrimination toward all sexual minorities has been alleged and described in a variety of reports. For example, analyses conducted by the Williams Institute at the University of California, Los Angeles (Goldberg, 2009), reveal that older lesbian couples have significantly lower income levels than comparably aged heterosexual couples, likely owing to employment discrimination over their lifetimes and the concomitant earnings disparities, reduced lifelong earnings, lower social security payments, and fewer opportunities to build pensions. Social security, for example, provides spousal, survival, and death benefits—none of which are available to same-sex couples, who are not recognized by federal law.

The challenges of discrimination exist within the older LGBT community as well. Some research has shown that older gay men feel ignored because of their age and believe that LGBT communities do not do enough to engage older people in social activities (Hostetler, 2004). Likewise, a nonacademic study (Bergling, 2004) examined the role of ageism in the gay male community, reporting high levels on the part of both younger and older gay men.

Discrimination and fear of discrimination are common and prominent themes in studies of LGBT aging. One study of 127 LGBT people aged 15–72 found that 33 percent of gay and lesbian respondents thought they would have to hide their sexual identity if they moved to a retirement home (Johnson et al., 2005). In focus group research conducted across Canada, Brotman and colleagues (2003) found that older gay men and lesbians (n = 21) often spoke of mistrust of the health and social service networks as a result of lifelong experiences of marginalization and oppression. Such experiences continued to the present day, with many instances of overt homophobia and ageism and covert experiences of neglect and invisibility being reported—both within the LGBT community and more broadly.

As previously noted, few studies have explicitly examined racial and ethnic groups in their samples. One exception is David and Knight (2008), who found in a study of 383 white and black gay men from across the adult life course that the older black gay men experienced significantly higher levels of ageism than the older white gay men and higher levels of perceived racism than the younger black gay men. The authors suggest that the differences in perceived racism may be a cohort difference, reflecting the views of society when the older men were coming of age. It is notable that these older black gay men did not experience higher levels of negative mental health outcomes.

The combined stigma of being elderly and transgender can serve as a strong traumatizing force, potentially exacerbating both forms of discrimination and stigma (Witten and Eyler, 2007). Studies of the particular experiences of stigma in this population appear to focus on the health care system and are reported later in the chapter.

Violence

Another area that is substantially underresearched is LGBT elders' experiences of violence. In a previously mentioned study involving LGB adults, D'Augelli and Grossman (2001) asked participants (n = 416, aged 60–91) about their lifetime experiences with violence based on their sexual orientation. They found that 63 percent reported verbal abuse, 29 percent had been threatened with violence, 16 percent had experienced assault, 12 percent had experienced assault with a weapon, and 11 percent had had an object thrown at them.

Systematic examination of the violence experienced by transgender elders has been inadequate, although several authors have commented that rates of violence and crime in this population are sufficiently acute to warrant consideration as a primary health priority for the transgender community (Xavier et al., 2007). A small, online survey of 30 transgender adults aged 50–70 revealed that 64.8 percent had experienced emotional or psychological abuse more than once in their lives (Cook-Daniels and Munson, 2010).

Substance Use

Tobacco and alcohol use appear to be greater among older LGB populations than among older heterosexuals (Gruskin et al., 2007; Tang et al.,

2004); the Virginia study of transgender adults, including a small proportion of older adults, reports similar findings (Xavier et al., 2007). No particular data on older transgender adults are available.

Using the Alcohol Use Disorders Identification Test, developed by the World Health Organization, with a previously mentioned sample of 416 LGB elders aged 60–91, Grossman and colleagues (2001) found that gay men had significantly higher levels of alcohol use and problem drinking than lesbians. Valanis and colleagues (2000) found that adult and lifetime lesbians, as well as bisexual women, in their sample had the lowest rates of never smoking and were more likely to be current smokers. They were also the most likely to use alcohol and to use more of it compared with the heterosexual and never sexual groups.

Using data from the Chicago Health and Life Experiences of Women Study, structured interviews were conducted with 447 adult women (aged 18–83) who self-identified as lesbians (48 percent non-Hispanic white, 28 percent non-Hispanic black, and 20 percent Latina). The researchers compared the prevalence of lifetime and 12-month drinking indicators across racial/ethnic groups and across four age groups (including those aged 51 and older, n = 74). Forty-five percent of women in the oldest group reported that they were light drinkers, while 19 percent reported being moderate drinkers and 8 percent being heavy drinkers. While findings from general population surveys have shown that women's rates of drinking tend to decrease with age, there were few differences across the age groups in this study (Hughes et al., 2006).

Childhood Abuse

In the research of Balsam and colleagues (2005), in which age was treated as a continuous variable, LGB participants were more likely than their heterosexual counterparts to report experiences of childhood sexual abuse; moreover, sexual-minority status significantly predicted all variables of childhood abuse. LGB participants reported higher levels of overall lifetime victimization than their heterosexual counterparts.

In D'Augelli and Grossman's (2001) research with 416 LGB adults aged 60 or older, the earlier a person was aware of her or his sexual orientation and first disclosed it to others, the more likely he or she was to report incidences of physical assault. Those who had been physically attacked spent more of their lives aware of their sexual orientation. These findings suggest that abuse and victimization may occur at an early age for LGB people. More than one-half (58 percent) of the convenience, online sample of transgender persons over age 50 mentioned earlier reported instances of sexual abuse (defined as "unwanted sexual touch") prior to age 19 (Cook-Daniels and Munson, 2010). In a life span sample of transgender persons,

Kenagy (2005) found a comparable percentage (53.8 percent) reporting that they had been forced to have sex; she also found that more than half of the 80 respondents to a question on physical violence reported a physical assault at some point in the course of their lives, with male-to-females being significantly more likely to have experienced abuse than female-to-males.

Protective Factors

In the MetLife (2006) survey, 38 percent of the 1,000 LGBT participants reported positive consequences in their lives as a result of being a sexual or gender minority. Positive aspects included strong character traits, resilience, and better support networks. Differences by race and ethnicity are worth noting, with Latino (51 percent) and black (43 percent) respondents being considerably more likely than the sample as a whole to report that their LGBT identity was beneficial as they aged (MetLife, 2006).

As noted earlier, a recent follow-up to this survey found that almost three-quarters of another national LGBT sample (n = 1,206) felt that "being LGBT has helped them prepare for aging." Among those who saw benefits, two broad categories of benefit were identified: personal/interpersonal strengths, including being more accepting of others, being more resilient, and having greater self-reliance, and overcoming adversity. Still, more than a quarter of respondents said their sexual orientation and/or gender identity had not helped them prepare for aging (MetLife, 2010).

Several authors have referred to such findings and interpretations as "crisis competence." Kimmel (1978) proposed that dealing with the crises of "family disruption, intensive feelings and sometimes alienation from family . . . will provide a perspective on major life crises . . . that buffers the person against later crises." Crisis competence embodies the development or enhancement of life skills as a result of having to deal with being a sexual minority and all that entails in a heterosexual society, perhaps placing older sexual minorities at an advantage, relative to heterosexuals, in confronting the issues and crises of aging. For example, recent findings from a community sample of 396 self-identified gay, lesbian, and bisexual people aged 18–59 found that those aged 40 and over scored in the upper tertile on more dimensions of social well-being compared with those younger than 40; older participants also scored higher than younger participants on coherence, acceptance, and contribution (Kertzner et al., 2009). It should be noted that these data are within-LGB comparisons and cannot be used to address whether these age-related gains in social well-being surpass those experienced by heterosexual older adults.

Social support has been identified as a potential protective factor in the lives of LGBT elders. Grossman and colleagues (2000) comment, for example, that the positive contributions of friends to individual well-being should be even stronger in the lives of older gay men and lesbians given that friends and the support they provide "can serve a unique function in mitigating the impact of stigmatization" (p. 171). Results of the qualitative study of de Vries and Hoctel (2006) with a sample of gay men and lesbians aged 55–81 support this proposition.

Certain socioeconomic factors may also be seen as protective. In a variety of studies and in at least one review of smaller community-based surveys (de Vries, 2006), education levels of LGBT older persons exceeded those of comparably aged heterosexual persons (the latter as reported in census data, given that heterosexual comparison groups are rare in LGBT research). This advantage has been noted elsewhere: Black and colleagues (2000) report similar findings in their analysis of data generated by the U.S. census. If education can be regarded as a proxy for problem solving, solution seeking, and action taking, as Lopata (1993) has suggested, such data provide some cause for optimism. As discussed in Chapter 2, however, the effect of education may not be the same across racial and ethnic groups; some groups may be less likely to disclose sexual orientation with increasing education (Kennamer et al., 2000).

Although research has not explicitly addressed the protective factors associated with transgender aging, Witten (2002) has proposed that, notwithstanding the increased medical risks that may accompany gender transition for older persons, certain physical exigencies of aging may facilitate social gender transition. Some theorists describe this as the normal unisex of later life (e.g., Gutmann, 1985), in which women and men are more physically similar than previously in the life course. Witten (2002) notes that these similarities include a loss of facial skin tone for men and reduced estrogens for women. The loss of muscle mass and increased body fat similarly render males and females more similar in later life. These changes may be seen as advantages for older transgender people, particularly those who begin the transition process in later life.

HEALTH SERVICES

Older adults tend to be the most frequent users of health care services in the United States. This is the case among LGBT populations as well; however, their use of health services may be complicated by trepidation and fear of discrimination.

Access and Utilization

As with early/middle adulthood (Chapter 5), limited attention has been paid to access to and utilization of health care among older LGBT persons. Data from the California Health Interview Study, one of the very few state-level health surveys to include information on LGBT persons, reveal that LGBT adults of all ages are much more likely than heterosexual adults to delay or not seek medical care; among respondents, 30 percent of transgender adults, 29 percent of LGB adults, and 17 percent of heterosexual adults delayed/did not seek care (Movement Advancement Project and Services and Advocacy for Gay, Lesbian, Bisexual and Transgender Elders, 2010). For older adults in particular, these findings are often attributed to a reluctance to disclose their sexual orientation or gender identity in health care settings for fear of discrimination and provider bias.

Age is infrequently considered as a variable in research on health care access or health insurance. A survey by the Transgender Law Center (Hartzell et al., 2009) of 646 transgender adults living in California, including 80 respondents over age 55, found that even when covered by insurance, 42 percent of respondents had delayed seeking care because they could not afford it, and 26 percent reported health conditions that had worsened because they postponed care. Some evidence from earlier studies suggests that older lesbians and bisexual women obtain fewer cervical cancer screenings (Price et al., 1996), and that many older gay men and older lesbians seek health care services less frequently than their heterosexual peers (Harrison and Silenzio, 1996).

In narrative comments collected in the previously described brief online survey by Cook-Daniels and Munson (2010), fear and shame emerged as reasons for not accessing available services. Kammerer and colleagues (1999), in their interview and focus group research with mainly midlife transgender persons, cite lack of insurance and lack of acceptance/fear of rejection as the primary reasons for either delaying or not seeking services. They report disparaging and transphobic comments from staff at homeless shelters (as well as from others seeking such services), as well as a general lack of services tailored to the particular needs of transgender persons.

In the life-course sample described by Kenagy (2005), more than one-quarter (26 percent) of the sample reported being denied medical services because they were transgender. Similar results are reported by Xavier and colleagues (2007) in their description of a life span sample of transgender persons in Virginia.

Quality of Care

While little research exists on the quality of care currently received by LGBT elders, a national survey found that fewer than half of LGBT people in midlife believe they will receive respectful care in old age (MetLife, 2006).

Using focus group data, researchers have explored the anticipated (Orel, 2006a) and actual (Brotman et al., 2003) discriminatory experiences older LGB adults have had within health care settings. In both cases, the authors suggest that discrimination (anticipated or actual) is associated with a decreased likelihood of seeking health care services (relative to comparably aged heterosexual women and men, as noted above). Observations from a variety of community groups and community-based needs surveys suggest that LGBT elders delay seeking health care for fear of discrimination and provider bias. The survey conducted by the Transgender Law Center, mentioned previously, found that 30 percent of respondents had delayed seeking treatment or preventive care because of disrespect or discrimination from providers (Hartzell et al., 2009). Witten (2002) notes that the apparent mismatch between genital anatomy and gender of presentation can result in disclosure; confusion; and perhaps difficulty in obtaining appropriate, sensitive health services at all levels, including long-term care.

Long-term care issues are particularly salient for older persons and especially so for LGBT elders, who are disproportionately without partners and children, the primary caregivers for older adults. Shanas (1980) describes the principle of substitution or, as Qureshi and Walker (1989) term it, the "hierarchy of normative obligation priorities," referring to the order in which individuals are called upon (and/or present themselves) to be providers of support or informal caregivers. The typical order is spouses first; followed closely thereafter by children (typically daughters and daughters-in-law); then by other, more distant relatives; and finally by friends. This order reflects traditional family patterns, rendering it significantly less applicable to the lives of aging LGBT individuals (Barker et al., 2006).

Although long-term care is often mentioned in the literature on LGBT aging, there are few empirical studies to reference. Fairchild and colleagues (1996) examined nursing home social workers' (n = 29) perceptions of staff attitudes toward residents' sexuality (inclusive of LGBT identification) in the facility in which they worked. Social workers characterized staff attitudes toward gay and lesbian residents as negative and reported that one nursing home avoided "the problem of homosexuality and lesbianism all together: 'We don't allow partners of the same sex into the home. . . . It's part of the admission requirements'" (p. 166). Some advocates who work with elderly LGBT residents caution that they may encounter considerable challenges, including hostile staff members and fellow patients; denial of visits from families of choice or from friends the staff does not approve of; refusal to allow same-sex partners to room together; and refusal to involve families of choice in medical decision making, even when legal directives are in place.

Some literature provides a glimpse of the issues surrounding the delivery of care for LGBT people. A report prepared by the Office of the New York City Public Advocate (2008) claims that the health care environment in New York City is both heterocentric (oriented toward heterosexual practices and roles) and gender-normative (oriented toward society's expectations of gender). Providers lack knowledge about health disparities affecting LGBT persons of all ages, and LGBT individuals experience hostility and discrimination in care. Medical forms often do not reflect patient diversity (e.g., gender identity, relationship status) or the breadth of patients' care networks. The report notes that LGBT persons often assume they are not welcome in an institution, and accordingly avoid or delay seeking care. The report recommends mandatory LGBT diversity training and the establishment of a zero tolerance discrimination policy.

A community needs assessment (Orel, 2006a) found that slightly more than half of LGB elders were dissatisfied with federal, state, and local services for older adults. They reported that these services failed to meet their unique needs. The same study found that LGB elders who had disclosed their sexual orientation to their physician believed they had a more open and trusting relationship as a result of the disclosure. Finally, small, mainly qualitative studies with transgender convenience samples that included elders have found that treatment facilities often are not prepared to accommodate transgender patients because of a lack of provider competence and strong segregation by gender (Clements et al., 1999; Kammerer et al., 1999; Nemoto et al., 2005).

CONTEXTUAL INFLUENCES

In addition to sociodemographic and familial factors, which influence the health of LGBT people across the life course, LGBT elders face a number of end-of-life issues.

Sociodemographic Factors

There is a paucity of research documenting the influences of race, ethnicity, geography, and socioeconomic status on older LGBT individuals.

Some studies do describe the racial categories that make up their samples. However, the results of these studies are rarely analyzed by racial or ethnic group because of insufficient data.

Similarly, geography has rarely been explicitly considered. Small qualitative studies have suggested some of the unique situational and support issues experienced by rural LGB elders (Comerford et al., 2004). King and Dabelko-Schoeny (2009) explored health care service utilization and support networks among 20 midlife and older LGB participants who lived in rural communities (all of whom were at least 40 years of age). Respondents described transportation difficulties, the lack of choices for care, problems with affordability of care, and the lack of connection and sense of belonging to a community. The authors conclude that the unique issues faced by LGB adults, such as isolation and the lack of informal support, make obstacles to aging in place difficult to overcome for LGB adults living in rural communities.

As noted earlier, differences in education between LGBT and heterosexual people have been observed in both small- and large-scale studies, particularly favoring lesbian and gay adults, including older adults. Recent analyses of the Massachusetts Behavioral Risk Factor Surveillance System surveys (Conron et al., 2010), inclusive of adults aged 18–64 and with no analysis by age, found that lesbian and gay adults were more likely than heterosexual and bisexual adults to have at least a 4-year college degree. Reported levels of education among samples of transgender persons vary, with some studies reporting comparable levels (e.g., Witten and Eyler, 1999) and some lower overall levels (e.g., Kenagy, 2005). Authors often note that the mechanisms by which samples are recruited have an impact on such results.

In contrast with differentials in education, studies have found that income levels among LGBT populations tend to be lower than those among the general population (the latter being based on U.S. census means [e.g., Adelman et al., 2006] or samples of the general population [e.g., MetLife, 2010]). Some researchers (e.g., de Vries, 2006) have commented on the apparent and surprising lack of association between education and income, suggesting that LGB persons may "settle" for lesser employment possibilities than those for which they might be qualified in order to remain in or seek out an LGBT-friendly workplace and/or community.

Familial Factors

As noted above with reference to caregiving, families, formally defined, play a significant role in the social support of elders; however, the presence of and access to biological and other legal kin is limited in the lives of LGBT elders. For example, a variety of studies have noted that LGBT elders, especially gay men, are much less likely than their heterosexual counterparts to have partners, both legally recognized and informally. As reported in the MetLife (2010) survey, 58 percent of LGBT participants had partners, compared with 72 percent of the general population. Grossman and colleagues (2000) found that just over half of the LGB older adults in their survey (n = 416) were not partnered.

Regional surveys of LGBT elders have found even more dramatic differences in partnering between older LGBT and heterosexual adults. In San Francisco, for example, more than 70 percent of gay and bisexual men and almost 50 percent of lesbian and bisexual women over age 65 reported not having a partner (Adelman et al., 2006). It is worth noting that partnered LGBT elders may have varying living arrangements. In the previously mentioned survey of older adults by Grossman and colleagues

(2000), for example, 62 percent of those with partners reported living with those partners.

Adult children are common sources of support and care for heterosexual older persons, as noted above; in contrast, LGBT elders are less likely to have children. In the MetLife (2006) survey, about 20 percent of LGBT participants reported being parents (MetLife, 2006). The San Francisco survey referenced above found that 72 percent of gay men and 43 percent of lesbians over age 65 reported having no children (Adelman et al., 2006). A national LGBT aging needs assessment conducted by the group Services and Advocacy for Gay, Lesbian, Bisexual, and Transgender Elders (SAGE) in 2003 found that LGBT elders were four times less likely to have children and grandchildren than non-LGBT older adults. Less likelihood of access to a partner and to children for later-life care significantly distinguishes the experiences of LGBT and heterosexual elders.

The potential and understudied role of sibling ties is highlighted in the MetLife (2010) report, wherein siblings figure significantly in support exchanges and in discussions about end of life.

Orel (2006b) presents findings from a qualitative study of 16 Midwestern U.S. self-identified lesbian (n = 12) and bisexual (n = 4) grandmothers recruited by local networks using snowball techniques. The study featured open-ended recorded, transcribed interviews lasting up to 120 minutes discussing the centrality of sexual orientation in the grandparent–grandchild relationship, including the role of grandparenthood for LB women, the formation of LB identity as a grandparent, the role of homonegativity, and the mediating role of the parents in the grandparent–grandchild relationship.

In a similarly qualitative manner, Fruhauf and colleagues (2009) explored the experiences of 11 gay grandfathers in western and Midwestern states. These interviews focused on coming out to grandchildren, the nature of the tie to the grandchild, and the role of adult children in the coming out process of the grandfather, along with associated fears of rejection. These examples stand at the forefront of a rich but as yet largely unexplored field of inquiry.

Among LGBT elders, social support networks have been shown to be associated with physical health (Grossman, 2006; Masini and Barrett, 2008). One source of support for LGBT individuals, including LGBT elders, is families of choice. Beeler and colleagues (1999) found that 89 percent of the older gay male and lesbian adults in their sample (n = 160, ages 45–90) had at least three friends they could turn to if they were experiencing a "serious problem." Nearly two-thirds (64 percent) of the 1,200 LGBT participants (aged 45–64) in the national MetLife (2010) survey agreed they had a "chosen family," defined by the survey as "a group of people to whom you are emotionally close and consider 'family' even though you are not biologically or legally related."

Given that these families of choice are often made up of friends, it is not surprising that friendship has a particularly complex and broad-based meaning for LGBT older persons. This observation is reflected in the thematic content analyses of the 53 gay men and lesbians interviewed by de Vries and Megathlin (2009) as compared with those of 106 heterosexual women and men, all aged 50–88 and recruited primarily through snowball techniques in the San Francisco Bay Area. In the MetLife (2010) study, older LGBT individuals were more likely than the heterosexual comparison group to report receiving emotional support from friends, living with friends, discussing end-of-life preferences with friends, and depending on friends as caregivers.

When de Vries and Hoctel (2006) conducted in-depth individual interviews on the meaning and experience of friendship in the San Francisco Bay Area, the majority of respondents reported feeling that friendships are more important to gay men and lesbians because their friends, for various reasons, become their family. For example, one man said, "I think for gay people—many of whom are disowned by their families because of their sexual orientation—their friendships are stronger" (p. 227). A woman noted, "So many of us have lost our original families—particularly older people, because of our sexuality. We need each other in a way that heterosexuals don't. We've led a life of nobody being there" (p. 227).

In the MetLife (2010) survey, LGBT participants (n = 1,201) aged 45–64 were slightly more likely than non-LGBT persons to have provided care to an adult friend or relative in the past 6 months (21 percent versus 17 percent). In the same survey, men were just as likely to be caregivers as women. Male caregivers actually reported more time spent as caregivers than their female counterparts.

Caregiving is an area in which large numbers of midlife and older gay men and lesbians have had significant experience: particularly in the early years of the AIDS epidemic, the provision of care for someone dying of AIDS was often the responsibility of members of the LGBT community (e.g., Mullan, 1998). Martin and Dean (1993) note that two important aspects of the epidemiology of AIDS-related bereavement are the experience of multiple losses and the occurrence of chronic bereavement. They found that almost 30 percent of their sample of bereaved gay men (n = 200) had experienced two or more deaths (of lovers, former lovers, or close friends) within a 12-month period (in 1987), and nearly half of the sample had experienced three or more deaths (not including deaths of social network members, acquaintances, or friends of friends). Such experiences may well both serve as a model for support in the later years and place some elder gay men (and perhaps LGBT persons in general) at risk for having outlived their networks of support.

Another aspect of social support is group membership. In the research of Grossman and colleagues (2000), LGB persons aged 60 and older belonged to many LGB organizations: about one-quarter (26 percent) belonged to one organization, 26 percent to two, 19 percent to three, and 20 percent to four or more. When asked about the number of LGB organizations whose events they regularly attended, 12 percent of respondents said none, 38 percent said one, 29 percent said two, 13 percent said three, and 8 percent said four or more.

Older LGBT adults participating in focus groups reported unanimously that their membership in the LGBT community was important, especially in helping them be comfortable with their sexual orientation (Shippy et al., 2004). Results of the MetLife (2010) survey were similar, with one exception: although 47 percent of lesbians, 44 percent of gay men, and 39 percent of transgender individuals said their LGBT identity was important to them, only about 25 percent of bisexuals said being LGBT was important in how they think about themselves.

Although the committee could find no published research describing the family relationships of transgender persons, Witten (2002) notes that family relationships (encompassing the full breadth of relationship types, including spousal, parenthood, grandparenthood, sibling, and other ties) may be reevaluated during and following an older person's "coming out" with a transgender and perhaps different gender identity. This observation raises the issue of relational quality and its effect on the well-being of older LGBT adults: What is the utility of relational ties in addressing the health-related needs of LGBT elders? The answer to this question is unknown, and this is a central issue meriting future research.

End-of-Life Issues

A host of older studies have drawn attention to the losses of loved ones to AIDS as endured by LBT and especially gay men during the 1980s and early 1990s and the enduring legacy of such trauma. Martin and Dean (1993) compare these AIDS-related loss experiences with "previously studied stressors, such as the experiences of concentration camp survivors and soldiers in combat" (p. 323). Schwartzberg (1992) notes the breadth and depth of experienced grief, writing that "survivors [grieve] not only for their most personal losses, but also for all the victims, for strangers, and for the loss of community and culture" (p. 424). This remains a context within which to consider the experiences of midlife and older LGBT persons and their approaches to their later and final years (de Vries, 2008). In a qualitative and observational report, Shernoff (1998) notes that gay widowers shared many of the same attributes and experiences as other widowers; he also cites unique characteristics, most of which he attributes to the lack of recognition of male couples in general and of the status of a gay man as widower in particular.

The MetLife (2006) study also inquired about end-of-life issues. Just over half of the study's 1,000 LGBT participants aged 40–61 had not yet prepared living wills or advance health care directives, documents spelling out the health care decisions they would want made for them should they become incapacitated. Only about two in five (43 percent) had assigned someone else decision-making authority through a legal document such as a durable power of attorney for health care or a health care proxy. For LGBT individuals, these legal and financial preparations for the end of life may be even more important than for heterosexual people, given the absence of legally recognized relationships and the greater reliance on "chosen families" who often are not recognized by health care institutions. Drawing on the MetLife (2006) data set, de Vries and colleagues (2009) found that older lesbian and gay adults (of any relationship status) residing in states in which same-sex relationships are not recognized were more likely to have prepared a will, living will, and durable power of attorney than participants residing in states in which such relationships are recognized. Similarly, those living in states with no recognition of same-sex relationships also expressed greater fear of dying in pain and being the object of discrimination because of their sexual orientation than those residing in states where same-sex relationships are recognized. State recognition was the only significant predictor of fear of dying alone in these analyses.

Riggle and colleagues (2005) studied the execution of five legal documents, including a will, living will, and durable power of attorney, as well as power of attorney for finances and hospital visitation authorization, among almost 400 LGBT adults. The sample included participants up to age 73, although the data were not analyzed with respect to age ranges. The authors found that, compared with single LGBT individuals, a higher percentage of LGBT couples had completed such documents. They interpreted these differences as reflecting an effort to formalize commitment in the couples' relationships and as associated evidence of their heightened awareness of legal status, rights or the absence thereof, and options.

SUMMARY OF KEY FINDINGS AND RESEARCH OPPORTUNITIES

Findings

Issues related to LGBT aging have not been well studied. From the limited research available, however, some key findings pertinent to this cohort can be drawn, which are presented below.

Mental Health Status

- Depression levels and suicidality appear to be elevated among older lesbians and gay men. Less research has been conducted in this area among bisexual and transgender elders.

Physical Health Status

- It appears that rates of hysterectomy, oral contraceptive use, and hormone replacement therapy may be similar for lesbians, bisexual women, and heterosexual women.
- Lesbians and bisexual women may have higher rates of breast cancer than heterosexual women.
- Data on whether lesbians have a higher risk for cardiovascular disease are conflicting.
- Limited research suggests that transgender elders may experience negative health outcomes as a result of long-term hormone use.
- HIV/AIDS impacts not only younger but also older LGBT individuals. However, few HIV prevention programs target older adults, a cohort that also has been deeply affected by the losses inflicted by AIDS.
- Disability among LGBT elders is a topic rarely considered in research.

Risk and Protective Factors

- LGBT elders experience stigma, discrimination, and victimization across the life course.
- Little research examines violence experienced by LGBT elders, but some studies suggest that LGBT elders report high rates of lifetime experiences with violence.
- Some research suggests that, compared with their heterosexual counterparts, LGB elders may have higher rates of tobacco and alcohol use. Research on tobacco and alcohol use among transgender elders is largely lacking.
- There is some evidence of crisis competence (resilience and perceived hardiness) within older LGBT populations; however, this concept is not yet well understood and has not been thoroughly researched.
- Very limited data suggest that education may play a protective role in the lives of some older LGBT people.

Health Services

- Limited research suggests that LGBT elders may be less likely to seek health services than the general population.

- Some research suggests that older LGBT individuals do not believe they will receive respectful care in old age and may delay seeking care for fear of discrimination.
- Long-term care for LGBT elders has not been the subject of many empirical studies.

Contextual Influences

- Research on the influence of sociodemographic characteristics on the health of LGBT elders is very limited.
- The role of families in the lives of older LGBT people has been underresearched. Lesbian and gay elders are less likely than their heterosexual peers to have children, and their other kinship ties are not well understood. Families of choice appear to be a source of support for LGBT people in later life.

Research Opportunities

While the above findings provide some information on the health status of LGBT elders, there is a dearth of data on a number of topics in this area. Even among the studies that exist, lesbians, gay men, bisexual men and women, and transgender people are not equitably represented. Very little is known about transgender and bisexual aging in particular. Similarly, more research has focused on the first part of later life, while almost no published research exists on LGBT populations aged 85 and above. In studies whose participants represent a wide range of ages, age is rarely considered as a factor. Thus, while the potential exists to better understand this cohort, researchers often miss this opportunity by failing to include age as a variable. Both cross-sectional and longitudinal research is especially needed to explore the demographic realities of LGBT aging in an intersectional and social ecology framework, to allow an understanding of the mechanisms of both risk and resilience in LGBT elders, and to identify appropriate interventions for working effectively with this cohort. These parameters could be brought to bear in research in the following areas:

- **Demographic and descriptive information,** including the percentage of elders who are LGBT and how that percentage varies by such demographic characteristics as race, ethnicity, socioeconomic status, geography, and religion; also, the general experiences and health status of older LGBT adults and how these vary by demographic characteristics, the percentage of LGBT elders who are parents, and the trajectory of LGBT identity and experiences (particular bisexual identity) over the life course.

- **Family and interpersonal relations**, including the experience of LGBT aging and family life (e.g., experiences with biological kin across generations, "chosen family" ties and relations), the effect of the greater likelihood of childlessness (particularly among older gay men), and experiences of grief and loss (including multiple losses); also intrafamily and domestic violence (e.g., caregiver/provider abuse, intimate partner violence) and anti-LGBT victimization.
- **Health services**, including barriers to access (particularly related to identity disclosure and interactions with providers), utilization rates, long-term care issues for older LGBT persons, quality of care received, and end-of-life issues (e.g., preparations, fears, and plans).
- **Mental health**, including depression and suicidality (about which little has been written), the effects of stigma and discrimination (over the course of a lifetime), and the experience of and preparations for late life among older LGBT persons.
- **Physical health**, including cancer rates, risks, and treatment (particularly for prostate cancer among older gay and bisexual men and transgender women and anal cancer among older men who have sex with men); the effects of long-term hormone use among older transgender persons; and the effects of disabilities among older LGBT persons.
- **Sexual and reproductive health**, including HIV rates and interventions (and the experience of aging with HIV) and sexual well-being and sexual dysfunction (particularly among older lesbians and transgender elders, about whom little is known).

REFERENCES

Adelman, M. 1990. Stigma, gay lifestyles, and adjustment to aging: A study of later-life gay men and lesbians. *Journal of Homosexuality* 20(3/4):7–32.

Adelman, M., L. Gurevich, B. de Vries, and J. Blando. 2006. Openhouse: Community building and research in the LGBT aging population. In *Lesbian, gay, bisexual, and transgender aging: Research and clinical perspectives*, edited by D. Kimmel, T. Rose, and S. David. New York: Columbia University Press.

Altekruse, S. F., C. L. Kosary, M. Krapcho, N. Neyman, R. Aminou, W. Waldron, J. Ruhl, N. Howlader, Z. Tatalovich, H. Cho, A. Mariotto, M. P. Eisner, D. R. Lewis, K. Cronin, H. S. Chen, E. J. Feuer, D. G. Stinchcomb, and B. K. Edwards. 2010. *SEER Cancer Statistics Review, 1975–2007*. Bethesda, MD: National Cancer Institute.

Asencio, M., T. Blank, L. Descartes, and A. Crawford. 2009. The prospect of prostate cancer: A challenge for gay men's sexualities as they age. *Sexuality Research & Social Policy: A Journal of the NSRC* 6(4):38–51.

Balsam, K. F., E. D. Rothblum, and T. P. Beauchaine. 2005. Victimization over the life span: A comparison of lesbian, gay, bisexual, and heterosexual siblings. *Journal of Consulting & Clinical Psychology* 73(3):477–487.

Baltes, P. B., U. M. Staudinger, and U. Lindenberger. 1999. Lifespan psychology: Theory and application to intellectual functioning. *Annual Review of Psychology* 50:471–507.

Barker, J. C. 2002. Neighbors, friends, and other nonkin caregivers of community-living dependent elders. *The Journals of Gerontology Series B: Psychological Sciences and Social Sciences* 57(3):S158–S167.

Barker, J. C., G. Herdt, and B. de Vries. 2006. Social support in the lives of lesbians and gay men at midlife and later. *Sexuality Research & Social Policy: A Journal of the NSRC* 3(2):1–23.

Bayer, R. 1987. *Homosexuality and American psychiatry: The politics of diagnosis* (revised ed.). Princeton, NJ: Princeton University Press.

Beeler, J. A., T. W. Rawls, G. Herdt, and B. J. Cohler. 1999. The needs of older lesbians and gay men in Chicago. *Journal of Gay & Lesbian Social Services* 9(1):31–49.

Bergling, T. 2004. *Reeling in the years: Gay men's perspectives on age and ageism*. New York: Harrington Park Press.

Black, D., G. Gates, S. Sanders, and L. Taylor. 2000. Demographics of the gay and lesbian population in the United States: Evidence from available systematic data sources. *Demography* 37(2):139–154.

Blanchard, R. 1989. The concept of autogynephilia and the typology of male gender dysphoria. *Journal of Nervous and Mental Disease* 177(10):616–623.

Blank, T. O. 2008. The challenge of prostate cancer: 'Half a man or a man and a half.' *Generations* 32(1):68–72.

Blank, T. O., M. Asencio, L. Descartes, and J. Griggs. 2009. Aging, health, and GLBTQ family and community life. *Journal of GLBT Family Studies* 5(1–2):9–34.

Bockting, W., and E. Avery, eds. 2005. *Transgender health and HIV prevention: Needs assessment studies from transgender communities across the United States*. New York: Haworth Medical Press.

Bockting, W. O., and E. Coleman. 2007. Developmental stages of the transgender coming out process: Toward an integrated identity. In *Handbook of transgender medicine and surgery*, edited by R. Ettner, S. Monstrey, and E. Evan. New York: Haworth Press.

Bradford, J., C. Ryan, and E. D. Rothblum. 1993. National lesbian health care survey: Implications for mental health care. *Journal of Consulting and Clinical Psychology* 62(2): 228–242.

Brotman, S., B. Ryan, and R. Cormier. 2003. The health and social service needs of gay and lesbian elders and their families in Canada. *Gerontologist* 43(2):192–202.

Brotman, S., B. Ryan, S. Collins, L. Chamberland, R. Cormier, D. Julien, E. Meyer, A. Peterkin, and B. Richard. 2007. Coming out to care: Caregivers of gay and lesbian seniors in Canada. *Gerontologist* 47(4):490–503.

Brown, L. B., G. R. Alley, S. Sarosy, G. Quarto, and T. Cook. 2001. Gay men: Aging well! *Journal of Gay & Lesbian Social Services: Issues in Practice, Policy & Research* 13(4):41–54.

Buhrich, N., and N. McConaghy. 1978. Two clinically discrete forms of transsexualism. *The British Journal of Psychiatry* 133:73–76.

Catania, J. A., D. Osmond, R. D. Stall, L. Pollack, J. P. Paul, S. Blower, D. Binson, J. A. Canchola, T. C. Mills, L. Fisher, K. H. Choi, T. Porco, C. Turner, J. Blair, J. Henne, L. L. Bye, and T. J. Coates. 2001. The continuing HIV epidemic among men who have sex with men. *American Journal of Public Health* 91(6):907–914.

CDC (Centers for Disease Control and Prevention). 2007. *Cases of HIV infection and AIDS in the United States and dependent areas, 2005*. Atlanta, GA: CDC.

CDC. 2010. *HIV and AIDS among gay and bisexual men*. Atlanta, GA: CDC.

Chin-Hong, P. V., E. Vittinghoff, R. D. Cranston, S. Buchbinder, D. Cohen, G. Colfax, M. Da Costa, T. Darragh, E. Hess, F. Judson, B. Koblin, M. Madison, and J. M. Palefsky. 2004. Age-specific prevalence of anal human papillomavirus infection in HIV-negative sexually active men who have sex with men: The EXPLORE study. *Journal of Infectious Diseases* 190(12):2070–2076.

Clements, K., K. Kitano, W. Wilkinson, and R. Marx. 1999. HIV prevention and health service needs of the transgender community in San Francisco. *International Journal of Transgenderism* 3(1/2):1.

Clements-Nolle, K., R. Marx, R. Guzman, and M. Katz. 2001. HIV prevalence, risk behaviors, health care use, and mental health status of transgender persons: Implications for public health intervention. *American Journal of Public Health* 91(6):915–921.

Clunis, D. M., K. Fredriksen-Goldsen, P. Freeman, and N. Nystrom. 2005. *Lives of lesbian elders*. New York: Haworth Press.

Cochran, S. D., and V. M. Mays. 2006. Estimating prevalence of mental and substance-using disorders among lesbians and gay men from existing national health data. In *Sexual orientation and mental health*, edited by A. M. Omoto and H. S. Kurtzman. Washington, DC: American Psychological Association. Pp. 143–165.

Comerford, S. A., M. M. Henson-Stroud, C. Sionainn, and E. Wheeler. 2004. Crone songs: Voices of lesbian elders on aging in a rural environment. *Affilia-Journal of Women and Social Work* 19(4):418–436.

Conron, K. J., M. J. Mimiaga, and S. J. Landers. 2010. A population-based study of sexual orientation identity and gender differences in adult health. *American Journal of Public Health* 100(10):1953–1960.

Cook-Daniels, L., and M. Munson. 2010. Sexual violence, elder abuse, and sexuality of transgender adults, age 50+: Results of three surveys. *Journal of GLBT Family Studies* 6(2):142–177.

D'Augelli, A., and A. Grossman. 2001. Disclosure of sexual orientation, victimization, and mental health among lesbian, gay, and bisexual older adults. *Journal of Interpersonal Violence* 16(10):1008–1027.

Dahl, M., J. L. Feldman, J. M. Goldberg, and A. Jaberi. 2006. Physical aspects of transgender endocrine therapy. *International Journal of Transgenderism* 9(3):111–134.

David, S., and B. G. Knight. 2008. Stress and coping among gay men: Age and ethnic differences. *Psychology and Aging* 23(1):62–69.

de Vries, B. 2006. Home at the end of the rainbow. *Generations* 29(4):64–69.

de Vries, B. 2008. Lesbian, gay, bisexual and transgender persons in later life. In *Encyclopedia of the life course and human development*, edited by D. S. Carr. Farmington Hills, MI: Cengage Learning, Inc. Pp. 161–165.

de Vries, B., and J. Blando. 2004. The study of gay and lesbian aging: Lessons for social gerontology. In *Gay and lesbian aging: Research and future directions*, edited by G. Herdt and B. de Vries. New York: Springer.

de Vries, B., and P. Hoctel. 2006. The family-friends of older gay men and lesbians. In *Sexual inequalities and social justice*, edited by N. Teunis and G. Herdt. Berkeley, CA: University of California Press. Pp. 213–232.

de Vries, B., and D. Megathlin. 2009. The meaning of friendship for gay men and lesbians in the second half of life. *Journal of GLBT Family Studies* 5(1):82–98.

de Vries, B., A. M. Mason, J. Quam, and Aquaviva. 2009. State recognition of same-sex relationships and preparations for end of life among lesbian and gay boomers. *Sexuality Research & Social Policy: A Journal of the NSRC* 6(1):90–101.

Department of Health and Human Services. 2010. *Medical management of older patients with HIV/AIDS (R21)*. http://grants.nih.gov/grants/guide/pa-files/pa-09-019.html (accessed February 28, 2011).

Doctor, R. F. 1988. *Transvestites and transsexuals: Towards a theory of cross-gender behavior*. New York: Plenum Press.

Doorn, C. D., J. Poortinga, and A. M. Verschoor. 1994. Cross-gender identity in transvestites and male transsexuals. *Archives of Sexual Behavior* 23(2):185–201.

Emerson, S. 1996. Stages of adjustment in family members of transgender individuals. *Journal of Family Psychotherapy* 7(3):1–12.

Eyler, A. E. 2007. Primary care of the gender-variant patient. In *Principles of transgender medicine and surgery*, edited by R. Ettner, S. Monstrey, and A. E. Eyler. New York: Haworth Press. Pp. 15–31.

Fairchild, S. K., G. E. Carrino, and M. Ramirez. 1996. Social workers' perceptions of staff attitudes toward resident sexuality in a random sample of New York state nursing homes: A pilot study. *Journal of Gerontological Social Work* 26(1):153–169.

Feldman, J. 2007. Preventive care of the transgendered patient: An evidence-based approach. In *Principles of transgender medicine and surgery*, edited by R. Ettner, S. Monstrey, and A. E. Eyler. New York: Haworth Press. Pp. 33–72.

Feldman, J. L., and J. M. Goldberg. 2007. Transgender primary medical care. *International Journal of Transgenderism* 9(3–4):3–34.

Fredriksen-Goldsen, K. I., and A. Muraco. 2010. Aging and sexual orientation: A 25-year review of the literature. *Research on Aging* 32(3):372–413.

Fredriksen-Goldsen, K. I., H. J. Kim, A. Muraco, and S. Mincer. 2009. Chronically ill midlife and older lesbians, gay men, and bisexuals and their informal caregivers: The impact of the social context. *Sexuality Research & Social Policy: A Journal of the NSRC* 6(4):52–64.

Fredriksen-Goldsen, K. I., H.-J. Kim, and J. Goldsen. 2011 (unpublished). *Resilience and disparities among lesbian, gay, bisexual and transgender older adults*. Institute for Multigenerational Health.

Fruhauf, C. A., N. A. Orel, and D. A. Jenkins. 2009. The coming-out process of gay grandfathers: Perceptions of their adult children's influence. *Journal of GLBT Family Studies* 5(1):99–118.

Garnets, L. D., and L. A. Peplau. 2006. Sexuality in the lives of aging lesbian and bisexual women. In *Lesbian, gay, bisexual, and transgender aging: Research and clinical perspectives*, edited by D. Kimmel, T. Rose, and S. David. New York: Columbia University Press. Pp. 70–90.

Goldberg, N. G. 2009. *The impact of inequality for same-sex partners in employer-sponsored retirement plans*. Los Angeles, CA: The Williams Institute.

Grossman, A. H. 2006. Physical and mental health of older lesbian, gay, and bisexual adults. In *Lesbian, gay, bisexual and transgender aging: Research and clinical perspectives*, edited by D. Kimmel, T. Rose and S. David. New York: Columbia University Press. Pp. 53–69.

Grossman, A. H., A. R. D'Augelli, and S. L. Hershberger. 2000. Social support networks of lesbian, gay, and bisexual adults 60 years of age and older. *The Journals of Gerontology: Series B: Psychological Sciences and Social Sciences* 3(3):171.

Grossman, A. H., A. R. D'Augelli, and T. S. O'Connell. 2001. Being lesbian, gay, bisexual, and 60 or older in North America. *Journal of Gay & Lesbian Social Services: Issues in Practice, Policy & Research* 13(4):23–40.

Grov, C., D. S. Bimbi, J. E. Nanin, and J. T. Parsons. 2006. Exploring racial and ethnic differences in recreational drug use among gay and bisexual men in New York City and Los Angeles. *Journal of Drug Education* 36(2):105–123.

Gruskin, E. P., G. L. Greenwood, M. Matevia, L. M. Pollack, and L. L. Bye. 2007. Disparities in smoking between the lesbian, gay, and bisexual population and the general population in California. *American Journal of Public Health* 97(8):1496–1502.

Gutmann, D. 1985. The parental imperative revisited: Towards a developmental psychology of adulthood and later life. *Contributions to Human Development* 14:31–60.

Harrison, A. E., and V. M. Silenzio. 1996. Comprehensive care of lesbian and gay patients and families. *Primary Care; Clinics in Office Practice* 23(1):31–46.

Hartzell, E., M. S. Frazer, K. Wertz, and M. Davis. 2009. *The state of transgender California: Results from the 2008 California Transgender Economic Health Survey*. San Francisco, CA: Transgender Law Center.

Herek, G. M., and L. D. Garnets. 2007. Sexual orientation and mental health. *Annual Review of Clinical Psychology* 3:353–375.

High, K. P., R. B. Effros, C. V. Fletcher, K. Gebo, J. B. Halter, W. R. Hazzard, F. M. Horne, R. E. Huebner, E. N. Janoff, A. C. Justice, D. Kuritzkes, S. G. Nayfield, S. F. Plaeger, K. E. Schmader, J. R. Ashworth, C. Campanelli, C. P. Clayton, B. Rada, and N. F. Woolard. 2008. Workshop on HIV infection and aging: What is known and future research directions. *Clinical Infectious Diseases* 47(4):542–553.

Hostetler, A. 2004. Old, gay and alone? The ecology of well-being among middle-aged and older single gay men. In *Gay and lesbian aging: Research and future directions*, edited by G. Herdt and B. de Vries. New York: Springer. Pp. 143–176.

Hughes, T. L., S. C. Wilsnack, L. A. Szalacha, T. Johnson, W. B. Bostwick, R. Seymour, F. Aranda, P. Benson, and K. E. Kinnison. 2006. Age and racial/ethnic differences in drinking and drinking-related problems in a community sample of lesbians. *Journal of Studies on Alcohol* 67(4):579–590.

Johnson, M. J., N. C. Jackson, J. K. Arnette, and S. D. Koffman. 2005. Gay and lesbian perceptions of discrimination in retirement care facilities. *Journal of Homosexuality* 49(2):83–102.

Kammerer, N., T. Mason, and M. Connors. 1999. Transgender health and social service needs in the context of HIV risk. *International Journal of Transgenderism* 3(1/2):1.

Karpiak, S. E., R. A. Shippy, and M. H. Cantor. 2006. *Research on older adults with HIV.* New York: AIDS Community Research Initiative of America.

Kehoe, M. 1989. *Lesbians over sixty speak for themselves.* New York: Harrington Park Press.

Kenagy, G. P. 2005. Transgender health: Findings from two needs assessment studies in Philadelphia. *Health & Social Work* 30(1):19–26.

Kenagy, G. P., and C. M. Hsieh. 2005. The risk less known: Female-to-male transgender persons' vulnerability to HIV infection. *AIDS Care* 17(2):195–207.

Kennamer, J. D., J. Honnold, J. Bradford, and M. Hendricks. 2000. Differences in disclosure of sexuality among African American and white gay/bisexual men: Implications for HIV/AIDS prevention. *AIDS Education & Prevention* 12(6):519–531.

Kertzner, R. M., I. H. Meyer, D. M. Frost, and M. J. Stirratt. 2009. Social and psychological well-being in lesbians, gay men, and bisexuals: The effects of race, gender, age, and sexual identity. *American Journal of Orthopsychiatry* 79(4):500–510.

Kimmel, D. C. 1978. Adult development and aging: A gay perspective. *Journal of Social Issues* 34(3):113–130.

King, M., J. Semlyen, S. S. Tai, H. Killaspy, D. Osborn, D. Popelyuk, and I. Nazareth. 2008. A systematic review of mental disorder, suicide, and deliberate self harm in lesbian, gay and bisexual people. *BMC Psychiatry* 8:70.

King, S., and H. Dabelko-Schoeny. 2009. "Quite frankly, I have doubts about remaining": Aging-in-place and health care access for rural midlife and older lesbian, gay, and bisexual individuals. *Journal of LGBT Health Research* 5(1):10–21.

Landen, M., J. Walinder, and B. Lundstrom. 1998. Clinical characteristics of a total cohort of female and male applicants for sex reassignment: A descriptive study. *Acta Psychiatrica Scandinavica* 97(3):189–194.

Lawrence, A. A. 2003. Factors associated with satisfaction or regret following male-to-female sex reassignment surgery. *Archives of Sexual Behavior* 32(4):299–315.

Lawrence, A. A. 2010. Sexual orientation versus age of onset as bases for typologies (subtypes) for gender identity disorder in adolescents and adults. *Archives of Sexual Behavior* 39(2):514–545.

Lee, J. A. 1987. The invisible lives of Canada's gray gays. In *Aging in Canada: Social perspectives*, edited by V. M. Marshall. Markham, Ontorio: Fitzhenry & Whitside. Pp. 138–155.

Lev, A. I. 2004. *Transgender emergence: Therapeutic guidelines for working with gender*. New York: Haworth Press.

Lindau, S. T., L. P. Schumm, E. O. Laumann, W. Levinson, C. A. O'Muircheartaigh, and L. J. Waite. 2007. A study of sexuality and health among older adults in the United States. *New England Journal of Medicine* 357(8):762–774.

Lopata, H. Z. 1993. The support system of American urban widows. In *Handbook of bereavement: Theory, research, and intervention*, edited by M. S. Stroebe, W. Stroebe, and R. O. Hansson. Cambridge, UK: Cambridge University Press. Pp. 381–396.

Martin, J. L., and L. Dean. 1993. Bereavement following death from AIDS: Unique problems, reactions, and special needs. In *Handbook of bereavement: Theory, research, and intervention,* edited by M. S. Stroebe, W. Stroebe, and R. O. Hansson. New York: Columbia University Press. Pp. 315–330.

Masini, B. E., and H. A. Barrett. 2008. Social support as a predictor of psychological and physical well-being and lifestyle in lesbian, gay, and bisexual adults aged 50 and over. *Journal of Gay & Lesbian Social Services* 20(1):91–110.

Massachusetts Department of Public Health. 2009. *The health of lesbian, gay, bisexual and transgender (LGBT) persons in Massachusetts: A survey of health issues comparing LGBT persons with their heterosexual and non-transgender counterparts.* Boston, MA: Massachusetts Department of Public Health.

McLaughlin, K. A., M. L. Hatzenbuehler, and K. M. Keyes. 2010. Responses to discrimination and psychiatric disorders among black, Hispanic, female, and lesbian, gay, and bisexual individuals. *American Journal of Public Health* 100(8):1477–1484.

MetLife. 2006. *Out and aging: The MetLife study of lesbian and gay baby boomers.* Westport, CT: MetLife Mature Market Institute.

MetLife. 2010. *Still out, still aging: The MetLife study of lesbian, gay, bisexual, and transgender baby boomers.* Westport, CT: MetLife Mature Market Institute.

Mills, T. C., J. Paul, R. Stall, L. Pollack, J. Canchola, Y. J. Chang, J. T. Moskowitz, and J. A. Catania. 2004. Distress and depression in men who have sex with men: The Urban Men's Health Study. *American Journal of Psychiatry* 161(2):278–285.

Möller, B., H. Schreier, A. Li, and G. Romer. 2009. Gender identity disorder in children and adolescents. *Current Problems in Pediatric & Adolescent Health Care* 39: 117–143.

Moore, E., A. Wisniewski, and A. Dobs. 2003. Endocrine treatment of transsexual people: A review of treatment regimens, outcomes, and adverse effects. *Journal of Clinical Endocrinology & Metabolism* 88(8):3467–3473.

Movement Advancement Project and Services and Advocacy for Gay, Lesbian, Bisexual and Transgender Elders. 2010. *Improving the lives of LGBT older adults.* http://www.sageusa.org/uploads/Advancing%20Equality%20for%20LGBT%20Elders%20%5BFINAL%20COMPRESSED%5D.pdf (accessed March 17, 2011).

Mullan, J. T. 1998. Aging and informal caregiving to people with HIV/AIDS. *Research on Aging* 20(6):712.

Nemoto, T., D. Operario, and J. G. Keatley. 2005. Health and social services for male-to-female transgender persons of color in San Francisco. *International Journal of Transgenderism* 8(2/3):5–19.

NIMH (National Institute of Mental Health). 2007. *Suicide in the U.S.: Statistics and prevention.* http://www.nimh.nih.gov/health/publications/suicide-in-the-us-statistics-and-prevention/index.shtml (accessed November 9, 2010).

Nuttbrock, L., S. Hwahng, W. Bockting, A. Rosenblum, M. Mason, M. Macri, and J. Becker. 2010. Psychiatric impact of gender-related abuse across the life course of male-to-female transgender persons. *Journal of Sex Research* 47(1):12–23.

Office of the New York City Public Advocate. 2008. *Improving lesbian, gay, bisexual and transgender access to healthcare at New York City health and hospitals corporation facilities.* New York: Office of the New York City Public Advocate.

Orel, N. 2006a. Community needs assessment: Documenting the need for affirmative services for LGB older adults. In *Lesbian, gay, bisexual, and transgender aging: Research and clinical perspectives*, edited by D. Kimmel, T. Rose, and S. David. New York: Columbia University Press. Pp. 227–246.

Orel, N. 2006b. Lesbian and bisexual women as grandparents: The centrality of sexual orientation in the grandparent-grandchild relationship. In *Lesbian, gay, bisexual, and transgender aging: Research and clinical perspectives*, edited by D. Kimmel, T. Rose, and S. David. New York: Columbia University Press. Pp. 175–194.

Paul, J. P., J. Catania, L. Pollack, J. Moskowitz, J. Canchola, T. Mills, D. Binson, and R. Stall. 2002. Suicide attempts among gay and bisexual men: Lifetime prevalence and antecedents. *American Journal of Public Health* 92(8):1338–1345.

Person, E., and L. Ovesey. 1974. The transsexual syndrome in males. I. Primary transsexualism. *American Journal of Psychotherapy* 28(1):4–20.

Price, J. H., A. N. Easton, S. K. Telljohann, and P. B. Wallace. 1996. Perceptions of cervical cancer and Pap smear screening behavior by women's sexual orientation. *Journal of Community Health* 21(2):89–105.

Qureshi, H., and A. Walker. 1989. *The caring relationship: Elderly people and their families.* Philadelphia, PA: Temple University Press.

Rawls, T. W. 2004. Disclosure and depression among older gay and homosexual men: Findings from the Urban Men's Health Study. In *Gay and lesbian aging: Research and future directions*, edited by G. Herdt and B. De Vries. New York: Springer. Pp. 117–141.

Riggle, E. D., S. S. Rostosky, R. A. Prather, and R. Hamrin. 2005. The execution of legal documents by sexual minority individuals. *Psychology, Public Policy, and Law* 11(1):138–163.

Roberts, S. A., S. L. Dibble, B. Nussey, and K. Casey. 2003. Cardiovascular disease risk in lesbian women. *Womens Health Issues* 13(4):167–174.

Scherrer, K. S. 2009. Images of sexuality and aging in gerontological literature. *Sexuality Research & Social Policy: A Journal of the NSRC* 6(4):5–12.

Schlesinger, B. 1996. The sexless years or sex rediscovered. *Journal of Gerontological Social Work* 26(1/2):117–131.

Schwartzberg, S. 1992. AIDS-related bereavement among gay men: The inadequacy of current theories of grief. *Psychotherapy* 29(3):422–429.

Shanas, E. 1980. Older people and their families: The new pioneers. *Journal of Marriage and Family* 42(1):9–15.

Shernoff, M. 1998. Gay widowers: Grieving in relation to trauma and social supports. *Journal of the Gay and Lesbian Medical Association* 2(1):27–34.

Shippy, R., M. H. Cantor, and M. Brennan. 2004. Social networks of aging gay men. *The Journal of Men's Studies* 13(1):107–120.

Statewide Office of Suicide Prevention. 2009. *Suicide prevention.* Tallahassee, FL: Statewide Office of Suicide Prevention.

Tang, H., G. L. Greenwood, D. W. Cowling, J. C. Lloyd, A. G. Roeseler, and D. G. Bal. 2004. Cigarette smoking among lesbians, gays, and bisexuals: How serious a problem? (United States). *Cancer Causes & Control* 15(8):797–803.

Valanis, B. G., D. J. Bowen, T. Bassford, E. Whitlock, P. Charney, and R. A. Carter. 2000. Sexual orientation and health: Comparisons in the women's health initiative sample. *Archives of Family Medicine* 9(9):843–853.

Van Kesteren, P. J. M., H. Asscheman, J. A. J. Megens, and L. J. G. Gooren. 1997. Mortality and morbidity in transsexual subjects treated with cross-sex hormones. *Clinical Endocrinology* 47(3):337-343.

Wahler, J. J., and S. G. Gabbay. 1997. Gay male aging. *Journal of Gay and Lesbian Social Services* 6(3):1-20.

Wallien, M. S. C., and P. T. Cohen-Kettenis. 2008. Psychosexual outcome of gender-dysphoric children. *Journal of the American Academy of Child & Adolescent Psychiatry* 47(12):1413–1423.

Williams, M. E., and P. A. Freeman. 2005. Transgender health: Implications for aging and caregiving. *Journal of Gay & Lesbian Social Services* 18(3/4):93–108.

Witten, T. M. 2002. Geriatric care and management issues for the transgender and intersex populations. *Geriatric Care Management Journal* 12(3):20–24.

Witten, T. M. 2009. Graceful exits: Intersection of aging, transgender identities, and the family/community. *Journal of GLBT Family Studies* 5(1/2):35–61.

Witten, T. M., and A. E. Eyler. 1999. Hate crimes and violence against the transgendered. *Peace Review* 11(3):461.

Witten, T. M., and A. E. Eyler. 2007. Transgender aging and the care of the elderly transgendered patient. In *Principles of transgender medicine and surgery*, edited by R. Ettner, S. Monstrey, and A. E. Eyler. New York: Haworth Press. Pp. 285–309.

Witten, T. M., and S. Whittle. 2004. Transpanthers: The graying of transgender and the law. *Deakin Law Review* 9(2):503–522.

Xavier, J. M., J. Bradford, and J. Honnold. 2007. *The health, health-related needs, and life-course experiences of transgender Virginians*. Richmond, VA: Virginia Department of Health.

Zaritsky, E., and S. L. Dibble. 2010. Risk factors for reproductive and breast cancers among older lesbians. *Journal of Women's Health* 19(1):125–131.

7

Recommendations

In accordance with its statement of task, the committee's primary recommendation is for a research agenda that will assist the National Institutes of Health (NIH) in enhancing its research efforts in the area of LGBT health. The committee also formulated recommendations in several areas that would advance understanding of LGBT health: data collection, methodological research, research training, and policy on research participation.

RESEARCH AGENDA

Recommendation 1. NIH should implement a research agenda designed to advance knowledge and understanding of LGBT health.

The committee believes that building the evidence base on LGBT health issues will not only benefit LGBT individuals but also provide new research on topics that affect heterosexual and non-gender-variant individuals as well. Given the large number of areas in LGBT health in which research is needed, the committee formulated a research agenda that reflects those areas of highest priority. Within each of these areas, the conceptual frameworks identified in Chapter 1 are evident as cross-cutting perspectives that should be considered. Figure 7-1 illustrates the interactions between the priority research areas identified by the committee and these cross-cutting perspectives.

As noted earlier in the report, although lesbians, gay men, bisexual men and women, and transgender people each are separate populations, they frequently are considered as a group. The primary driving force behind

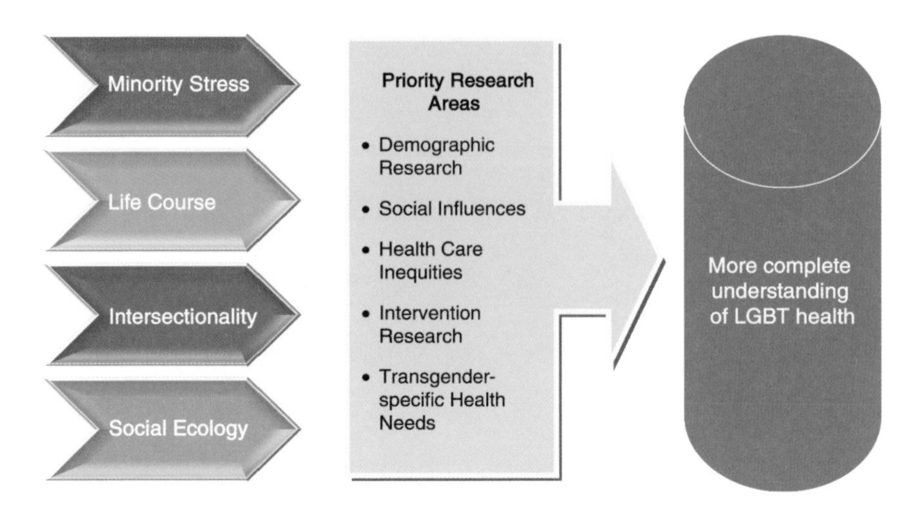

FIGURE 7-1 Research agenda. A number of different conceptual perspectives can be applied to priority areas of research in order to further the evidence base for LGBT health issues.

combining these populations is that they are nonheterosexual or gender nonconforming and are frequently stigmatized as a consequence. These populations also are often combined in some way for research purposes. For example, researchers frequently merge lesbians, gay men, and bisexual people into a group labeled "nonheterosexual." Similarly, in some HIV research, study participants are combined in a single category that may include gay men, bisexual men, transgender women, and men who do not identify as any of the above but still have sex with other men. Combining these populations in this way obscures differences among them.

Given that lesbians, gay men, bisexual women and men, and transgender people are in fact separate populations, it is important to note that most of the research on these populations has focused on lesbians and gay men. Much less research has been conducted on bisexual and transgender people. The committee therefore recommends research that focuses on these populations.

Cross-Cutting Perspectives

Chapter 1 introduces four conceptual frameworks that are useful for understanding the health of LGBT people: the minority stress model, a life-course perspective, intersectionality, and social ecology. In this report's review of the existing literature, these frameworks are present to greater and lesser degrees, sometimes implicit and sometimes explicit. They are introduced once again here as cross-cutting perspectives that should be pursued in research on each of the priority areas identified by the committee. Each of these perspectives is discussed in turn below, followed by a discussion of each of the priority areas. It is important to note that these perspectives represent a current but probably partial list that the committee believes would be brought to bear profitably in the study of LGBT health. Other perspectives not yet named or published may well serve this enterprise in the future in ways yet to be determined.

A Minority Stress Perspective

As the minority stress model illustrates, sexual and gender minorities are subjected to chronic stress as a result of their stigmatization as a minority group. Minority stress processes are both proximal (subjective) and distal (objective); they are also external (enacted stigma) and internal (felt stigma, self-stigma) (see Chapter 2). The shared and common experience of stigma and the influences and impact of minority stress should be considered as central to LGBT health in addressing all of the areas on the committee's recommended research agenda.

A Life-Course Perspective

The committee drew on life-course theory because it serves as a framework for understanding a range of health issues that occur throughout life. The influence of cohort and age differences on health needs must be recognized. Longitudinal cohort studies, which are largely absent from LGBT research, are an excellent way of gaining insight into health issues by following participants over a period of time. Such studies would be useful for understanding many health issues related to sexual and gender minorities, including the development of gender-variant youth in their social contexts, the effects of pathways to family formation on the health of sexual and gender minorities, men who have sex with men in the context of HIV, identity as an LGBT person (i.e., member of a sexual and/or gender minority) over the life course, and changes in patterns of substance use over time.

In addition to longitudinal cohort studies, there is a particular need for more research focused on later life. The committee also encourages the analysis of data with age as a factor or variable in studies encompassing a broad age range that crosses over cohorts and into later life.

An Intersectional Perspective

The concept of intersectionality emphasizes that sexual- or gender-minority status is just one of many factors that influence the lives and health of individuals. Contextual factors, and therefore life experiences, vary greatly among LGBT populations. However, research examining the health status of LGBT people that takes account of this diversity is still rare. There is a need to understand the role of geography, race, ethnicity, socioeconomic status, and other factors, as well as the combined effect of their interaction, in the health status of LGBT people. Thus, multiple identities should be considered in research on LGBT health.

A Social Ecological Perspective

The social ecology model illustrates that an individual influences and in turn is influenced by the social environment, including the family, other relationships, the community, culture, and society at large. Thus, one's community and social circumstances affect one's health, and integrating these multiple levels into research will provide a richer understanding of LGBT health. For example, community-based participatory research stresses the collaboration and partnership between the community and the researcher, often resulting in the community's sense of investment in the research. Whether examining mechanisms of risk or designing and testing interventions, researchers should consider both individuals and the contexts in which they live.

Research Areas

While recognizing that many areas in the field of LGBT health are in need of and deserve more attention, the committee also understands the importance of identifying priorities for research. Therefore, the committee identified the following areas as being especially important in taking an early step toward building a solid evidence base and as being likely to make the greatest contributions to the field at this point in time: demographic research, social influences on the lives of LGBT people, inequities in health care, intervention studies, and transgender-specific health needs. As noted, the cross-cutting perspectives described above should be considered across these areas.

Demographic Research

To better understand the health needs of sexual and gender minorities, more data on these populations are needed, beginning with demographic data. In the broadest sense, this means that more demographic information about lesbian, gay, bisexual, and transgender people across the life course is needed. However, there is also a pressing need for a better demographic understanding of the subpopulations that make up the LGBT community as a whole. Only with a better understanding of the racial, ethnic, geographic, and other demographic variations within the larger LGBT community can the health needs of all LGBT individuals be clarified and addressed.

Social Influences on the Lives of LGBT People

Many social structures—such as biological families, families of choice, marriages/partnerships, friends, schools, workplaces, and community organizations—can be sources of either stress or support for LGBT people. These social structures and the roles they play in the lives of LGBT people are underresearched. For example, little attention has been paid to the potentially positive role families and other social structures can play in the lives of LGBT adolescents. The role of parenthood in adult development among LGBT people also is not well understood. Similarly, how biological families and families of choice affect LGBT elders has not yet been studied in any detail. Recognizing that social support plays an important role in mental health, the committee believes that research examining the formation and experiences of families among LGBT individuals, as well as other social influences, would contribute to a fuller understanding of LGBT health.

Inequities in Health Care

LGBT individuals face barriers to equitable health care that can have a profound impact on their overall well-being (see Chapter 2). Lack of health insurance, fear of discrimination from providers, lack of providers who are well trained in the health needs of LGBT individuals, and dissatisfaction with services can all limit the extent to which sexual and gender minorities access health services. More research on LGBT health inequities is needed. Understanding the experiences of LGBT individuals seeking care, outcome disparities, provider attitudes and education, and ways in which the care environment could be improved would provide a solid base from which to address these inequities.

Intervention Research

Research is needed to develop and test the effectiveness of interventions designed to address health inequities experienced by LGBT populations. Studies focused on increasing access to care or addressing the mental or physical conditions that lead to impaired health among LGBT individuals would assist in reducing these inequities. For example, interventions are needed to identify and test effective ways of reducing homelessness among LGBT youth and reaching transgender people at risk of HIV infection. In many cases, it may be clear that a negative health outcome exists, but the underlying mechanisms of risk have not been identified. Conducting research on the mechanisms of risk among selected populations would help in developing appropriate interventions. Another approach might consist of modifying existing interventions from other areas, such as interventions addressing bullying and eating disorders.

A growing body of research examines the use of technology for delivering interventions. Some studies have used text messaging as a means of communicating preventive health information or interventions, while others have used geographic information systems to examine various risk factors and determine where to direct resources and interventions. The committee believes that as communication technology continues to evolve, it may hold potential for extending interventions to difficult-to-reach LGBT populations and that its use for this purpose warrants further research.

Transgender-Specific Health Needs

All aspects of the evidence base for transgender-specific health care need to be expanded. Research methods that will yield the data needed to inform decisions about transgender-specific health should be developed. In addition, there is a need for more research on the health implications of hormone use (e.g., randomized controlled trials of puberty-delaying hormones, masculinizing and feminizing hormone therapies, and the consequences of long-term hormone use). More research would also help inform the discussion around the diagnosis of gender identity disorder. Currently, this diagnosis forms the basis for access of transgender people to procedures that may be medically necessary for many of these individuals. Studies on transition-related care and body modification and an evaluation of the *Standards of Care* for the treatment of gender identity disorder would contribute to this discussion.

Research Gaps and Opportunities

The above research agenda is drawn from the myriad of research opportunities that exist in the field of LGBT health. All of the priority research areas identified by the committee represent multiple opportunities for research that extend across the life course. Some of the areas focus on specific populations or fields, while others encompass types of research or particular contexts. The committee is recommending this research agenda to address the most pressing needs for advancing knowledge and understanding of LGBT health.

As part of the process of creating this research agenda, the committee was asked to identify research gaps and opportunities in the area of LGBT health. After completing its review of the available literature, the committee found that the idea of identifying research gaps was not particularly useful in the context of this study. When identifying research gaps, one sets out to review a body of evidence that needs additional work on a selected number of topics. In the case of LGBT health, however, the committee found that the body of evidence assembled to date is sparse, and the work ahead must be more substantial than simply filling in gaps. While some research has been conducted in a number of areas pertaining to LGBT health, most areas are lacking research altogether or require considerable additional work. As an analogy, one might say that work has begun on a foundation, but it is not yet complete, and without a substantive foundation, it will be difficult to construct an understanding of LGBT health needs. In terms of opportunities, this means that there are many research questions that remain unanswered. At the end of Chapters 2 through 6, some key areas that are missing from the literature are noted. Table 7-1 lists many of the research opportunities that exist across the life course (presented in alphabetical order and not necessarily in order of importance). Although this is not an exhaustive listing, conducting effective and rigorous research in any of these areas will contribute to the body of evidence that is needed in the field of LGBT health.

DATA COLLECTION

Recommendation 2. Data on sexual orientation and gender identity should be collected in federally funded surveys administered by the Department of Health and Human Services and in other relevant federally funded surveys.

The need for demographic data is reflected in the above research agenda. Collecting data on sexual orientation and gender identity in federally funded surveys would generate these data. While the Department of Health and Human Services administers a number of surveys that relate directly to health, other federal agencies also administer surveys that could provide information on a number of dimensions that affect health. For example, recognizing the interaction between social and economic circumstances and health, data from social and economic surveys could provide valuable information on the context for health disparities experienced by LGBT people. Similarly, surveys on crime and victimization, housing, and families would provide data on variables that relate to the health of sexual and gender minorities.

Like race and ethnicity data, data on sexual and gender minorities should be included in the battery of demographic information that is collected in federally funded surveys. This data collection would be aided

TABLE 7-1 Research Opportunities for Studying Lesbian, Gay, Bisexual, and Transgender Health Across the Life Course

	Childhood/ Adolescence	Early/ Middle Adulthood	Later Adulthood
Demographic and Descriptive Information	• Percentage of adolescents who are LGBT • How the percentage of LGBT adolescents varies by demographic characteristics such as race, ethnicity, socioeconomic status, geography, and religion • General experiences and health status of LGBT adolescents and how these vary by demographic characteristics	• Percentage of adults who are LGBT • How the percentage of LGBT adults varies by demographic characteristics such as race, ethnicity, socioeconomic status, geography, and religion • General experiences and health status of LGBT adults and how these vary by demographic characteristics • Percentage of LGBT adults who are parents	• Percentage of elders who are LGBT • How the percentage of LGBT elders varies by demographic characteristics such as race, ethnicity, socioeconomic status, geography, and religion • General experiences and health status of LGBT elders and how these vary by demographic characteristics • Percentage of LGBT elders who are parents • The trajectory of LGBT identity and experiences (bisexual identities in particular) over the life course
Family and Interpersonal Relations	• Family life of LGBT youth from diverse backgrounds (e.g., race/ethnicity, socio-economic status) • School and social life concomitants of LGBT identity and attraction • Protective factors at the individual, interactional (family, school, peers), and systems levels • Patterns and experiences of homelessness among LGBT youth • Intrafamily and domestic violence (e.g., sexual abuse, abuse by parents, intimate partner violence) • Anti-LGBT victimization	• Effect of the greater likelihood of childlessness among LGBT adults • The experience of parenting (with a particular focus on the experiences of gay male and bisexual parents, largely absent from the research literature) • The experience and prevalence of "chosen families" • Intrafamily and domestic violence (e.g., interpersonal violence, including intimate partner violence) • Anti-LGBT victimization	• Effect of the greater likelihood of childlessness among LGBT elders (particularly among older gay men) • The experience of LGBT aging and family life (e.g., experiences with biological kin across generations; "chosen family" ties and relations) • Experiences of grief and loss (including multiple losses) • Intrafamily and domestic violence (e.g., caregiver/ provider abuse, intimate partner violence) • Anti-LGBT victimization

	Childhood/ Adolescence	Early/ Middle Adulthood	Later Adulthood
Health Services	• Barriers to access (particularly related to identity disclosure and interactions with providers) • Utilization rates • Quality of care received	• Barriers to access (particularly related to identity disclosure and interactions with providers) • Utilization rates • Quality of care received	• Barriers to access (particularly related to identity disclosure and interactions with providers) • Utilization rates • Quality of care received • Long-term care issues of older LGBT persons • End-of-life issues (e.g., preparations, fears, and plans)
Mental Health	• Diagnosis of disorders among LGBT youth • Depression and suicidality • Effects of stigma and discrimination • Identity-related issues • Eating disorders	• Depression and suicidality (particularly unknown among transgender adults) • Effects of stigma and discrimination (particularly unknown among bisexual adults) • Eating disorders	• Depression and suicidality • Effects of stigma and discrimination (over the course of a lifetime) • The experience of and preparations for late life among older LGBT persons
Physical Health	• Substance use (including smoking and alcohol abuse) • Obesity	• Substance use (particularly among transgender individuals) • Obesity (particularly among lesbians and bisexual women) • Cancer rates, risks, and treatment (e.g., breast cancer among lesbians and bisexual women; anal cancer rates and evaluations of screening effectiveness among men who have sex with men; cancer among transgender adults in general, about which very little is known) • Cardiovascular disease among all LGBT adults	• Cancer rates, risks, and treatment (particularly prostate cancer among older gay and bisexual men and transgender women, and anal cancer rates among older men who have sex with men) • Effects of long-term hormone use among older transgender persons • Effects of disabilities among older LGBT persons

continued

TABLE 7-1 Continued

	Childhood/ Adolescence	Early/ Middle Adulthood	Later Adulthood
Sexual and Reproductive Health	• HIV rates and interventions (with a focus on natural history studies of high-risk groups) • Sexually transmitted infections • Sexual development • Sexual and reproductive health and risk behaviors	• HIV rates and interventions (particularly addressing racial disparities) • Fertility, infertility, and reproductive health issues • Reproductive technology and its use	• HIV rates and interventions (and the experience of aging with HIV) • Sexual well-being and sexual dysfunction (particularly among older lesbians and transgender elders, about whom little is known)

NOTE: Research in these areas should, to the extent possible, encompass key themes identified throughout this report, including the role of stigma and discrimination; commonalities and differences across racial, ethnic, gender, and other subpopulations (including the ways in which these overlap); and the life-course, community, and cultural contexts in which the phenomena occur

by the development of standardized measures for sexual orientation and gender identity (see Recommendation 4 below).

In contrast to surveys that collect data at a certain point in time, longitudinal studies allow for the collection of data over a period of years. At NIH, data on sexual orientation and gender identity are already being collected in the National Longitudinal Study of Adolescent Health. The collection of these data should be extended to other longitudinal studies. These data collection efforts could be expected to generate national, population-level data that could be used to glean information on LGBT populations in general, as well as to explore characteristics of LGBT subpopulations.

In addition, including variables to measure sexual orientation and gender identity in a variety of studies (e.g., through the addition of appropriate questions on gender identity and sexual orientation to the demographic section of questionnaires) would generate much-needed data on LGBT populations that could assist in assembling a reliable body of evidence regarding their health status.

Recommendation 3. Data on sexual orientation and gender identity should be collected in electronic health records.

The Office of the National Coordinator for Health Information Technology within the Department of Health and Human Services should include the collection of data on sexual orientation and gender identity as part of its meaningful-use objectives for electronic health records. One of the meaningful-use objectives is Record Demographics, including preferred language, gender, race, ethnicity, and date of birth. Sexual orientation and gender identity could be included in the required set of demographic data. However, the collection of such data will need to be performed with adequate privacy and security protections. While all data collected in electronic health records are subjected to high levels of privacy and security protection, overseen by the Office of the National Coordinator, information on sexual orientation and gender identity could be perceived by some as being more sensitive than other information.

At present, some barriers exist to collecting useful data on sexual orientation and gender identity through electronic health records. These barriers include possible discomfort on the part of health care workers with asking questions about sexual orientation and gender identity, a lack of knowledge by providers of how to elicit this information, and some hesitancy on the part of patients to disclose this information. While recognizing that obstacles to the collection of meaningful data on sexual orientation and gender identity exist, the committee encourages the Office of the National Coordinator to begin planning for the collection of these data as part of the required set of demographic data for electronic health records. Detailed patient-level data such as those found in electronic health records could provide a rich source of information about LGBT populations and subpopulations.

METHODOLOGICAL RESEARCH

Recommendation 4. NIH should support the development and standardization of sexual orientation and gender identity measures.

NIH should support the rigorous development of valid, reliable measures for the collection of data on sexual orientation and gender identity. This call for additional research on measures does not mean that measures do not exist. Existing measures of sexual orientation and gender identity are used differently in various studies depending on the research question. This is an appropriate practice, and researchers should be able to use measures as they see fit. At this time, however, there is no generally accepted and well-validated set of questions that can cover a variety of situations, including studies among different age cohorts, surveys that focus on topics other than sexual behavior, and research in which participants may not understand terms such as "gender identity." Developing and validating suitable measures would make it easier for researchers to collect data on sexual orientation and gender identity.

One of the greatest challenges to synthesizing scientific knowledge about the health of sexual and gender minorities has been the lack of standardized measures in federal surveys. The development and adoption of standardized measures for use in federal surveys would assist in the collection and analysis of data from large-scale sample surveys and advance the evidence base on LGBT health.

Recommendation 5. NIH should support methodological research that relates to LGBT health.

NIH should support research that will assist in addressing the methodological challenges associated with conducting research on LGBT health. Particularly helpful would be studies aimed at developing innovative ways to conduct research with small and difficult-to-reach populations; overcoming challenges involved in combining multiple data sets to obtain a sample with sufficient numbers of sexual- and gender-minority respondents to permit analysis; and determining the best ways to collect information on sexual and gender minorities in research, health care, and other settings.

RESEARCH TRAINING

Recommendation 6. A comprehensive research training approach should be created to strengthen LGBT health research at NIH.

The committee recognizes that, in addition to its well-developed training program, NIH supports a variety of training activities through research grants. However, the field of sexuality research in general has been neglected and, at times, marginalized. Currently, there are limited opportunities for conducting NIH-sponsored research on LGBT health. To create a more robust cadre of researchers in LGBT health, NIH should expand its existing research training framework for both intramural and extramural training. Three audiences should be targeted: researchers who are working with or considering working with LGBT populations, other researchers who may not be aware of LGBT health issues, and NIH staff.

In its intramural training program, NIH should develop postdoctoral training opportunities in the area of LGBT research (for example, research on youth and families). Similarly, NIH should expand the curriculum of its postbaccalaureate NIH Academy to include LGBT-specific issues in addition to the racial and ethnic disparities that are currently studied within the program. To implement these research training activities, NIH should increase its capacity to provide on-site experts as mentors for researchers examining LGBT health issues.

As part of a broad effort to raise awareness about LGBT health issues, NIH should conduct intramural training on these issues with researchers who are not specifically studying LGBT populations. LGBT health issues cut across a large number of research topics. An awareness of LGBT health issues among researchers focusing on these topics would assist them in finding appropriate opportunities to include LGBT study participants (see Recommendation 7 below). Additionally, training these researchers to collect data on sexual orientation and gender identity effectively would expand the body of knowledge about LGBT health and more broadly inform understanding of the diverse experiences of human development.

Within its existing extramural program, NIH should increase the number of individual awards offered to researchers studying LGBT health issues, including postdoctoral, graduate student, and career awards. In addition, the current loan repayment program should be expanded to assist students who choose to study LGBT health issues. In particular, the development of researchers of color who will study LGBT health should be encouraged.

At the institutional level, NIH should create multisite training programs designed to allow students to gain expertise in LGBT health research from a number of different institutions. A similar model has been used in family psychology. The benefit of such a program is that it would draw upon the knowledge of multiple centers and expose students to opportunities afforded by various training sites. Similarly, the idea of centers of excellence for LGBT health research should be explored. Like multisite training programs, these centers would allow researchers to be trained in various sites rather than having to be trained at NIH.

Finally, NIH should provide its employees with recurring training on LGBT research issues. While many project officers at NIH are knowledgeable about LGBT issues, NIH would benefit as an institution if all staff had a firm understanding of the key issues in LGBT health research.

POLICY ON RESEARCH PARTICIPATION

Recommendation 7. NIH should encourage grant applicants to address explicitly the inclusion or exclusion of sexual and gender minorities in their samples.

Using the NIH policy on the inclusion of women and minorities in clinical research as a model, NIH should encourage grant applicants to address explicitly the extent to which their proposed sample includes or excludes sexual and gender minorities. Researchers would thereby be prompted to consider the scientific implications of including or excluding sexual and gender minorities and whether these groups will be included in sufficient numbers to permit meaningful analyses.

Appendix A

Study Activities

The committee held data-gathering sessions that were open to the public at four of its five meetings. Three of these meetings were held in Washington, DC, and one in San Francisco, California. The open-session agendas of the public meetings are below.

MEETING ONE

Committee on Lesbian, Gay, Bisexual and Transgender
(LGBT) Health Issues and Research Gaps and Opportunities
February 1, 2010
Keck Building of the National Academies
500 Fifth Street, NW
Washington, DC

9:30 a.m.–11:00 a.m.	**Sponsor's Charge to the Committee** *Raynard Kington, M.D., Ph.D.* *Deputy Director* *National Institutes of Health*
11:00 a.m.–11:30 a.m.	**Presentations** *Michael Adams* *Executive Director* *Services and Advocacy for GLBT Elders (SAGE)*

	Eliza Byard, Ph.D. *Executive Director* *Gay, Lesbian, Straight Education Network (GLSEN)* *Jason S. Schneider, M.D.* *Immediate Past President* *Gay and Lesbian Medical Association*
11:30 a.m.–12:00 p.m.	**Panel Discussion with Presenters**
1:00 p.m.–1:50 p.m.	**Presentations** *Rebecca Fox* *Director* *The National Coalition for LGBT Health* *Leslie J. Calman, Ph.D.* *Executive Director* *Mautner Project: The National Lesbian Health Organization* *Mara Keisling* *Executive Director* *The National Center for Transgender Equality* *Jaime M. Grant* *Director* *Policy Institute of the National Gay and Lesbian Task Force* *Tom Sullivan* *Deputy Director* *HRC Family Project* *Human Rights Campaign*
1:50 p.m.–2:20 p.m.	**Panel Discussion with Presenters**
2:20 p.m.–2:30 p.m.	**Break**
2:30 p.m.–3:00 p.m.	**Presentations** *Saul Levin, M.D., M.P.A.* *Vice President, Science, Medicine and Public Health* *American Medical Association*

Gal Mayer, M.D.
Vice Chair, AMA–GLBT Advisory Committee
Medical Director, Callen–Lorde Community Health Center

Clinton W. Anderson, Ph.D.
Director, LGBT Concerns Office, and Associate Executive Director, Public Interest Directorate
American Psychological Association

Patrick M. High, Dr.P.H.
Chair, LGBT Caucus of Public Health Professionals
American Public Health Association

3:00 p.m.–3:30 p.m. **Panel Discussion with Presenters**

3:30 p.m.–4:00 p.m. **Open Comments from Public**

MEETING TWO

Committee on Lesbian, Gay, Bisexual and Transgender (LGBT) Health Issues and Research Gaps and Opportunities
March 22, 2010
Lecture Room of the National Academy of Sciences
2101 Constitution Avenue, NW
Washington, DC

9:30 a.m. **Welcome**

9:35 a.m.–10:20 a.m. **Demographics/Data Collection**
Gary J. Gates, Ph.D.
Williams Distinguished Scholar
The Williams Institute
University of California, Los Angeles School of Law

Martin O'Connell, Ph.D.
Chief, Fertility and Family Statistics Branch
Housing and Household Economic Statistics Division
U.S. Bureau of the Census

Randall L. Sell, Sc.D.
Associate Professor
Department of Community Health and Prevention
Drexel University School of Public Health

10:20 a.m.–10:30 a.m.	**Break**
10:30 a.m.–11:15 a.m.	**Current LGBT Research Supported by NIH** *Raynard S. Kington, M.D., Ph.D.* *Deputy Director* *National Institutes of Health* *U.S. Department of Health and Human Services*
11:15 a.m.–12:15 p.m.	**LGBT Research in Minority Populations** *Margaret Rosario, Ph.D.* *Professor of Clinical Psychology, Cognitive Neuroscience, and Social/Personality Psychology* *Department of Psychology* *The City University of New York* *Alicia Matthews, Ph.D.* *Associate Professor* *Department of Health Systems Science* *University of Illinois at Chicago College of Nursing* *David H. Chae, Sc.D., M.A.* *Assistant Professor* *Department of Behavioral Sciences and Health Education* *Emory University, Rollins School of Public Health* *Karina L. Walters, M.S.W., Ph.D.* *William P. and Ruth Gerberding Endowed Professor* *University of Washington School of Social Work*
12:15 p.m.–1:15 p.m.	**Lunch**
1:15 p.m.–1:45 p.m.	**Mental Health: Stress and Protective Factors** *Ilan H. Meyer, Ph.D.* *Associate Professor of Clinical Sociomedical Sciences and Deputy Chair for MPH Programs* *Mailman School of Public Health* *Columbia University* *Lisa Bowleg, Ph.D.* *Associate Professor* *Department of Community Health and Prevention* *Drexel University School of Public Health*

1:45 p.m.–2:00 p.m. **Individual Perspective**
Tiffany M. Joslyn, J.D.
Nonprofit Lawyer and LGBT Activist

2:00 p.m.–2:45 p.m. **Open Comments from Public**

MEETING THREE

Committee on Lesbian, Gay, Bisexual and Transgender (LGBT) Health Issues and Research Gaps and Opportunities
May 20, 2010
Parc55 Hotel
55 Cyril Magnin Street
San Francisco, California

8:55 a.m. **Welcome**

9:00 a.m.–10:00 a.m. **Transgender Health Panel**
Jae Sevelius, Ph.D.
Assistant Professor
Center for AIDS Prevention Studies, University of California, San Francisco

Sean Saifa M. Wall
Project Manager
The MASAI Project

Jamison Green
Primary Care Protocols Manager
Center of Excellence for Transgender Health, University of California, San Francisco

Joel Baum, M.S.
Director
Gender Spectrum Education and Training

10:00 a.m.–10:30 a.m. **LGBT Health Perspectives**
Beth Teper
Executive Director
COLAGE: People with a Lesbian, Gay, Bisexual, Transgender or Queer Parent

	Laura Rifkin *Founder* *Fabled Asp*
10:30 a.m.–10:45 a.m.	**Break**
10:45 a.m.–11:45 a.m.	**LGBT Health Perspectives** *Nancy Flaxman* *Consultant, LGBT Aging Issues* *Tania Israel, Ph.D.* *Associate Professor* *Department of Counseling, Clinical, and School Psychology* *University of California, Santa Barbara* *Rafael Diaz, Ph.D.* *Professor of Ethnic Studies* *San Francisco State University*
11:45 a.m.–12:30 p.m.	**Open Comments from Public**

MEETING FOUR

Committee on Lesbian, Gay, Bisexual and Transgender (LGBT) Health Issues and Research Gaps and Opportunities
August 11, 2010
Washington, DC

9:00 a.m.–10:00 a.m.	**Presentation on Research Training Activities at NIH** *Sharon Milgram, Ph.D.* *Director, Office of Intramural Training and Education* *Office of the Director, NIH* *Rodney Ulane, Ph.D.* *Training Officer and Director, Division of Scientific Program* *Office of Extramural Research, NIH*

B

Literature Review

For this study, the committee conducted an extensive review of the literature using Medline, PsycInfo, and the Social Science Citation Index. The committee did not limit itself to those documents identified through this search, but included other references as well. These searches initially yielded more than 6,000 citations. Given that not all of the relevant literature was published in national peer-reviewed journals, the committee developed an approach to use of the literature that is described in Chapter 1. Below is a listing of the terms used to search Medline, PsycInfo, and the Social Science Citation Index.

Terms defining the populations of interest:

- bisexuality or heterosexuality or homosexuality or homosexuality, male or homosexuality, female
- "gender minorit*"
- "homophob*"
- "men who have sex with men"
- "sex* identity"
- "sex* minorit*"
- "sex* orientation"
- "transgender"
- transsexualism
- transvestism
- "women who have sex with women"

Terms used to search within the results set of the above terms combined:

- adolescent development (limited to those aged 18 and below)
- adolescent health services (limited to those aged 18 and below)
- adolescent medicine (limited to those aged 18 and below)
- adolescent psychiatry (limited to those aged 18 and below)
- adolescent psychology (limited to those aged 18 and below)
- age distribution or censuses
- age factors or age distribution
- continental population groups or ethnic groups
- crime victims
- cultural characteristics or cultural diversity
- "delivery of health care" or health care disparities
- demography
- depression
- emergency medical care or patient care or community health services or mental health services
- epidemiologic methods or data collection or epidemiologic study characteristics or clinical trials or epidemiologic research design
- family characteristics
- family or family relations or nuclear family or single-parent family
- geography or urban health or urbanization
- health services accessibility
- health status
- health status indicators
- human development or child development
- introductory journal articles
- mental disorders
- mental health
- "outcome and process assessment (health care)" or "outcome assessment (health care)"
- population dynamics
- population or rural population or suburban population or urban population
- prejudice or health status disparities
- research
- risk assessment
- risk factors
- risk reduction behavior or risk-taking
- rural health or suburban health
- rural health services or suburban health services
- social behavior or aggression or social identification or social isolation or stereotyping

- social environment
- social perception or social change
- socioeconomic factors
- suicide
- treatment outcome or treatment failure
- utilization or use of health care
- violence or domestic violence

- AIDS or Acquired Immunodeficiency Syndrome
- HIV (Including a number of subheadings)

- sexually transmitted diseases (including a number of subheadings)

- anxiety disorders
- cancer or neoplasms
- cardiovascular diseases
- "disparities"
- health personnel
- hypertension
- jurisprudence or patient advocacy
- minority groups
- mood disorders
- obesity
- patient care
- public policy
- "substance abuse" or substance-related disorders

- health care surveys
- health surveys
- "methodological"
- population surveillance
- questionnaires
- research design

C

Glossary

ACASI—Audio computer-assisted self-interviews (ACASIs) allow participants to view a survey on a computer and hear a recorded voice stating the questions. Participants enter their answers on the computer.

Autogynephilic—Being sexually aroused by the thought or image of oneself as a woman (Blanchard, 1989).

Behaviorally bisexual women—Women who have sex with both men and women.

Bisexual—One whose sexual or romantic attractions and behaviors are directed at members of both sexes to a significant degree.

Body mass index—A statistical measure of the weight of a person scaled according to height, used to estimate whether a person is underweight or overweight. BMI is weight in kilograms divided by the square of height in meters (kg/m^2) (WHO, 2006).

Coming out—Coming out of the closet, or coming out, is a figure of speech for lesbian, gay, bisexual, and transgender (LGBT) people's disclosure of their sexual orientation and/or gender identity (Riley, 2010).

Cross-dresser (or transvestite)—Refers to an individual who wears clothes and adopts behaviors associated with the other sex for emotional or sexual gratification, and who may live part time in the cross-gender role.

Discrimination—Differential treatment of a person because of group membership, such as sexual- or gender-minority status.

Disorders of sex development—Congenital conditions in which the development of chromosomal, gonadal, or anatomic sex is atypical (Lee et al., 2006).

Drag queen or king—An individual who cross-dresses in women's or men's clothing, adopts a hyperfeminine or hypermasculine presentation, and appears part time in the cross-gender role.

Gay—An attraction and/or behavior focused exclusively or mainly on members of the same sex or gender identity; a personal or social identity based on one's same-sex attractions and membership in a sexual-minority community.

Gender dysphoria—A term for distress resulting from conflicting gender identity and sex of assignment (Cohen-Kettenis and Gooren, 1999; Murad et al., 2010).

Gender expression—Characteristics in appearance, personality, and behavior culturally defined as masculine or feminine.

Gender identity—One's basic sense of being a man, woman, or other gender (such as transgender) (Bockting, 1999).

Gender role conformity—The extent to which an individual's gender expression adheres to the cultural norms prescribed for people of his or her sex.

Gender role nonconformity—Nonconformity with prevailing norms of gender expression.

Gender-variant children—Children who are gender role nonconforming.

Heterosexual—Refers to individuals who identify as "heterosexual" or "straight" or whose sexual or romantic attractions and behaviors focus exclusively or mainly on members of the other sex or gender identity.

Homophobia—A term used broadly to refer to various manifestations of sexual stigma, sexual prejudice, and self-stigma based on one's homosexual or bisexual orientation.

Homosexual—As an adjective, used to refer to same-sex attraction, sexual behavior, or sexual orientation identity; as a noun, used as an identity label by some persons whose sexual attractions and behaviors are exclusively or mainly directed to people of their same sex.

Intersectionality—A theory used to analyze how social and cultural categories intertwine (Knudsen, 2006).

Intersex—A term used for people who are born with external and/or internal genitalia that vary from typical male or female genitalia, or a chromosomal pattern that varies from XX (female) or XY (male).

Intimate partner violence—Physical, sexual, or psychological harm inflicted by a current or former partner or spouse (CDC, 2006).

Lesbian—As an adjective, used to refer to female same-sex attraction and sexual behavior; as a noun, used as a sexual orientation identity label by women whose sexual attractions and behaviors are exclusively or mainly directed to other women.

Nulliparity—The condition of being nulliparous, or not bearing offspring.

Queer—In contemporary usage, an inclusive, unifying sociopolitical, self-affirming umbrella term for people who are gay; lesbian; bisexual; pansexual; transgender; transsexual; intersexual; genderqueer; or of any other nonheterosexual sexuality, sexual anatomy, or gender identity.[1] Historically, a term of derision for gay, lesbian, and bisexual people.

Real life experience—With respect to transgender persons, denotes living full time in the preferred gender role.

Serostatus (or HIV serostatus)—Blood test results indicating the presence or absence of antibodies the immune system creates to fight HIV. A seropositive status indicates that a person has antibodies to fight HIV and is HIV-positive.[2]

Sex—(1) Generally understood as a biological construct, referring to the genetic, hormonal, anatomical, and physiological characteristics of males or females. Sex is typically assigned at birth based on the appearance of the external genitalia. Only when this appearance is ambiguous are other indicators of sex assessed to determine the most appropriate sex assignment. (2) All phenomena associated with erotic arousal or sensual stimulation of the genitalia or other erogenous zones, usually (but not always) leading to orgasm.

Sexual orientation—Encompasses attraction, behavior, and identity. Most researchers studying sexual orientation have defined it operationally in terms of one or more of the following components. Defined in terms of *behavior*, sexual orientation refers to an enduring pattern of sexual or romantic activity with men, women, or both sexes. Defined in terms of *attraction* (or desire), it denotes an enduring pattern of experiencing sexual or romantic feelings for men, women, or both sexes. Identity encompasses both personal identity and social identity. Defined in terms of *personal identity*, sexual orientation refers to a conception of the self based on one's enduring pattern of sexual and romantic attractions and behaviors toward men, women, or both sexes. Defined in terms of *social* (or collective) *identity*, it refers to a sense of membership in a social group based on a shared sexual orientation and a linkage of one's self-esteem to that group.

Stigma—The inferior status, negative regard, and relative powerlessness that society collectively assigns to individuals and groups that are associated with various conditions, statuses, and attributes.

Transgender—Refers to individuals who cross or transcend culturally defined categories of gender (Bockting, 1999).

Transgenderist—An individual who lives full time in the cross-gender role and who may also take hormones, but does not desire sex reassignment surgery.

---

[1] See http://www.algbtical.org/2A%20QUEER.htm.

[2] See http://highered.mcgraw-hill.com/sites/0072972653/student_view0/chapter23/glossary.html.

Transsexual—An individual who strongly identifies with the other sex and seeks hormones and/or sex reassignment surgery to feminize or masculinize the body; may live full time in the cross-gender role.

Two spirit—Adopted in 1990 at the third annual spiritual gathering of GLBT Natives, the term derives from the northern Algonquin word *niizh manitoag,* meaning "two spirits," and refers to the inclusion of both feminine and masculine components in one individual (Anguksuar, 1997).

Vaginoplasty—A surgical procedure to construct a vagina.

REFERENCES

Anguksuar, L. R. 1997. A postcolonial perspective on western [mis]conceptions of the cosmos and the restoration of indigenous taxonomies. In *Two-spirit people: Native American gender identity, sexuality, and spirituality*, edited by S.E. Jacobs, W. Thomas, and S. Lang. Chicago, IL: University of Illinois Press. Pp. 217–222.

Blanchard, R. 1989. The concept of autogynephilia and the typology of male gender dysphoria. *The Journal of Nervous and Mental Disease* 177:616–623.

Bockting, W. O. 1999. From construction to context: Gender through the eyes of the transgendered. *SIECUS Report* 1(Oct./Nov.):3–7.

CDC (Centers for Disease Control and Prevention). 2006. *Understanding intimate partner violence.* http://www.cdc.gov/ncipc/dvp/ipv_factsheet.pdf (accessed October 13, 2010).

Cohen-Kettenis, P. T., and L. J. G. Gooren. 1999. Transsexualism: A review of etiology, diagnosis and treatment. *Journal of Psychosomatic Research* 46(4):315–333.

Knudsen, S.V. 2006. Intersectionality—A theoretical inspiration in the analysis of minority cultures and identities in textbooks. Paper presented at Eighth International Conference on Learning and Educational Media, October 26–29, 2005, Caen, France.

Lee, P. A., C. P. Houk, S. F. Ahmed, and I. A. Hughes. 2006. Consensus statement on management of intersex disorders. *Pediatrics* 118(2):e488–500.

Murad, M. H., M. B. Elamin, M. Z. Garcia, R. J. Mullan, A. Murad, P. J. Erwin, and V. M. Montori. 2010. Hormonal therapy and sex reassignment: A systematic review and meta-analysis of quality of life and psychosocial outcomes. *Clinical Endocrinology* 72(2): 214–231.

Riley, B. H. 2010. GLB adolescent's "coming out." *Journal of Child & Adolescent Psychiatric Nursing* 23(1):3–10.

WHO (World Health Organization). 2006. *BMI classification.* http://apps.who.int/bmi/index.jsp?introPage=intro_3.html (accessed October 29, 2010).

D

Biosketches of Committee Members and Staff

Robert Graham, M.D. (*Chair*), is professor of family medicine and Robert and Myfanwy Smith Endowed Chair in the Department of Family Medicine at the University of Cincinnati, School of Medicine, a position he has held since March 2005. Dr. Graham was previously associated with the discipline of family medicine as executive vice president/CEO of the American Academy of Family Physicians (AAFP) (1985–2000), head of the Academy's Foundation (1988–1997), and administrative officer of the Society of Teachers of Family Medicine (1973–1975). In addition to his activities in family medicine, Dr. Graham has held a number of leadership positions in the federal health sector, including the position of administrator of the Health Resources and Services Administration (HRSA) (1981–1985), during which time he also held the rank of rear admiral in the Commissioned Corps of the U.S. Public Health Service and served as an assistant surgeon general. He also served in senior positions at the Agency for Healthcare Research and Quality (2001–2004), the Health Resources Administration (1976–1979), and the Health Services and Mental Health Administration (1970–1973). From 1979 to 1980, he served as a professional staff member of the U.S. Senate Subcommittee on Health. Throughout his career, Dr. Graham has spoken extensively and written about a number of critical topics in health policy, such as health care reform and the need for universal health insurance coverage, federal health workforce policy, and the organizational characteristics of effective health systems. Dr. Graham's contributions and expertise in health policy have been recognized by his election to the National Academy of Sciences, Institute of Medicine (IOM), and his selection as board chair of the bipartisan Alliance of Health Reform. His current areas of interest are leadership development, organizational change, and universal health insurance coverage. Dr. Graham is a graduate of Earlham College, Richmond, Indiana (1965), and the University of Kansas School of Medicine in Kansas City, Kansas (1970).

Bobbie A. Berkowitz, Ph.D, RN, CNAA, FAAN, is currently dean and Mary O'Neil Mundinger Professor of Nursing at Columbia University School of Nursing and senior vice president of the Columbia University Medical Center. She was previously Alumni Endowed Professor of Nursing and chair of the Department of Psychosocial and Community Health at the University of Washington School of Nursing and adjunct professor in the School of Public Health and Community Medicine. In addition, she served as a consulting professor with Duke University and the University of California, Davis. Dr. Berkowitz directed the National Institutes of Health (NIH)/National Institute of Nursing Research (NINR)–funded Center for the Advancement of Health Disparities Research and the National Program Office for the Robert Wood Johnson Foundation (RWJF)–funded Turning Point Initiative. She joined the faculty at the University of Washington after having served as deputy secretary for the Washington State Department of Health and chief of nursing services for the Seattle-King County Department of Public Health. Dr. Berkowitz has been a member of the Washington State Board of Health, the Washington Health Care Commission, and the board of the American Academy of Nursing and chaired the board of trustees of Group Health Cooperative. She serves on a number of editorial boards, including those of the *Journal of Public Health Management and Practice* and *American Journal of Public Health, Policy, Politics, and Nursing Practice*, and as associate editor of *Nursing Outlook*. Dr. Berkowitz is an elected fellow in the American Academy of Nursing and an elected member of the IOM. She holds a Ph.D. in nursing science from Case Western Reserve University and master of nursing and bachelor of science in nursing degrees from the University of Washington. Her areas of expertise and research include public health systems and health equity.

Robert Wm. Blum, M.D., M.P.H., Ph.D., is William H. Gates, Sr. Professor and chair of the Department of Population, Family and Reproductive Health, Johns Hopkins Bloomberg School of Public Health. He has edited two books and has written nearly 250 journal articles, book chapters, and special reports. Dr. Blum's research interests include adolescent sexuality, chronic illness, and international adolescent health. In July 2007, he was named director of the Johns Hopkins Urban Health Institute. He is a past president of the Society for Adolescent Medicine, has served on the American Board of Pediatrics, was a charter member of the Sub-Board of Adolescent Medicine, is a past chair of the Alan Guttmacher Institute board of directors, and served as chair of the National Academy of Sciences Committee on Adolescent Health and Development. He is a consultant to The World Bank and UNICEF, as well as the World Health Organization, where he has served on the Technical Advisory Group of the Child and Adolescent Health Department, as well as the Scientific and Technical Advisory Group of the Human Reproductive Program. Dr. Blum has been awarded the Society for Adolescent Medicine's Outstanding Achievement Award (1993), and in 1998 was the recipient of the American Public Health Association's Herbert Needleman Award "for scientific achievement and courageous advocacy" on behalf of children and youth. He received an M.D. from Howard University College of Medicine, as well as an M.P.H. in maternal and child health and a Ph.D. in health policy at the University of Minnesota. Dr. Blum is an elected a member of the IOM.

Walter O. Bockting, Ph.D., is associate professor and coordinator of Transgender Health Services, Program in Human Sexuality, Department of Family Medicine and Community Health, University of Minnesota Medical School. He also is a founding member of the university's Leo Fung Center for Congenital Adrenal Hyperplasia (CAH) and Disorders of Sex Development. Dr. Bockting has more than 20 years of direct clinical experience serving the transgender population. Currently, he leads a multidisciplinary team providing tailored health services to transgender children, adolescents, and adults and their families. Dr. Bockting teaches medical students, physicians, and psychologists to work competently with this population. His research has focused on the sexual health of various sexual- and ethnic-minority populations, and has been funded by the American Foundation for AIDS Research, the Minnesota Department of Health, the Centers for Disease Control and Prevention (CDC), and NIH. He currently is conducting a randomized controlled trial to study the efficacy of an Internet-based, transgender-specific health promotion intervention. Dr. Bockting has edited five volumes, including *Transgender Health and HIV Prevention* (Haworth Press, 2005) and *Guidelines for Transgender Care* (Haworth Press, 2007), and has published numerous peer-reviewed journal articles. He is editor of the *International Journal of Transgenderism.* A frequent consultant, Dr. Bockting has served on the American Psychological Association's Task Force on Gender Identity, Gender Variance, and Intersex Issues. He is the 2009–2011 president of the World Professional Association for Transgender Health.

Judith Bradford, Ph.D., is director of the Center for Population Research in Lesbian, Gay, Bisexual and Transgender (LGBT) Health, funded by the Eunice Kennedy Shriver National Institute for Child Health and Human Development (NICHD) at The Fenway Institute (TFI). She co-chairs TFI with Kenneth Mayer, M.D., and is professor emeritus in the Institute of

Women's Health at Virginia Commonwealth University (VCU). Since 2001, Dr. Bradford has worked with Fenway Community Health to expand its sexual- and gender-minority health research and to develop TFI as its research, provider training and education, and policy division. As associate director/director of the VCU Survey and Evaluation Research Laboratory for 24 years, she built divisions for social and health policy research and for community-based research. During this time, she taught courses, chaired the Health Policy concentration in the Center for Public Policy, and directed doctoral dissertations. Dr. Bradford has participated in LGBT health research since 1984, working with public health programs and community-based organizations to conduct studies on sexual and gender minorities and racial minority communities and to translate results into programs to reduce health disparities. She was a committee member for the IOM's 1997–1999 study of lesbian health research priorities, a founding member of the National Coalition of LGBT Health, and a board member of the Gay and Lesbian Medical Association. Dr. Bradford has been recognized for her work by a number of organizations, including Mautner Project, the Gay and Lesbian Medical Association, the Richmond Healthy Start Initiative, and the Lesbian Health and Research Center.

Brian de Vries, Ph.D., is professor of gerontology at San Francisco State University. He received his doctorate in life span developmental psychology from the University of British Columbia in 1988 and was a postdoctoral fellow at both Simon Fraser University in Vancouver and the University of Southern California. He is a fellow of the Gerontological Society of America and a member of the board of the American Society on Aging and co-chair of its LGBT Aging Issues Network constituent group. Dr. de Vries is editor of the academic journal *Sexuality Research and Social Policy*; he is former associate editor of *The International Journal of Aging and Human Development* (2000–2006). He has served as guest editor of *Omega: Journal of Death and Dying* (1997 and 2004) and as guest co-editor of *Generations* (2001). In addition, he has edited four books, including *Gay and Lesbian Aging* (2004). He is currently editing a special issue of the *Journal of Homosexuality* on community-based needs assessments of LGBT elders. Dr. de Vries has authored or coauthored more than 80 journal articles and book chapters and has made more than 125 presentations to professional audiences on a variety of topics, such as the social and psychological well-being of midlife and older LGBT persons, friendship and social support in the lives of older gay men and lesbians, and end-of-life issues and bereavement within LGBT populations.

Robert Garofalo, M.D., M.P.H., is director of Adolescent HIV Services at Children's Memorial Hospital, and associate professor of pediatrics and preventive medicine at Northwestern University's Feinberg School of Medicine. Dr. Garofalo received his B.S. from Duke University (1988), his M.D. from New York University School of Medicine (1992), and his M.P.H. from the Harvard School of Public Health (1999). He completed a pediatric internship and residency at Children's Hospital of Philadelphia, and then the Dyson Pediatric Advocacy Fellowship and a fellowship in adolescent medicine at Harvard Medical School/Boston Children's Hospital. Dr. Garofalo's clinical and academic career has been devoted to community-based health and the care of both HIV-infected adolescents and other at-risk teen populations, such as LGBT youth. He is a past president of the Gay and Lesbian Medical Association. He has written a number of peer-reviewed articles and other publications on HIV and the health risks facing LGBT youth. Dr. Garofalo is currently the principal investigator for a number of federally funded research projects for HIV-positive adolescents, LGBT youth, and other at-risk youth populations.

Gregory M. Herek, Ph.D., is professor of psychology at the University of California, Davis. His work focuses broadly on sexual orientation, HIV/AIDS, prejudice and stigma, and public policy related to these topics. His empirical research has included studies of sexual prejudice and stigma in the U.S. population and among sexual minorities; the prevalence and psychological sequelae of hate crimes against lesbians, gay men, and bisexuals; and the nature of AIDS-related stigma and its impact on people with HIV/AIDS. A fellow of the American Psychological Association (APA) and the Association for Psychological Science, Dr. Herek received the 1996 APA Award for Distinguished Contributions to Psychology in the Public Interest and the 2006 Kurt Lewin Memorial Award from the Society for the Psychological Study of Social Issues (APA Division 9). He is the 2009 recipient of the Distinguished Service Award from the Society for the Psychological Study of Lesbian, Gay, Bisexual, and Transgender Issues (APA Division 44). His other honors include the 1999 and 1989 awards for Distinguished Scientific Contributions from APA Division 44 and the 1992 Outstanding Achievement Award from the APA Committee on Lesbian and Gay Concerns. Dr. Herek is past chairperson of the APA Committee on Lesbian and Gay Concerns. He also served on the APA Task Force on Avoiding Heterosexist Bias in Research and the APA Task Force on AIDS. He received his Ph.D. in social psychology from the University of California, Davis, and was a postdoctoral fellow at Yale University.

Elizabeth A. Howell, M.D., M.P.P., is associate professor in the Departments of Health Evidence and Policy, Obstetrics, Gynecology, and Reproductive Science, and Psychiatry at the Mount Sinai School of Medicine. She conducts research on racial/ethnic disparities in health and health care in maternal and child health, barriers to mental health care for low-income women of color, and quality of care. She currently is running two NIH-funded randomized controlled trials aimed at reducing postpartum depression among majority and minority mothers in New York City. Dr. Howell also has conducted studies on racial/ethnic disparities in treatment of cervical cancer, disparities in infant mortality rates in New York City, and quality of care in women's health. She is a fellow of the American College of Obstetricians and Gynecologists (ACOG) and currently serves on the ACOG Committee on Health Care for Underserved Women. Dr. Howell received her undergraduate degree from Stanford University and her medical and public policy degrees at Harvard Medical School and the Harvard Kennedy School of Government. She received her residency training at Cornell/New York Hospital and is a board-certified obstetrician gynecologist. Dr. Howell received her training in clinical epidemiology as a Robert Wood Johnson Clinical Scholar at Yale Medical School.

Daniel Kasprzyk, Ph.D., is vice president, senior fellow, and director of the Center for Excellence in Survey Research at National Opinion Research Center (NORC) at the University of Chicago. Prior to his appointment at NORC, he was director of statistical services at Mathematica Policy Research, Inc. Dr. Kasprzyk has more than 25 years of experience in managing large-scale sample surveys in a variety of topic areas, including holding various positions on the staff of the Survey of Income and Program Participation at the Census Bureau and carrying out methodological research associated with federal survey programs. He has particular expertise in nonsampling error issues in surveys. Prior to his private-sector positions, Dr. Kasprzyk was program director of the elementary and secondary sample survey studies program at the National Center for Education Statistics, where he was responsible for the Schools and Staffing Survey system. He was a member of the Organization for Economic Cooperation and Development committee that, among other responsibilities, developed and reported school and teacher data for cross-country comparisons. He served as the U.S. Department of Education's liaison to the National Academy of Sciences Panel on Estimates of Poverty for Small Geographic Areas and was a member of the National Academy of Sciences Panel to Review the National Children's Study Research Plan. Dr. Kasprzyk chaired the American Statistical Association's (ASA) Sections on Survey Research Methods and on Social Statistics, as well as serving as officer for other sections of the ASA and for the Washington Statistical Society, a Chapter of the ASA. He served for 20 years on the Office of Management and Budget's Federal Committee on Statistical Methodology; he is an elected member of the International Statistical Institute and fellow and former vice president of the ASA. He currently serves as associate editor for the *Journal of Official Statistics and*

Survey Methodology. Dr. Kasprzyk received his Ph.D. in mathematical statistics from The George Washington University.

Harvey J. Makadon, M.D., is clinical professor of medicine at Harvard Medical School and director of professional education and training at The Fenway Institute, Fenway Health, in Boston. He has been a local and national leader in care for vulnerable populations, with a particular focus on LGBT communities and people with HIV/AIDS. He is lead editor of *The Fenway Guide to LGBT Health*, published by the American College of Physicians in 2007—the first text for health care professionals published on this topic in the United States. Dr. Makadon has written numerous articles and reviews on HIV care and education. He edited a text, *HIV*, published by the American College of Physicians in April 2000. A third edition was published in 2007. The first Indian edition of the book came out in 2004, with a special focus on care in resource-limited countries.

Charlotte J. Patterson, Ph.D., is a professor in the Department of Psychology and in the Center for Children, Families, and the Law at the University of Virginia. Since receiving her Ph.D. in psychology from Stanford University, Dr. Patterson has pursued research on children's personal and social development in the context of family, peer, and school environments. In recent years, much of her work has focused on child development in lesbian- and gay-parented families. Dr. Patterson has served as director of the Bay Area Families Study, a study of psychosocial development among children who were born to or adopted by lesbian mothers, and as codirector of the Contemporary Families Study, which examined psychosocial adjustment among children born via donor insemination to lesbian and heterosexual parents. Recently, she has worked with data on adolescents with same-sex parents from the National Longitudinal Study of Adolescent Health (Add Health) and has collected new data for a variety of additional studies of sexual-minority families. Dr. Patterson has won a number of awards, including a Distinguished Scientific Contributions Award from the Society for Psychological Study of Lesbian, Gay and Bisexual Issues (APA Division 44); an Outstanding Achievement Award from the APA's Committee on Lesbian, Gay, and Bisexual Concerns; and the Carolyn Attneave Diversity Award from APA Division 43 (Family Psychology) for contributions that advance the understanding of diversity and its integration into family psychology. During the 2005–2006 academic year, Dr. Patterson served as president of the Society for Psychological Study of Lesbian and Gay Issues (APA Division 44), and in 2009 she won the APA's Award for Distinguished Contributions to Research in Public Policy.

John L. Peterson, Ph.D., is professor of psychology at Georgia State University. He joined the faculty at Georgia State as associate professor in

1994 following his position as a research psychologist at the University of California, San Francisco, in the Department of Medicine and the Center for AIDS Prevention Studies. His research expertise focuses on the social determinants and cultural factors associated with racial disparity in HIV infection among African American gay and bisexual men, as well as the social, psychological, and structural determinants of HIV risk reduction in randomized trials. Dr. Peterson has published extensively on HIV/AIDS in the leading behavioral science and public health journals and is coeditor of the *Handbook of HIV Prevention*. He has served on several editorial boards, including those of the *American Journal of Community Psychology* and *AIDS and Behavior*, and has frequently served as an expert consultant to CDC's Division of HIV/AIDS. Dr. Peterson's expertise also includes research on the perpetration of aggression toward gays and lesbians, with emphasis on the sociocultural and psychological factors that influence verbal and physical assaults on lesbians and gay men. Dr. Peterson is a fellow of the APA and the Society for Community Research and Action. He also serves on the NIH Office of AIDS Research, Behavioral and Social Science Planning Group. He received his Ph.D. in psychology from the University of Michigan.

Caitlin C. Ryan, Ph.D., ACSW, is director of the Family Acceptance Project at the Marian Wright Edelman Institute at San Francisco State University. She is a clinical social worker who has worked on LGBT health and mental health since the 1970s and on AIDS since 1982. Dr. Ryan received her clinical training with children and adolescents at Smith College School for Social Work in inpatient and community mental health programs and began her social work career in school-based psychoeducational settings. She pioneered community-based AIDS services at the beginning of the epidemic, initiated the first major study to identify lesbian health needs in the early 1980s, and has worked to implement quality care for LGBT youth since the early 1990s. Dr. Ryan founded the Family Acceptance Project—a research, intervention, and policy initiative—in 2002 to promote family support, decrease risk, and improve well-being for LGBT youth. Her book *Lesbian and Gay Youth: Care and Counseling*—the first comprehensive guide to health and mental health care for lesbian and gay youth—was written as a follow-up to the federal government's first conference on the primary care needs of lesbian and gay youth, which she coordinated for the Health Resources and Services Administration. Her work has been acknowledged by many groups, including the National Association of People with AIDS. In 1988 she was named Social Worker of the Year by the National Association of Social Workers for her leadership and contributions on the AIDS epidemic and social change. She was named Researcher of the Year by the Lesbian Health and Research Center at the University of California, San

Francisco, for her pioneering work in lesbian health. Dr. Ryan also received the Distinguished Scientific Contribution Award from the APA, Division 44, for directing critical research on LGBT youth and families.

Mark A. Schuster, M.D., Ph.D., is William Berenberg Professor of Pediatrics at Harvard Medical School and chief of general pediatrics and vice chair for health policy in the Department of Medicine at Children's Hospital Boston. Previously, he held similar positions at the University of California, Los Angeles (UCLA), and served as director of health promotion and disease prevention at RAND, where he held the RAND Distinguished Chair in Health Promotion. In addition, he was founding director of the UCLA/RAND Center for Adolescent Health Promotion, a prevention research center funded by CDC. Dr. Schuster has a long history of conducting research on child, adolescent, and family health issues with funding from NIH and CDC. He is also funded by the Agency for Healthcare Research and Quality to lead the Children's Hospital Boston Center of Excellence for Quality Measurement. His research has covered wide-ranging topics, including LGBT health and health care, adolescent sexual behavior, HIV prevention, and access to care for people with HIV. He was co-author of *Everything You Never Wanted Your Kids to Know About Sex (But Were Afraid They'd Ask): The Secrets to Surviving Your Child's Sexual Development from Birth to the Teens* and co-editor of *Child Rearing in America: Challenges Facing Parents of Young Children*. Dr. Schuster received his B.A. summa cum laude from Yale, his M.D. from Harvard Medical School, his M.P.P. from the Kennedy School of Government at Harvard, and his Ph.D. from the Pardee Rand Graduate School. He performed his pediatrics residency at Children's Hospital Boston and a fellowship with the Robert Wood Johnson Clinical Scholars Program at UCLA and RAND. He is the 2003 winner of the Nemours Child Health Services Research Award from AcademyHealth for a young investigator and the 2009 winner of the Academic Pediatric Association Research Award for career achievement.

Lowell J. Taylor, Ph.D., is professor of economics at the H. John Heinz III College, Carnegie Mellon University. He has been on the Heinz College faculty since 1990. Dr. Taylor holds an M.A. in statistics and an M.A. in economics from the University of Michigan; he earned his Ph.D. in economics in 1989, also at the University of Michigan. He has taught in the economics department at the University of Texas at Austin and has been a visiting professor in the economics department at the University of California, Berkeley. In 2000 he worked as senior economist for President Clinton's Council of Economic Advisers. He also served on the National Research Council Committee to Review the Scientists and Engineers Statistical Database System (SESTAT) 2000 Decade Design. Dr. Taylor's general research interests are labor markets, economic incentives within firms, and economic demography. His papers span a wide range of topics, including the causes of racial disparity in U.S. labor markets, the economics of lesbian and gay families, and the economics of health care delivery. He is co-author of the first paper on the lesbian and gay population ever to appear in the flagship journal *Demography.* His work has also appeared in leading economics and statistics journals, including the *American Economic Review*, *Quarterly Journal of Economics*, *Journal of Political Economy*, and *Journal of the American Statistical Association.*

Ruth Enid Zambrana, Ph.D., M.S.W., is professor in the Department of Women's Studies; director of the Consortium on Race, Gender and Ethnicity; and former interim director of the U.S. Latino Studies Initiative (2007–2009) at the University of Maryland, College Park. She is also adjunct professor of family medicine at the University of Maryland Baltimore, School of Medicine, Department of Family Medicine. Dr. Zambrana's work focuses on the intersections of gender, race/ethnicity, socioeconomic status, and other contextual variables in health disparities and social inequality, with an emphasis on Latino populations. Her emerging scholarship is on racial/ethnic inequalities in women's health, knowledge production, and public policy. Co-authored books include *Health Issues in the Latino Community* (2001); *Drawing from the Data: Working Effectively with Latino Families* (2003); and an anthology (2008) entitled *Emerging Intersections: Race, Class, and Gender in Theory, Policy, and Practice.* She has published extensively in her field and has served on several editorial boards, including those of the *American Journal of Public Health* and *Journal of Health Care for the Poor and Underserved.* She has served on several national and state boards and committees and as a member of the CDC Agenda Committee, Office of Public Health Research, Health Information Services and Health Equity Champions Workgroups (2005) and the State of Maryland Governor's Transition Task Force on Higher Education (2006). She received her Ph.D. in sociology from Boston University and her M.S.W. from the University of Pennsylvania.

Study Staff

Monica N. Feit, Ph.D., M.P.H., is a senior program officer at the IOM. Prior to joining the IOM, Dr. Feit spent a year as the American Public Health Association's government fellow, working for the Senate Committee on Health, Education, Labor and Pensions on the Subcommittee on Children and Families. She received her M.P.H. from Columbia University and her Ph.D. from London South Bank University and has a broad background in public health and extensive experience in international health. She has worked with a variety of nongovernmental organizations in Niger, as country director of Project HOPE in Bosnia-Herzegovina, and with the Medical Research Council of South Africa in its Environment and Health Research Unit.

Joshua Joseph, J.D., is an associate program officer with the IOM's Board on the Health of Select Populations. He received his J.D. from American University's Washington College of Law in 2008 and is licensed to practice law in New York and New Jersey. Within the legal field, he has performed a variety of research and writing tasks, assisted indigent clients as a pro bono attorney, and worked on policy issues and regulatory affairs. He received his B.A. in economics with a minor in psychology from the University of Pennsylvania in 2005. His current interests include public health, health policy, and regulatory law.

Jon Q. Sanders is a veteran program associate with the Board on the Health of Select Populations at the IOM. He received his B.A. in anthropology with a minor in geosciences from Trinity University and recently completed the program management certification at George Mason University. In his 10 years with the National Academies, Mr. Sanders has worked on a variety of projects on topics ranging from childhood obesity to national security. He is coauthor of *Sitting Down at the Table: Mediation and Resolution of Water Conflicts* (2001). His research interests include public health, emergency management, and environmental decision making.

Karen Anderson, Ph.D., is senior program officer in the IOM. She is responsible for the Roundtable on the Promotion of Health Equity and the Elimination of Health Disparities. She earned a Ph.D. in experimental psychology from the University of Pittsburgh. Her professional experience includes a range of positions involving the intersection of social science and public health research and public policy, including positions with the U.S. House of Representatives, the APA, and Howard University. Dr. Anderson is an adjunct professor of pediatrics in the college of medicine at Howard University. She has expertise in child health disparities, adolescent development, reproductive health issues, HIV/AIDS, LGBT issues, early childhood education and development, and education policy.

Frederick (Rick) Erdtmann, M.P.H., M.D., is currently director of the Board on the Health of Select Populations and the Medical Follow-up Agency at the IOM. Prior to joining the IOM he was a career military physician in the U.S. Army. While in the military, he served as chief of several large departments of preventive medicine at U.S. installations at home and overseas. He also was commander of the military community hospital at Ft. Carson, Colorado, and later served as hospital commander for the Walter Reed Army Medical Center. He had several assignments at the Army Surgeon General's Office, working on military health care policies. He received his undergraduate degree from Bucknell University and an M.P.H. from the University of California, Berkeley. He is a graduate of Temple University Medical School and is board certified in the specialty of preventive medicine.

Sarah Isquick is a third-year medical student at Case Western Reserve University School of Medicine. She received a B.S. in English literature from the University of Michigan. She contributed to the report as a Christine Mirzayan Science and Technology Policy Fellow at the National Academies. Upon receiving her M.D., she aspires to identify and redress health disparities by conducting outcomes-based research and working in policy. Some of her passions include LGBT health, reproductive and sexual health, and patient safety. At Case Western Reserve University School of Medicine, she works to educate other students and faculty by organizing lectures and film screenings on relevant issues in medicine, as well as advocacy events and letter writing campaigns.

Index

[Page numbers followed by *b, f*, or *t* refer to boxed text, figures, or tables, respectively.]

A

B

F

G

I

J

K

L

M

N

O

P

Q

R

S

T

U

V